Family Nurse Practitioner

CERTIFICATION PREP EXAMS
Fourth Edition

Family Nurse Practitioner

CERTIFICATION PREP EXAMS

Fourth Edition

Amelie Hollier, MSN, APRN, BC, FNP
Mari J. Wirfs, MN, PhD, BC, FNP

 Advanced Practice Education Associates
APEA

Family Nurse Practitioner
Certification Prep Exams
Fourth Edition

Practice Tests and Questions
with Rationales

Amelie Hollier, MSN, APRN, BC, FNP
Mari J. Wirfs, MN, PhD, BC, FNP

Publisher: Advanced Practice Education Associates, Inc.
103 Darwin Circle
Lafayette, LA 70508 U.S.A.

Printed in the United States of America.

ISBN 978-1-892418-11-1

The Authors

Amelie Hollier, MSN, APRN, BC, FNP is a nationally certified family nurse practitioner. She is president and CEO of Advanced Practice Education Associates (APEA). She is in full-time clinical practice at St. Clare's Employee Health Service at Our Lady of Lourdes Regional Medical Center in Lafayette, Louisiana. She has co-authored 10 books for primary care nurse practitioners. She travels extensively throughout the U.S. presenting on-site certification exam review courses and lecturing on advanced pharmacology and primary care topics to professional APRN groups.

Mari J. Wirfs, MN, PhD, BC, FNP is a nationally certified family nurse practitioner. She is Professor and Director, William Carey College School of Nursing, New Orleans, Louisiana and is a primary care provider in part-time private practice at the New Orleans Baptist Theological Seminary. She has over 30 years of experience in nursing education, has co-authored 5 books for primary care nurse practitioners, and is a frequent guest lecturer on a variety of advanced practice topics to professional APRN groups.

Preface

FNP Certification Prep Exams contains review questions and practice examinations intended to assist future family and adult nurse practitioners to prepare for national certification examinations. Nurse practitioner students will also find it invaluable for evaluation of their knowledge level. Also included is a chapter on study skills and test-taking strategies to maximize the test-taker's potential for success.

The authors' recommendation for the most effective use of this book is to first review a specific subject area independently, then answer the questions that correlate with that subject. If it is determined that certain topics are unfamiliar, then these areas may need further attention. After sufficient reading and review in all areas, a practice exam can be taken. The practice examinations will help to determine strengths and weaknesses in both knowledge and clinical application.

FNP Certification Prep Exams contains multiple choice, competency-based, questions intended to test the student's knowledge and ability to apply that knowledge in clinical situations. Content areas covered in the exams are health promotion, disease prevention, diagnosis and management of acute and chronic illnesses across the life span, the research process, and professional issues.

The test items in this book were written by practicing, certified, family nurse practitioners, and were reviewed by family nurse practitioners, faculty, and students.

A variety of current resources, from the clinical practice, educational, and research literature, were used in the development the items and rationales. A listing of these resources is located in the back of this book.

A sincere effort has been made to provide readers with current, accurate, and comprehensive information. If the reader has any questions or comments, the authors welcome communications via e-mail at *questions@apea.com*.

Contents

Study Skills

Plan ahead. Determine the total content that needs to be reviewed, and then allow yourself adequate time to prepare. Develop a reasonable study schedule *now* in order to avoid cramming. Research has demonstrated that short daily study periods are more productive than marathon cramming sessions. Divide the content into small sections that are not overwhelming. Set your study goals, and then set out to accomplish those goals. An effective way to achieve daily goals is to use an index card on which the tasks to complete are listed. The most important point to make is this: *Don't procrastinate!*

Outline the content to be learned. Use the practice questions in this book to familiarize yourself with the content. There will be areas identified that need very little further review, and areas identified that need extensive study. Begin by skimming and scanning all material for the session of study, then delve deeper. Remember to focus mainly on major concepts, avoiding becoming bogged down by details.

Decide how much time you can spend each day or week. Consider what time of day you study best. Pay attention to your biological clock. At the end of each study session, take a little time to summarize what you have learned, including important concepts.

Be versatile. Use a variety of resources, allowing all of your senses to help you learn. There are books, videotapes, computer programs, review tests, audio tapes, review courses, review books, and journals available. Organize a weekly study group with a few classmates. Hearing information and explaining to another (audio-learning) is a valuable adjunct to hearing and writing information (visual learning). Discover what method of learning works best for you, and enjoy the process.

A quiet atmosphere with minimal distractions facilitates concentration. Find a quiet place to study.

New information must be reviewed continually in order to **build strong memory traces.** The more frequently information is recalled, the more firmly it becomes etched in the memory.

Motivate yourself. Remember your personal goal, whether it is personal fulfillment, a more successful future, a career change, or something more altruistic in nature. Goals serve as incentives for work. The desire to reach a goal is a powerful motivator.

Test-Taking Strategies

Develop the ability to relax. After you have prepared for an examination, you do not want anxiety to impair your performance. Get enough rest the night before the test. Relaxation exercises such as deep breathing, progressive muscle relaxation, and guided imagery, can have positive effects.

Develop your test-taking skills through practice. Remember, the items are designed to test your knowledge and ability to apply the knowledge. Ask yourself what the purpose of the question is, and answer with that purpose in mind.

Practice. Use the sample tests. Read question stems carefully, becoming aware of the specific information requested, and identifying key words. Develop the habit of looking out for negative stems, which can be tricky. Examples of negative stems are "EXCEPT," "NOT," "LEAST," "INCORRECT," and "FALSE."

After you first read a question, try to answer it without looking at the multiple-choice options.

Evaluate each answer choice as if it were a "True-False" question. If the answer is true, include it in your options. If it is false, eliminate it. Eliminate obvious distractors, leaving fewer options from which to identify the correct answer. Again, beware of negative stems where the correct answer choice is the option that is *false*.

Base your answers on **principles of nursing practice** for the general population, unless the stem specifies otherwise.

If a particular item has you stumped, **make an educated guess** and move on. You can return to it later, if time allows. Attempt every question, but keep moving on. Pace yourself. Remember, there is no penalty for wrong answers. Guess if you have no idea, but answer every question.

Allow ample time to arrive on time at the test site. It is a good idea to make a practice run to the test site if you are not familiar with the area.

Listen to all instructions, and **read** all directions.

Try to **avoid becoming distracted** by those who finish the test before you. Work at your own pace. Finishing the examination first is not the objective.

Be aware of pitfalls. One major pitfall is the tendency to rely on past experience. Although certification examinations are practice-based, all practitioners may not follow standards of nursing practice.

Record your answers carefully. If you skip a question, be sure to mark the question so that you can come back to it.

Think positively! Maintain confidence. Continue to put forth your best effort and don't give up.

Check your work. After the test, as you review your answers, try not to make changes unless you are reasonably certain your original response was incorrect. Research has shown that when in doubt, the first answer choice is most likely to be the correct response.

We hope that this book will help future advanced practice registered nurses to meet the challenge of transition from student to practitioner. The challenge to constantly maintain current knowledge, enabling us to provide continuous expert nursing care, should never end.

Further Reading

Korchek, N., & Sides, M. B. (2002). *Nurse's guide to successful test taking* (4th ed.). Philadelphia: Lippincott.

Rooney, R., & Lipuma, A. (1992). *Learn to be the master student: How to develop self-confidence and effective study skills.* Silver Springs, CO: Maydale.

NOTE TO STUDENTS:

A special format has been created to assist with studying. The answers and rationales to the following items can be found on the reverse side of the question page. Merely fold the answer page back onto the question page and the answers will line up on the same line as the questions.

Cardiovascular Disorders

b 1. Four weeks ago, a 44-year-old patient's blood pressures were consistently 160 mmHg systolic and 100-110 mmHg diastolic. He started taking a low-dose beta-blocker and reports feeling "much better now." His blood pressure today is 145/95. What is the most appropriate action?

   a. Continue the beta-blocker for 4 more weeks and re-assess.
   b. Add a low-dose diuretic.
   c. Increase the dosage of beta-blocker.
   d. Choose a drug from a different class.

a 2. Acute rheumatic fever is an inflammatory disease which can follow infection with:

   a. Group A *Streptococcus.*
   b. *Staphylococcus aureus.*
   c. *β*-hemolytic *Streptococcus.*
   d. *Streptococcus pyogenes.*

a 3. A patient is taking an ACE inhibitor for blood pressure control. The nurse practitioner decides to add a diuretic. Which of the following is the best choice?

   a. A thiazide diuretic
   b. A loop diuretic
   c. A potassium-sparing diuretic
   d. Either a or b

c 4. An elderly patient is being seen in the clinic for complaint of "weak spells" relieved by sitting or lying down. How should the nurse practitioner proceed with the physical examination?

   a. Assist the patient to a standing position and take her blood pressure.
   b. Assess the patient's cranial nerves.
   c. Compare the patient's blood pressure lying first, then sitting, and then standing.
   d. Compare the amplitude of the patient's radial and pedal pulses.

a 5. Of the following lesions, which is associated with cyanosis?

   a. Tetralogy of Fallot
   b. Aortic stenosis
   c. Pulmonic stenosis
   d. Ventricular septal defect (VSD)

1. *b* The patient's blood pressure has improved but remains elevated. Waiting 4 additional weeks will not likely result in a further blood pressure reduction. In light of the recommendations from JNC VII and the findings of the ALLHAT study, adding a low dose diuretic is appropriate.

2. *a* Acute rheumatic fever follows infection with Group A *Streptococcus*. This disease can exhibit cardiac, joint, brain, and skin manifestations. This organism is one of the reasons streptococcal pharyngitis is treated with an antibiotic. Associated heart murmurs are typically mitral and aortic regurgitation, and a mid-diastolic murmur termed the Carey-Coombs murmur.

3. *a* *ACE* inhibitors are potassium-sparing. Thiazide diuretics are potassium-wasting. Thus, an ACE inhibitor together with a thiazide diuretic is a good combination. A potassium-sparing diuretic coupled with an ACE inhibitor can lead to hyperkalemia. Loop diuretics are a potassium wasting but are a common second choice for treatment of hypertension. Loop diuretics are more potent than thiazide diuretics and may lead to excessive diuresis resulting in dehydration and reduction in blood volume.

4. *c* Orthostatic hypotension should be included early in the differential diagnosis. This is documented by recording the patient's blood pressure in 3 different positions from supine to standing. A decrease in blood pressure ≥ 20 mmHg associated with position change is highly suggestive of orthostatic hypotension.

5. *a* Tetralogy of Fallot, hypoplastic right ventricle with pulmonary or tricuspid atresia, transposition of the great vessels, and complicated coarctation of the aorta are cardiac conditions associated with cyanosis.

a 6. Congenital heart disorders usually present at:

a. birth, infancy, or in childhood.
b. birth only.
c. birth and infancy.
d. any time after birth.

a 7. A manifestation of congenital heart disease in a child without previous symptoms may be:

a. growth delay.
b. increased bruising.
c. an immunization reaction.
d. frequent injuries.

a 8. In the initial evaluation of a patient with new onset hypertension, the nurse practitioner should:

a. look for correctable causes.
b. start medication to lower the blood pressure.
c. start the patient on a low-sodium diet.
d. discuss a low-cholesterol diet with the patient.

b 9. A 55-year-old patient has a work-up for hypertension and is noted to have elevated BUN and creatinine. Which of the following should the nurse practitioner suspect?

a. Pheochromocytoma
b. Renal disease
c. Diabetes
d. Dehydration

c 10. A patient has been taking enalapril (Vasotec®) for a period of 4 months for treatment of CHF. She has developed a nonproductive cough associated with this ACE inhibitor. The nurse practitioner knows that:

a. prescribing a different ACE inhibitor may alleviate the problem.
b. this may indicate worsening of the CHF.
c. the cough should subside 1 to 4 days after discontinuing the drug.
d. the patient's potassium is probably elevated.

6. *a*   A common misconception is that congenital disorders always present at birth. They can present at various times throughout childhood and are classified as cyanotic or acyanotic. Cardiac disorders in infants and children may be acquired from rheumatic fever or Kawasaki syndrome. It is rare for congenital heart disorders to present later than childhood.

7. *a*   Other clinical manifestations of congenital heart disease in children may include exercise intolerance, tachycardia, clubbing of the fingers and toes, irritability, and frequent napping.

8. *a*   Although 92 to 95% of hypertension in the US is primary or essential hypertension, patient history, physical exam, and laboratory tests should be completed to determine correctable causes. Some correctable causes include renal disease, adrenal hypertension, acromegaly, hypercalcemia, oral contraceptive use, coarctation of the aorta, and drug abuse.

9. *b*   The lone finding of elevated serum BUN and creatinine should direct the nurse practitioner to complete a detailed work-up for renal insufficiency. If an abdominal bruit is present, the nurse practitioner might suspect renal artery stenosis. The finding of bilateral abdominal masses might indicate polycystic kidney disease. The nurse practitioner would appropriately consider physician referral in all of these cases.

10. *c*   Cough has been associated with all ACE inhibitors, although the incidence is variable among them. Prescribing a different drug in the same class may not alleviate the problem. The actual incidence of cough ranges from 5 to 25% but is reported in lower numbers (0.5 to 3%) by drug manufacturers.

b _____ 11. A cashier complains of dull ache and pressure sensation in her lower legs. It is relieved by leg elevation. She occasionally has edema in her lower legs at the end of the day. What is the most likely cause of these problems?

    a. Congestive heart failure
    b. Varicose veins
    c. Deep vein thrombosis
    d. Arterial insufficiency

C _____ 12. The intervention that will provide the most relief for a patient with aching varicose veins is to:

    a. wear support stockings.
    b. avoid prolonged sitting.
    c. elevate her legs periodically.
    d. take 1 baby aspirin daily.

a _____ 13. Which of the following is a secondary cause of hyperlipidemia?

    a. Uncontrolled diabetes mellitus
    b. Family history
    c. Recent dietary excess and weight gain
    d. Lack of exercise

C _____ 14. A 70-year-old man who walks 2 miles every day complains of pain in his left calf when he is walking. The problem has gotten gradually worse and now he is unable to complete his 2-mile walk. What question asked during the history, if answered affirmatively, would suggest a diagnosis of arteriosclerosis obliterans?

    a. "Are you wearing your usual shoes?"
    b. "Do you also have chest pain when you have leg pain?"
    c. "Is your leg pain relieved by rest?"
    d. "Do you ever have the same pain in the other leg?"

b _____ 15. Of the following signs and symptoms of congestive heart failure (CHF), the earliest clinical manifestation is:

    a. peripheral edema.
    b. weight gain.
    c. shortness of breath.
    d. nocturnal dyspnea.

11. *b* Based on her complaints and what she says provides relief, the most likely cause of the patient's complaints is varicose veins. Varicose veins are more common in women and often there is a family history. Her work as a cashier (probably standing for hours in one place) contributes to her condition. Support hose will probably help her symptoms.

12. *c* The intervention that will provide the greatest relief for this patient is elevating the legs periodically. Use of support stockings will prolong the length of time she is able to stand in place, but will not provide relief after her legs begin aching. Support stockings should be applied prior to getting out of bed.

13. *a* Insulin resistance or deficiency, as seen in diabetes mellitus, is a secondary cause of hyperlipidemia. Other secondary causes include hypothyroidism, obstructive liver disease, and uremia.

14. *c* Arteriosclerosis obliterans is most common in the 6th and 7th decades of life and presents with pain or cramping in a lower extremity during exercise. The most common sites of plaque formation are the femoral and popliteal arteries (found in 80 to 90% of patients with symptoms). Pain or discomfort is distal to the site of blockage and is relieved with rest. Patients with intermittent claudication should be advised to walk to the point of leg pain, stop and rest until the leg pain is relieved, and then continue walking again.

15. *b* The earliest and most sensitive indication of CHF is weight gain. The other clinical manifestations listed present after the weight gain.

_a_ 16. A 70-year-old man complains of tightness in his chest while cutting firewood. It disappears quickly if he stops chopping. He denies shortness of breath, his cholesterol level is less than 200 mg/dL, and he is a non-smoker. What is the most appropriate action for the nurse practitioner to take with this patient?

    a. Treat the complaints as "cardiac" in origin until proven otherwise.
    b. Consider a gastrointestinal workup to rule out GERD.
    c. Consider arthritis and order chest and spinal x-rays.
    d. Encourage the patient to chop fewer pieces of wood at a time.

_a_ 17. A patient has been started on bisoprolol (Zebeta®) for hypertension and has taken a morning dose for 2 days. He calls the clinic this morning and reports extreme fatigue since leaving home. How should the nurse practitioner respond?

    a. Have him return to the office to check his blood pressure and heart rate.
    b. Have him take the medicine at bedtime.
    c. Because this is expected, have him return at his next scheduled visit.
    d. Ask him if he has been drinking grapefruit juice with his medicine.

_c_ 18. Which of the following heart murmurs warrants the greatest concern?

    a. Systolic murmur
    b. Venous hum murmur
    c. Diastolic murmur
    d. Flow murmur

_b_ 19. The most common adverse side effect of drugs taken to lower low-density lipoprotein (LDL) cholesterol is:

    a. headache.
    b. gastrointestinal symptoms.
    c. joint aches and pains.
    d. elevated hepatic enzymes.

_a_ 20. Which of the following is the best means to assess coagulation status in a patient receiving warfarin (Coumadin®) therapy?

    a. INR
    b. PT
    c. PTT
    d. Clotting studies

16. *a* Although the patient does not appear to have any other risk factors for coronary disease, he is 70 years old and male. Chest pain should always be considered cardiac in origin until proven otherwise. Reflux and arthritis are common causes of chest pain, but should only be considered after cardiac causes have been ruled out.

17. *a* Fatigue is a common complaint after initiation of a beta-blocker. However, the patient's complaint of "extreme fatigue" following the first 2 doses could be due to hypotension and bradycardia. The patient should be advised to return to the office for assessment of his blood pressure and heart rate. Grapefruit juice increases the bioavailability of calcium channel blockers and, therefore, exacerbates their antihypertensive effect. Bisoprolol (Zebeta®) is a beta-blocker.

18. *c* A diastolic murmur should always be considered abnormal. From the newborn period through adolescence, different murmurs can be auscultated which are considered normal. Any murmur that is associated with a thrill or is louder than Grade II/VI, should be referred for further investigation.

19. *b* Fibric acid, nicotinic acid, bile acid sequestrants, and HMG CoA-reductase inhibitors ("statins") most commonly cause GI symptoms and/or diarrhea. In addition, nicotinic acid may cause flushing and hyperglycemia. Usually these effects diminish over time. Elevated hepatic enzymes and arthralgias occur *infrequently*, but may be caused by taking a "statin."

20. *a* INR, international normalized ratio, is a value calculated from the PT. It is considered the most accurate measure of a patient's clotting status when the patient is taking warfarin (Coumadin®).

d **21.** The nurse practitioner works in a clinic for the homeless. A 69-year-old male has been seen twice in the last 2 months. His previous blood pressures were 182/80 and 176/82. What should the nurse practitioner do today?

    a. Discuss dietary changes.
    b. Prescribe a thiazide diuretic.
    c. Prescribe a beta-blocker.
    d. Prescribe a long-acting calcium channel blocker.

a **22.** In a young patient with multiple days of fever > 100.4°F (38° C), Kawasaki syndrome must be suspected. Of the following, the most life-threatening sequelae of Kawasaki syndrome are:

    a. cardiovascular complications.
    b. respiratory complications.
    c. neurological complications.
    d. hematological complications.

C **23.** A very active elderly patient has a documented diagnosis of arteriosclerosis obliterans. Common expected lower extremity physical exam findings include:

    a. decreased pulses proximal to the blockage and weeping ulcers.
    b. pain relieved with leg elevation and decreased leg hair growth.
    c. cool skin temperature and thickened toenails.
    d. dependent edema and brawny skin color.

d **24.** A patient with elevated lipids has been started on lovastatin (Mevacor®). After 3 weeks of therapy, he calls to report generalized muscle aches. The nurse practitioner should suspect:

    a. a drug interaction.
    b. hepatic dysfunction.
    c. hypersensitivity to lovastatin.
    d. rhabdomyolysis.

d **25.** A patient's creatinine kinase (CK) is 2 to 3 times higher than normal. The nurse practitioner should:

    a. suspect a myocardial infarction.
    b. question the patient regarding illicit drug use.
    c. order a serum lactate dehydrogenase (LDH).
    d. order a serum CK-MB level and re-evaluate.

21. *d* The patient is exhibiting isolated systolic hypertension (ISH), commonly found in the elderly and associated with loss of vascular compliance. The drug of choice for ISH is a long-acting dihydropyridine calcium channel blocker, such as amlodipine (Norvasc®) or nifedipine (Procardia®). Thiazide diuretics are a good choice for the elderly with hypertension, but the average systolic decrease is only 10 to 15 mmHg and, therefore, would not be the best choice for this patient.

22. *a* Kawasaki syndrome can lead to meningitis, jaundice, hepatitis, and other serious complications. However, cardiac complications are probably the most dangerous. There may be prolonged PR or QT intervals and/or there may be ST and T wave changes. Echocardiography and electrocardiography determine the extent of the cardiac consequences of Kawasaki syndrome.

23. *c* Important lower extremity findings in patients with arteriosclerosis obliterans are decreased or absent pulses distal to the site of blockage, hair loss, pallor, and/or dependent rubor. Ulcerations or gangrene may be present if impairment of blood flow is severe. The most common finding in all forms of the disease is decreased or diminished pedal pulses.

24. *d* Rhabdomyolysis with renal dysfunction secondary to myoglobinuria has occurred with some statins. Though rare, myalgias and muscle weakness signal possible serious problems. The statin should be discontinued immediately if CPK elevations are noted.

25. *d* An elevated creatinine kinase (CK) is not diagnostic of myocardial infarction (MI). MB bands are specific for myocardial smooth muscle damage. If these are elevated, the patient may have had a very recent MI. Troponin-1 biomarker should also be considered because it is more sensitive and specific in diagnosis of an acute MI. CK may be elevated from an intramuscular injection, surgery, or any type of extensive skeletal muscle trauma.

_d_   26. The murmur of aortic stenosis often radiates to the:

    a. apex of the heart.
    b. left axilla.
    c. mitral valve.
    d. carotid artery.

26. *d*   Degenerative aortic stenosis (AS) predominates in the elderly. This is due to a stiffened and thickened aortic valve. An increase in the pressure gradient increases the intensity of the murmur and causes it to radiate to the carotid artery. Obesity or COPD may soften the intensity of the murmur. However, usually the louder the murmur of AS, the more serious the problem.

Dermatological Disorders

b 1. Acne vulgaris is an inflammatory disorder of the:

   a. hair follicles.
   b. sebaceous glands.
   c. dermal layer.
   d. stratum corneum.

d 2. Which agent is most effective for the treatment of nodulocystic acne?

   a. benzoyl peroxide
   b. retinoic acid (Retin-A®)
   c. Topical minocycline
   d. isotretinoin (Accutane®)

c 3. A 35-year-old man presents with radicular pain followed by the appearance of grouped vesicles consisting of about 15 lesions across 3 different thoracic dermatomes. He complains of pain, burning, and itching. The nurse practitioner should suspect:

   a. a common case of shingles and prescribe an analgesic and an antiviral agent.
   b. a complicated case of shingles and prescribe acyclovir (Zovirax®), an analgesic, and a topical cortisone cream.
   c. *herpes zoster* and consider that this patient may be immunocompromised.
   d. a recurrence of chickenpox and treat the patient's symptoms.

b 4. Impetigo and folliculitis are usually successfully treated with:

   a. systemic antibiotics.
   b. topical antibiotics.
   c. topical steroid creams.
   d. cleansing and debridement.

b 5. A 40-year-old female with history of frequent sun exposure presents with a multicolored lesion on her back. It has irregular borders and is about 11 mm in diameter. What should the nurse practitioner suspect?

   a. Squamous cell carcinoma
   b. Malignant melanoma
   c. A common nevus
   d. Basal cell carcinoma

1. *b*   Acne is an inflammatory disorder of the sebaceous glands that presents as pustules, papules, and comedones. Enzymes from the causative organism, *Propionibacterium acnes*, mix with sebum causing irritation. Open comedones are "blackheads" and closed comedones are "whiteheads."

2. *d*   Isotretinoin (Accutane®) is a systemic agent indicated for treatment of severe inflammatory acne. Guidelines for its use must be clearly understood by the patient. A woman of childbearing age must use an effective method of contraception because isotretinoin is highly teratogenic.

3. *c*   The condition described is *herpes zoster*. The presence of more than ten lesions across more than one dermatome may indicate dissemination of this viral illness. It is most frequently seen in patients who are immuno-compromised. *Herpes zoster* usually is not common in persons 15 to 35 years-of-age. It is usually seen in patients 50 years-of-age and older. Topical steroids are contraindicated.

4. *b*   Simple cases of impetigo and folliculitis are not usually deep skin infections and, therefore, are amenable to topical antibiotic therapy. This is especially true if the topical antibiotics are used in conjunction with cleansing, which decreases bacterial colonization. Systemic antibiotics are appropriate for patients with extensive skin involvement. Extensive impetigo is sometimes referred to as "Indian fire."

5. *b*   Malignant melanoma has a propensity for the sun-exposed areas of the back. Recognition of suspicious lesions may be facilitated by using the ABCD mnemonic. *A*-asymmetry; *B*-irregular border; *C*-color variegation; and *D*-diameter greater than a pencil eraser tip or 6 mm; *E*-enlarging. This patient should be referred to a dermatologist or surgeon immediately for biopsy of the lesion.

6. A third-grader presents with several honey-colored crusts on her face. Her mother reports that she has had these for a few days and now her younger sister has them also. What is this patient's diagnosis and treatment of choice?

   a. Impetigo; treat with either topical or systemic antibiotics
   b. Ecthyma; treat with either topical or systemic antibiotics
   c. Erysipelas; treat with systemic antibiotics and steroids
   d. Folliculitis; treat with systemic or topical steroids

7. A 60-year-old male diabetic patient presents with redness, tenderness, and edema of the left lateral aspect of his face. His left eyelid is grossly edematous. He reports history of a toothache in the past week which "is better". His temperature is 100°F (38.3°C) and pulse is 102 bpm. The most appropriate initial action is to:

   a. start an oral antibiotic, refer the patient to a dentist immediately, and follow up within 3 days.
   b. order mandibular x-rays and question the patient about physical abuse.
   c. start an oral antibiotic, mouth swishes with an oral anti-infective, and an analgesic.
   d. initiate a parenteral antibiotic and consider hospital admission.

8. A 55-year-old man is diagnosed with basal cell carcinoma. The nurse practitioner correctly tells him:

   a. "It is the most common cause of death in patients with skin cancer."
   b. "It can be cured with surgical excision or radiation therapy."
   c. "It is a slow growing skin cancer that rarely undergoes malignant changes."
   d. "It can be cured using 5-fluorouracil cream twice daily for 2 to 4 weeks."

9. A 70-year-old patient presents with a slightly raised, scaly, erythematous patch on her forehead. She admits to having been a "sun worshipper." The nurse practitioner suspects actinic keratosis. This lesion is a precursor to:

   a. squamous cell carcinoma.
   b. basal cell carcinoma.
   c. malignant melanoma.
   d. acne vulgaris.

6. *a*   Honey-colored crusted lesions are typical of impetigo. Depending on the extent of the infection, it can be successfully treated with either a topical antibiotic, such as mupirocin (Bactroban®), or systemic antibiotics may be indicated if the lesions are more extensive. It is very contagious, so it is not surprising that this patient's younger sister has the condition also.

7. *d*   The condition described in this patient is facial cellulitis. A previous history of toothache with resolution is characteristic of pulpitis that can spread to adjacent areas and apparently has done so in this patient. This condition may be life threatening in young, healthy patients. This patient is a 60 year old with diabetes. This patient must be treated aggressively and hospitalization with IV/IM antibiotic therapy should be considered. A dental consult is also appropriate because tooth extraction could be necessary.

8. *b*   Basal cell carcinoma is the most common cause of skin cancer in humans with risk being proportional to sun exposure. This cancerous lesion rarely causes death, but can be disfiguring. Recurrence rate is high; hence, the reason for annual exams after a basal cell carcinoma lesion has been discovered. The cure rate is about 95%.

9. *a*   Actinic keratosis is often more easily palpated than visualized because of its light color and sandpaper texture. It is commonly felt or seen on sun-exposed areas in light-skinned people. If it is on the lips, it may present in an area of leukoplakia.

10. An adult presents with tinea corporis. Which item below is a risk factor for its development?

    a. Topical steroid use
    b. Topical antibiotic use
    c. A recent laceration
    d. Cold climates

11. A 3 year old has worn a new pair of plastic sandals at the beach. When her mother takes them off, she notices the straps of the sandals have left red marks and the child complains of itching and burning in the area of redness. What is the most likely diagnosis and how should the nurse practitioner manage the problem?

    a. Contact dermatitis; the mother should have the child wait until the rash is gone before wearing the sandals again.
    b. Contact dermatitis; the mother should not allow the child to wear these sandals again.
    c. Sunburn; the mother should apply sunscreen before allowing the child to play in the sun.
    d. Allergic reaction to the sand and heat; topical cortisone cream and Calamine® lotion are indicated.

12. The nurse practitioner diagnoses eczema on the face of a 2 year old. The patient's mother explains that she is embarrassed to take the child in public because her face is so red and dry. She asks for a "strong" cortisone cream so the eczema will clear rapidly. The nurse practitioner knows that:

    a. a high potency cortisone preparation applied to the face will shorten the duration of the eczema flare-up.
    b. a high potency cortisone cream on the face will only be helpful if used in conjunction with a hydrating lotion.
    c. a high potency cortisone cream is not recommended for use on children under 3 years-of-age.
    d. a high potency cortisone cream may cause atrophy, telangiectasia, purpura, or striae if used on the face.

10. *a*   Risk factors for acquiring tinea corporis include contact with infected animals, personal contact with infected persons, contact with contaminated fomites, immunosuppression, and temperate or tropical climate.

11. *b*   This is a case of classic contact dermatitis. When the skin is exposed to an irritant, the stratum corneum is disrupted, the underlying epidermis is injured, and an inflammatory reaction ensues. Plastic is a common precipitant of this kind of reaction. The child should avoid exposure to known skin irritants.

12. *d*   Regardless of the patient's age, only low-potency cortisone formulations should be used on the face, dorsum of the hands, and scrotum. Fluorinated steroids may cause rosacea on the face.

_a_ 13. A 6-year-old African-American child has a round alopecic patch on his scalp. There is scaling of the lesion and broken hair shafts. What is this child's diagnosis and what is the most appropriate nurse practitioner action?

    a. Tinea capitis; the child should be started on oral griseofulvin daily for 6 weeks

    b. Tinea capitis; the child should be started on a topical antifungal

    c. Trichotillomania; this patient should be referred for counseling

    d. Alopecia areata, topical steroids will be helpful

_a_ 14. A 16-year-old basketball player complains of itching in the crural folds, buttocks, and upper thighs. The lesions are well demarcated and are half-moon shaped. The area is red, irritated, and there are small breaks in the skin from scratching. What is this patient's diagnosis and how should it be treated?

    a. Tinea cruris; treat with a topical antifungal cream

    b. Eczema; treat with a topical steroid

    c. Scabies; treat with permethrin (Nix®) cream

    d. Syphilis; treat with penicillin

_a_ 15. A 45 year old with diabetes has had itching and burning lesions between her toes for 2 months. Scrapings of the lesions confirm the diagnosis tinea pedis. What is the best initial treatment option for this patient?

    a. Prescribe an antifungal powder for application between her toes and in her shoes and a topical prescription strength antifungal cream for other affected areas. Monitor for a secondary bacterial infection.

    b. Prescribe an oral antifungal for 4 to 12 weeks. Monitor BUN and creatinine at 1 week, 2 weeks, and every month thereafter.

    c. Prescribe an oral antifungal for 4 to 12 weeks. Monitor liver enzymes, BUN, and creatinine at 1 week, 2 weeks, and every month thereafter.

    d. Prescribe a prescription-strength antifungal/steroid combination cream. Monitor for a secondary bacterial infection.

13. *a* Tinea capitis is particularly prevalent in urban African-American children between the ages of 3 and 9 years. Topical antifungal agents are ineffective with tinea capitis. Oral griseofulvin is the drug of choice. Tinea capitis rarely occurs in adults.

14. *a* Tinea cruris ("jock itch") commonly occurs in patients from wearing wet or damp clothing. Application of steroids will cause the lesions to change in appearance and spread rapidly. Tinea cruris does not involve the penis or scrotum. Frequent exposure to the air (e.g., wearing boxer shorts) aids resolution and reduces recurrence.

15. *a* If the patient follows the treatment plan as outlined in choice *a*, she should get some relief in a couple of weeks and resolution in 4 to 6 weeks. She should also monitor for a secondary bacterial infection. She has diabetes and may have poor circulation; thus, resolution of this problem might be more difficult. If this course of treatment fails, the nurse practitioner should consider oral antifungal therapy with monitoring of liver enzymes. There should be no need to monitor BUN/Cr just because the patient is taking an oral antifungal.

16. A 23-year-old college student presents to the campus health clinic with a generalized rash on her trunk. The lesions are oriented in a Christmas tree pattern and are mildly pruritic. She describes a "round ringworm" that appeared about 1 week ago, but now has disappeared. What is this patient's diagnosis and how should she be treated?

    a. Tinea corporis; treat with a topical antifungal cream for 10 to 14 days
    b. Secondary syphilis; treat with penicillin
    c. Viral exanthem; no specific treatment is needed except rest and fluids
    d. Pityriasis rosea; treat with an oral antipruritic

17. A teenager has pruritic lesions with an erythematous base and silvery scales on his knees. What's the most likely diagnosis?

    a. Eczema
    b. Psoriasis
    c. Reiter's disease
    d. Lichen planus

18. Which of the following is *not* a form of diaper dermatitis?

    a. Contact dermatitis
    b. Candidiasis diaper rash
    c. Atopic diaper dermatitis
    d. Acrodermatitis enteropathica

19. A good sunscreen lotion or sunblock may contain all of the following components. Which provides the *least* protection against the sun's harmful rays?

    a. Zinc oxide
    b. The benzophenones
    c. Para-aminobenzoic acid (PABA)
    d. Lanolin

16. *d*   Pityriasis rosea occurs most frequently in persons aged 10 to 35 years. A "herald patch", which resembles a single ringworm lesion, often precedes the eruption by 1 to 30 days (but usually 7 days). The eruption consists of multiple macules progressing to papules that are parallel to each other on the trunk in a "Christmas tree" distribution. Treatment is symptomatic.

17. *b*   Psoriasis is a chronic, proliferative, epidermal disease with remissions and exacerbations. Flare-ups are related to environmental and systemic factors. There are many clinical forms of psoriasis. Silvery scales on red plaques is one clinical presentation. There is a genetic predisposition to this disease. Males and females are affected equally.

18. *d*   Diaper rash collectively can encompass 1 or several dermatoses. There are many types: friction, irritation, allergic, atopic, seborrheic, and candidal. Typically, candidal infections are beefy red with satellite lesions. Acrodermatitis enteropathica is a dermatitis due to zinc deficiency.

19. *d*   Lanolin is a moisturizer that provides no protection against the sun's harmful rays. Sunscreen components like the benzophenones protect against the ultraviolet light in the A range; PABA or PABA esters provide protection against ultraviolet light in the B range. Sunblocks, such as zinc oxide, scatter light and are especially useful on susceptible areas of the face, ears, and lips.

20. A male patient presents 36 hours after having been bitten on the arm during a fight with his spouse. His wound is swollen, red, with discolored exudate and a 5 cm tissue tear. Which action by the nurse practitioner is *least* appropriate at this time?

    a. Administer 0.5 ml tetanus toxoid vaccine if it has been > 5 years since his last tetanus booster.
    b. Prescribe amoxicillin-clavulanate (Augmentin®) and collect a swab specimen for culture and sensitivity.
    c. Suture the torn tissue to facilitate speedy healing.
    d. Prescribe an antibiotic ointment for application with twice a day dressing changes.

21. A patient states that he was bitten by a brown recluse spider. Which statement regarding brown recluse spider bites is *incorrect*?

    a. Erythema, widening of the macule at the puncture site, and tissue necrosis characterize this bite.
    b. A person is usually not aware of having been bitten.
    c. Within 12 hours after the bite, systemic symptoms may occur.
    d. Tissue necrosis can begin as early as 4 hours after a bite and may take weeks or months to heal.

22. A mother and 3 children, ranging in ages from 9 months to 4 years, are diagnosed with scabies. What is the drug of choice for treating this family?

    a. lindane (Kwell®) cream or lotion
    b. permethrin (Nix®) cream
    c. thiabendazole (Mintezol®) suspension
    d. selenium sulfide (Selsun®)

23. A young child is suspected of having pediculosis. The nurse practitioner examines the hair of the child with a Wood's lamp. The nurse practitioner would expect to see:

    a. adult lice glowing fluorescent green.
    b. no adult lice, but blue fluorescence where the adults have laid eggs.
    c. nits that fluoresce white and gray.
    d. no fluorescence unless there are live nits.

20. *c*   Infection is likely because of the discolored exudate from the wound. It would be inappropriate to suture a wound when it is apparent there is an infectious process.

21. *b*   The bite of a recluse spider produces an immediate, sharp, stinging pain. Application of ice and avoidance of exercise is recommended immediately after the bite. Application of local heat is contraindicated. A Td booster is indicated if the patient has not received one within the past 5 years.

22. *b*   Lindane should not be used to treat scabies in pregnant women, infants, or toddlers. A safer choice for the mother and young children is 5% permethrin. The cream or lotion is spread over the entire body (below the head for children and adults, and over the head and body of infants and toddlers). The cream or lotion should be removed by bathing in 8 to 14 hours. A re-application 48 hours later may be indicated.

23. *c*   Live eggs (nits) fluoresce white and empty nits fluoresce gray. Nits are found on the hair shafts and are difficult to remove. They are most often found on the back of the head, behind the ears, and nape of the neck.

_C_ 24. With Cat-scratch disease, the infected person:

    a. is contagious and should be isolated from others for 3 days.
    b. should be treated with antibiotics for 7 to 14 days.
    c. should be assessed for Hodgkin's, infectious mononucleosis, and other causes of regional lymphadenitis.
    d. may have an intermittent murmur that disappears in the prone position.

_d_ 25. A 2 year old has temperature of 102°F (38.8°C) without other symptoms. The patient's mother has amoxicillin left over from another illness 3 months ago. She gives the child amoxicillin for 2 days. The fever continues for another day and suddenly disappears, but then a maculopapular rash emerges. What is the most likely condition?

    a. Drug rash
    b. Rubella
    c. Fifth disease
    d. Roseola

_b_ 26. An 18 year old female applying for college admission presents to the health clinic because evidence of rubella vaccination is required for admission. The nurse practitioner orders a rubella titer. The result indicates negative serologic evidence of rubella antibody. The nurse practitioner should:

    a. tell her that serologic evidence demonstrates she is immune to rubella and that she probably had the disease as a child.
    b. administer the vaccination after a negative pregnancy test and advise her to avoid pregnancy for 28 days.
    c. tell her she needs the immunization and can get it today if her pregnancy test is negative.
    d. administer the rubella vaccination after a negative pregnancy test and advise her not to get pregnant for at least 6 months.

_d_ 27. A 4-year-old presents to the clinic with circumoral pallor and intense red eruptions on both cheeks which appeared last night. The child has low-grade fever but no other symptoms. What is the most likely diagnosis?

    a. Scarlet fever
    b. Chicken pox
    c. Roseola
    d. Fifth disease

24. *c*   With Cat-scratch disease, the patient typically has regional lymphadenitis following inoculation by a cat, kitten, or other animal. Other causes of lymphadenitis must be ruled out, including pharyngitis, solid tumors, Kawasaki disease, tuberculosis, dental abscess, and otitis media. Isolation is not necessary. Antibiotic therapy is controversial.

25. *d*   Roseola infantum or exanthem subitum commonly occurs in children 6 months to 4 years-of-age. It is unlikely that amoxicillin caused the rash because it was discontinued for 24 hours before the rash emerged. High fever, then sudden temperature decrease with emergence of a maculopapular rash is classic roseola.

26. *b*   Administration of rubella vaccination during pregnancy is absolutely contraindicated because of the possible teratogenic effects of rubella on the developing fetus. The earlier in the pregnancy the fetus is exposed, the greater the potential for congenital anomalies. Regardless of the actual time of gestational development in which the fetus is exposed, the infant may be chronically ill.

27. *d*   The eruptive rash of Fifth disease appears on the cheeks and forehead and looks like the child has been slapped; hence, the name "slapped cheek" disease. This is a viral infection that starts on the face, but by the next day appears as a maculopapular rash on the extremities. It finally spreads to the trunk and distal extremities leaving a lace-like appearance. A prodrome with malaise and fever occurs occasionally.

a 28. A 3-year-old child is brought to the health clinic. Her immunizations are up to date and she has been healthy. She has a fine maculopapular rash from head to toe, has been coughing, and has had fever for 3 days. No one she has had contact with has similar symptoms. The mother is concerned that the child has measles. The nurse practitioner explains that:

    a. measles is a disease that usually occurs in outbreaks and is rare in an immunized child.

    b. there is specific medication to treat measles that should be started immediately.

    c. measles usually occurs in young adults in the 2nd or 3rd decade of life.

    d. measles can cause severe birth defects in unborn babies and the mother has now been exposed.

c 29. A 6 year old had an acute onset of fever, pharyngitis, and headache 2 days ago. Today, he presents with cervical lymphadenopathy and sandpaper-textured rash everywhere except on his face. A rapid streptococcal antigen test is positive. The remainder of the assessment is unremarkable. What are the most likely diagnosis and the most appropriate action?

    a. Rubeola; treat symptomatically

    b. Kawasaki disease; consult a physician immediately

    c. Scarlet fever; initiate antibiotic treatment

    d. Toxic shock syndrome; consult a physician immediately

a 30. A child has just scalded her index finger with hot water at home. The mother calls the nurse practitioner within 5 minutes of the injury. All of the following are appropriate instructions for the mother regarding care of the patient with a 2nd degree burn *except*:

    a. applying butter, cooking oil, or lanolin for pain relief.

    b. flushing the area with cool water for about 5 to 10 minutes and then applying silver sulfadiazine.

    c. tetanus prophylaxis is indicated if not received within the past 5 years.

    d. medicate the child for pain as needed with an over-the-counter analgesic.

28. *a* Measles is an acute, highly contagious, viral illness characterized by fever, the presence of cough, coryza, or conjunctivitis, and a maculopapular rash. This child may have measles, but it seems unlikely considering his immunization status and the fact that no other children he has been in contact with are sick.

29. *c* This disease is due to infection with Group A *β*-hemolytic *Streptococcus*. The rash is thought to be due to a systemic reaction to the toxin produced by the microorganism. The rash fades with pressure and ultimately desquamates. A deep, non-blanching rash on the flexor surfaces of the skin is referred to as "Pastia lines."

30. *a* Flushing a 1st or 2nd degree burn with cool water is appropriate to prevent further thermal injury and to provide pain relief. Oil should never be applied to a burn injury. Consider physician consultation for burns in patients who are under 10 years-of-age and over 50 years-of-age. Physician referral is recommended for all 3rd degree burns, for 2nd and 3rd degree burns involving more than 10% of the body surface area, any deep thickness burns more than 2% of the body surface area, and burns involving the face.

Endocrine Disorders

_b_ 1. Diagnostic criteria for diabetes include:

1. a fasting glucose ≥ 200 mg/dL.
2. a random nonfasting plasma glucose ≥ 200 mg/dL.
3. an 8 hour fasting plasma glucose ≥ 126 mg/dL.

   a. 1, 2, 3   c. 1, 3
   b. 2, 3   d. 1, 2

_d_ 2. Which of the following patients most warrants screening for hypothyroidism?

   a. A young adult female with postpartum depression lasting 2 weeks
   b. A patient taking a thyroid replacement preparation
   c. A 40 year old male with unexplained tremors
   d. An elderly female with recent onset of mental dysfunction

_a_ 3. A patient taking levothyroxine is being over-replaced. What condition is he at risk for?

   a. Osteoporosis
   b. Constipation
   c. Depression
   d. Exophthalmia

_d_ 4. Which of the following is _not_ a risk factor associated with the development of syndrome X and type 2 diabetes mellitus?

   a. Hypertriglyceridemia and low high-density lipoprotein
   b. Gestational diabetes and polycystic ovarian syndrome
   c. Hispanic, African-American, Native-American, and Pacific Islander ethnicity
   d. Postprandial hypoglycemia

_b_ 5. What is the most common cause of Cushing's syndrome?

   a. Excessive ACTH production
   b. Administration of a glucocorticoid or ACTH
   c. Pituitary adenoma or a non-pituitary ACTH-producing tumor
   d. Autonomous cortisol production from adrenal tissue

1. *b* Since the year 2000, diagnostic criteria established by the American Diabetes Association include: numbers 2 and 3. Either abnormal value must be confirmed by repeating the test on another day. Choice *a* is an abnormal value, but it is not a diagnostic criterion.

2. *d* Screening whole populations for hypothyroidism is not warranted. There is a high prevalence of hypothyroidism among the elderly with cognitive impairment.

3. *a* Over replacement is common in the U.S., but should be avoided because patients are at increased risk for osteoporosis and atrial arrhythmias, especially atrial fibrillation. The average dose required for replacement in a young or middle aged adult is 1.6 mcg/kg ideal body weight. Needs are increased by 45% during pregnancy and are decreased after 65 years-of-age.

4. *d* Postprandial hyperglycemia, hypertriglyceridemia, low HDL, truncal obesity, and Hispanic, African-American, Native-American, and Pacific Islander ethnicity are risk factors for developing syndrome X and type 2 diabetes mellitus.

5. *b* Iatrogenic Cushing's syndrome is the most common type. Exogenous glucocorticoid administration produces a Cushing's syndrome that is reversible by discontinuation of the medication.

d 6.   Which of the following is *not* a characteristic of type 2 diabetes mellitus?

   a.   Insulin resistance
   b.   High body mass index
   c.   Central obesity
   d.   Unexplained weight loss

C 7.   What diabetic complications result from hyperglycemia?

   1.   Retinopathy
   2.   Hypertension resistant to treatment
   3.   Peripheral neuropathy
   4.   Accelerated atherogenesis

   a.   1, 2, 3
   b.   2, 3, 4
   c.   1, 3, 4
   d.   1, 2, 4

C 8.   A patient has been diagnosed with hypothyroidism and thyroid hormone replacement therapy is prescribed. How long should the nurse practitioner wait before checking the patient's TSH?

   a.   1 weeks
   b.   2 weeks
   c.   4 weeks
   d.   8 weeks

a 9.   A patient presents with dehydration, hypotension, and fever. Laboratory testing reveals hyponatremia, hyperkalemia, and hypoglycemia. These imbalances are corrected, but the patient returns 6 weeks later with the same symptoms and hyperpigmentation, weakness, anorexia, fatigue, and weight loss. What action(s) should the nurse practitioner take?

   a.   Obtain a thorough history and physical, and check serum cortisol and ACTH levels.
   b.   Obtain a diet history and check CBC and FBS.
   c.   Provide nutritional guidance and have the patient return in 1 month.
   d.   Consult home health for intravenous administration of fluids and electrolytes.

6. *d*   Type 2 diabetes mellitus is characterized by insulin resistance and, consequently, decreased peripheral glucose utilization. Patients with type 2 diabetes mellitus typically have a high body mass index (BMI) with central (truncal) obesity. The pathophysiology of type 1 diabetes mellitus is pancreatic beta cell destruction, accounting for the relative absence of insulin.

7. *c*   All of the choices are directly attributable to prolonged hyperglycemic states except hypertension. The current state of knowledge is unable to explain resistant hypertension in patients with diabetes.

8. *c*   The half-life of levothyroxine, the treatment of choice for thyroid replacement, is 7 days. It takes 4-5 half-lives for a drug to reach steady state. The TSH should be measured at steady state which is 28-35 days for levothyroxine. Therefore, the health care provider should wait 4-5 weeks before checking the patient's TSH.

9. *a*   These are the signs and symptoms of acute and chronic adrenal insufficiency. A thorough history, including medications, will help to determine the cause. Primary adrenal insufficiency (Addison's disease) is usually an autoimmune disorder. It can also be caused by infection. Secondary adrenocortical insufficiency is most often due to withdrawal of a glucocorticoid medication. It may also involve a tumor or trauma. Simultaneous low serum cortisol and high ACTH are diagnostic for primary adrenal insufficiency. This patient should receive an endocrinology consult.

a 10. A 30-year-old female patient presents to the clinic with heat intolerance, tremors, nervousness, and weight loss inconsistent with increased appetite. Which test would be most likely to confirm the suspected diagnosis?

    a. A serum thyroid stimulating hormone (TSH) level
    b. Follicle stimulating hormone (FSH)
    c. A urine drug screen
    d. The Hamilton Anxiety Scale

a 11. A child with type 1 diabetes mellitus has experienced excessive hunger, weight gain, and increasing hyperglycemia. The Somogyi effect is suspected. What steps should be taken to diagnose and treat this condition?

    a. Decrease the evening insulin dose and check capillary blood glucose (CBG) at 2:00 am.
    b. Instruct the child's parents on physical activities to help with weight loss.
    c. Increase the evening insulin dose and check the CBG at 2:00 am.
    d. Refer the child for instruction on a strict diabetic diet.

d 12. A child with type 1 diabetes mellitus brings in a glucose diary indicating consistent morning hyperglycemia. How can the nurse practitioner differentiate the Somogyi effect from dawn phenomenon?

    a. Experiment with a smaller insulin dose in the evenings.
    b. Increase the insulin dose and liberalize the child's diet.
    c. Check HbA_{1C} today and again in 3 months.
    d. Instruct the parent to monitor the blood glucose at 2:00 am.

a 13. An eight-year-old male patient's height has gradually fallen from the 70th percentile to the 5th percentile on the growth chart over the last 3 years. His parents are average height. CBC, UA, stool for occult blood, ova and parasites, chemistries and thyroid function tests are all normal. What intervention is appropriate?

    a. Refer the patient to a pediatric endocrinologist now.
    b. Recommend a daily multivitamin.
    c. Observe the patient's growth for 1 year.
    d. Obtain further diagnostic assessments such as growth hormone and bone age.

10. *a*   These are the classic signs and symptoms of hyperthyroidism. The absence of detectable serum thyroid stimulating hormone (TSH) is the screening and diagnostic test for hyperthyroidism.

11. *a*   The Somogyi effect, more common in children, occurs when there is rebound hyperglycemia following a hypoglycemic period. Rapid changes in plasma glucose occur over a short period of time. Hunger and weight gain in the presence of hyperglycemia are clues that this is occurring. If the Somogyi effect is suspected, the correct action is to decrease the evening insulin dose to reduce the likelihood of 1am hypoglycemia and check a capillary blood glucose at 1:00 or 2:00 am.

12. *d*   Dawn phenomenon is an early morning rise in plasma glucose. It indicates a need for increased insulin. The Somogyi effect is a rise in plasma glucose in response to hypoglycemia. It is usually accompanied by weight gain and hunger and is corrected by decreasing the evening insulin dose. A series of 3 morning measurements of blood glucose will differentiate between the 2 conditions.

13. *a*   Diagnostic assessment of a child with suspected growth hormone deficiency should be referred to a pediatric endocrinologist. Treatment should not be delayed. The younger the child is when treatment is begun, the greater the benefit.

_C_ 14. An obese hyperlipidemic patient, newly diagnosed with type 2 diabetes mellitus, has fasting blood glucose values 180 to 250 mg/dL. What is the most appropriate initial treatment to consider?

    a. A low-calorie diet and exercise
    b. Sliding-scale NPH insulin every 12 hours
    c. An oral hypoglycemic agent
    d. Sliding-scale regular insulin every 6 hours

_b_ 15. In which of the following presentations is further diagnostic testing *not* warranted?

    a. Bilateral gynecomastia in a pre-pubertal male of average weight; Tanner stage 1
    b. Bilateral gynecomastia in a 13 year old male with normal testicular size and volume
    c. Recent onset gynecomastia in a 20 year old male with breast tenderness
    d. Unilateral breast mass which is 5 centimeters in diameter

_C_ 16. What information should patients with diabetes and their families receive about hypoglycemia?

    a. Hypoglycemia is a rare complication.
    b. Hypoglycemia requires professional medical treatment.
    c. Hypoglycemia is serious, dangerous, and can be fatal if not treated quickly.
    d. Hypoglycemia occurs only as a result of insulin overdose.

_b_ 17. The most common presentation of thyroid cancer is:

    a. generalized enlargement of the thyroid gland.
    b. a solitary thyroid nodule.
    c. a multinodular goiter.
    d. abnormal thyroid function tests.

_C_ 18. Which patient would profit most from screening for type 2 diabetes?

    a. A 30 year old female with unintended weight loss
    b. A 25 year old male with family history of type 1 diabetes
    c. An obese female with recurrent vaginitis
    d. 50 year old hyperlipidemic male

14. *c* It is unlikely that this patient will have an adequate decrease in blood sugar with diet and exercise alone. This patient will likely respond best to an oral agent (or combination of agents) along with diet and exercise. Beginning therapy with insulin is not usually indicated unless FBS is extremely high and quick control is needed.

15. *b* There is a high prevalence of benign enlargement of the male breast during puberty. Gynecomastia results from excess estrogen and is more common in obese boys due to excessive conversion of androgen to estrogen in fatty tissue. The testicles should appear normal in size and volume for Tanner stage.

16. *c* Although hypoglycemia is common in type 1 diabetes mellitus, it is a serious life-threatening condition, and should be treated quickly. A conscious patient should be given a simple carbohydrate by mouth. If the patient is unconscious, parenteral glucagon may be used. Hypoglycemia may occur as a result of skipping a meal, unexpected exercise, or no apparent reason.

17. *b* Most thyroid cancer presents as a solitary nodule; however, it may coexist with other conditions that cause goiter. Abnormal thyroid function tests tend to support a non-malignant cause of goiter.

18. *c* Screening is of greatest value in patients with risk factors and/or symptoms. The most common risk factors are obesity (> 20% over ideal body weight), family history, age > 40 years plus one other risk factor, history of gestational diabetes or delivery of a macrosomic infant, the "3 Ps," and recurrent skin, vaginal, or urinary tract infection. The patient in item *c* has 2 risk factors. Family history of type 1 diabetes mellitus does not increase the risk of developing type 2 diabetes mellitus.

_b_____ 19. According to the American Diabetes Association, what minimum fasting plasma glucose level (confirmed on a subsequent day) warrants a diagnosis of diabetes mellitus?

    a. 121 mg/dL
    b. 126 mg/dL
    c. 130 mg/dL
    d. 140 mg/dL

_d_____ 20. Which terms does the American Diabetes Association (ADA) recommend to designate the types of diabetes mellitus?

    a. Non-insulin dependent diabetes (NIDDM) and insulin dependent diabetes (IDDM)
    b. Diabetes mellitus type I and type II
    c. Juvenile-onset diabetes and adult-onset diabetes
    d. Type 1 and type 2 diabetes mellitus

_c_____ 21. Which factors are associated with high risk for foot complications in a patient with diabetes mellitus?

    1. Obesity
    2. Abnormal nails
    3. Abnormal gait
    4. Poorly controlled lipids

    a. 1, 2, 3
    b. 2, 3, 4
    c. 2, 3
    d. 1, 4

_c_____ 22. What information should a 42-year-old patient with newly diagnosed diabetes receive about exercise?

    a. Buy good walking shoes with support and a flexible sole.
    b. Exercise at least 5 days per week.
    c. Snack before exercise.
    d. Do not exercise if your blood sugar is greater than 180 mg/dL.

19. *b* In June 1997, the American Diabetes Association (ADA) and the World Health Organization(WHO), acting on the advice of an expert panel, lowered the fasting plasma glucose from 140 mg/dL to 126 mg/dL for the diagnosis of diabetes. The ADA considers the fasting plasma glucose to be the most reliable diagnostic test for diabetes mellitus.

20. *d* The ADA recommends using the terms type 1 diabetes mellitus (T1DM) and type 2 diabetes mellitus (T2DM). Type 1 diabetes mellitus is characterized by total pancreatic beta cell failure. Type 2 diabetes mellitus is generally characterized by insulin resistance. Previous designations have included non-insulin dependent (NIDDM) and insulin dependent (IDDM), juvenile onset and adult onset, and type I and type II.

21. *c* The feet of patients with diabetes should be examined annually (if low-risk) or at each visit (if high risk) to detect problems and avoid the need for amputation. High risk characteristics are abnormal nails and skin, abnormal gait, structural deformity, neuropathy, history of foot ulcers or skin infections. Obesity without neuropathy does not increase the risk of foot complications.

22. *c* A diabetic patient should snack prior to exercise to avoid hypoglycemia. Exercise should be done "most days of the week," but not if glucose levels are greater than 300 mg/dL because exercise may worsen the hyperglycemia if insufficient insulin is available. Generally, exercise improves cardiovascular fitness and increases insulin secretion and glucose utilization.

C 23. Which medication below would be safest for an elderly diabetic patient if
     hypoglycemia is a major concern?

     a. tolbutamide (Orinase®)
     b. glipizide (Glucotrol® XL)
     c. metformin (Glucophage®-XR)
     d. chlorpropamide (Diabinese®)

b 24. A patient newly diagnosed with type 2 diabetes mellitus is having only
     postprandial glucose elevations. The best choice for treatment is:

     a. metformin (Glucophage®-XR).
     b. acarbose (Precose®).
     c. rosiglitazone (Avandia®).
     d. glipizide (Glucotrol® XL).

a 25. Which of the following is the target set by the American Diabetes
     Association (ADA) for diabetes control?

     a. Fasting blood glucose < 126 mg/dL in the absence of metabolic stress
     b. 2-hour postprandial glucose between 140 and 200 mg/dL
     c. Fasting blood glucose 80 to 120 mg/dL and bedtime glucose 100 to
         140 mg/dL
     d. HbA_{1C} 7.5% on random sample

b 26. Which of the following are most commonly observed in patients with type
     2 diabetes mellitus?

     1. Beta cell destruction
     2. High body mass
     3. Central obesity
     4. Unexplained weight loss

     a. 1, 2, 3   c. 1, 4
     b. 2, 3   d. 1, 3, 4

b 27. Retinal microaneurysms in a patient with diabetes resemble:

     a. cotton wool spots.
     b. small red dots.
     c. fuzzy white blots.
     d. blurred orange lines.

23. *c* Metformin does not cause hypoglycemia if given as monotherapy. It works by decreasing hepatic glucose production and increasing peripheral glucose utilization. Orinase® and Glucotrol® XL both have a 4 hour half-life and inactive metabolites and are good choices for the elderly if Glucophage®-XR cannot be tolerated or if a sulfonylurea is needed in addition to Glucophage®-XR. The half-life of Diabinese® is about 36 hours but does not require hepatic metabolism.

24. *b* Precose® is an excellent choice because it slows carbohydrate absorption from the GI tract and decreases postprandial glucose elevations. It is taken before meals.

25. *a* Target values set by the American Diabetes Association include fasting glucose less than 126 mg/dL and $HbA_{1C} < 6.5$ %.

26. *b* Type 2 diabetes mellitus is characterized by decreased peripheral glucose utilization, increased hepatic glucose production, and insufficient pancreatic insulin secretion. The majority of patients with type 2 diabetes mellitus have high body mass and central (truncal) obesity. The pathophysiology underlying type 1 diabetes mellitus is pancreatic beta cell destruction and accounts for the relative absence of insulin that is seen in type 1 diabetes mellitus.

27. *b* Retinal microaneurysms appear as small, red dots. Exudates appear as cotton wool spots. Both of these findings are associated with diabetic retinopathy. The patient may not be aware of a problem because, unless there is involvement of the macula, vision may not be impaired.

28. A diabetic patient is taking low-dose enalapril (Vasotec®) for hypertension. A record of the patient's blood pressure over 4 weeks ranges from 130 to 142 mmHg systolic and 75 to 85 mmHg diastolic. How should the nurse practitioner respond?

    a. Change to a different class of antihypertensive medication to get better control.
    b. Increase the dosage of the current BP medication.
    c. Continue the current medication and dosage for 4 more weeks.
    d. Add a beta-blocker to the current medication regimen.

 29. Microalbuminuria is a measure of:

    a. total urinary protein.
    b. late renal compromise in a diabetic patient.
    c. early glycemic abnormality.
    d. protein lost into the urine.

 30. The most accurate measure of diabetes control is:

    a. avoidance of micro- and macro-vascular complications.
    b. insulin sensitivity.
    c. early morning glucose levels.
    d. HbA_{1C}.

28. *b* The drug of choice for blood pressure management in a patient with diabetes is an ACE inhibitor (enalapril is an ACE inhibitor) or an angiotensin receptor blocker (ARB). Target blood pressure for a diabetic patient is less than 130/80 mmHg. This patient would benefit from a further reduction in blood pressure, so increasing the current dosage of enalapril is the most reasonable option. Clearly, many diabetics will require 3 or more drugs to achieve goal blood pressure.

29. *d* Albumin is a protein excreted into the urine in small amounts. Hence, the term, microalbuminuria. It is the most sensitive indicator of early renal compromise in a patient with diabetes.

30. *d* HbA$_{1C}$ is an average of blood glucose concentration as measured from red blood cells. The average life of a RBC is 90 to 120 days. Therefore, HbA$_{1C}$ reflects the average blood glucose concentration over the previous 90 to 120 days.

Eye, Ear, Nose, and Throat Disorders

1. Which choice below is *least* effective for alleviating symptoms of the common cold?

    a. Antihistamines
    b. Oral decongestants
    c. Topical decongestants
    d. Antipyretics

2. A 65 year old patient comes to the health clinic in October for an influenza vaccination. He has never had one before. A "yes" response to which of the following questions, may contraindicate influenza vaccine administration?

    a. "Are you allergic to penicillin?"
    b. "Did you ever have a reaction to the MMR vaccine?"
    c. "Are you allergic to eggs?"
    d. "Have you taken an antibiotic in the past week?"

3. Group A β-hemolytic streptococcal (GABHS) pharyngitis is most common in which age group?

    a. Under 3 years-of-age
    b. Preschool children
    c. 6 to 12 years-of-age
    d. Adolescents

4. A child complains that his "throat hurts" with swallowing. His voice is very "throaty" and he is hyperextending his neck to talk. Examination reveals asymmetrical swelling of his tonsils. His uvula is deviated to the left. What is the most likely diagnosis?

    a. Peritonsillar abscess
    b. Thyroiditis
    c. Mononucleosis
    d. Epiglottitis

1. *a*   There is no histaminic component to a viral infection; therefore, antihistamines have no purpose in the treatment of the common cold. They are commonly used by patients for relief of symptoms but they have no proven beneficial effect. Rhinovirus is the most common cause of the common cold.

2. *c*   The influenza vaccine should NOT be administered to patients who have a known "anaphylactic hypersensitivity" to eggs. Less severe reactions to eggs should not contraindicate vaccine administration. Vaccines should NOT be administered to patients who have an acute febrile illness, but concurrent antibiotic treatment is not a contraindication to receiving the influenza vaccine.

3. *c*   GABHS is the organism responsible for post-streptococcal rheumatic fever; therefore, it is important to recognize and treat early. The diagnosis is rare in children under 3 years-of-age. GABHS infection tends to occur most frequently in the colder months, between September and April.

4. *a*   This can be a complication of pharyngitis due to failure to seek treatment or a failure to treat. Peritonsillar or retropharyngeal abscess is a reason for immediate physician or emergency department referral due to the potential danger of airway obstruction and need for drainage of the abscess. In younger patients, drooling may be evident.

5. An 8-year-old presents to the health clinic with history of acute onset severe sore throat and respiratory distress with stridor in the last 2 hours. The child's history is positive for fever and pharyngitis for 2 days. What is the most likely diagnosis?

    a. Mononucleosis
    b. Asthma
    c. Respiratory syncytial virus (RSV)
    d. Epiglottitis

6. A 4-year-old presents with complaints of sore throat and fever for 2 days. He has multiple vesiculated ulcerations on his tonsils and uvula. There are no other remarkable findings. What is the most likely diagnosis?

    a. Viral pharyngitis
    b. Herpangina
    c. Epiglottitis
    d. Tonsillitis

7. Hand-foot-and-mouth disease can be distinguished from herpangina by the:

    a. causative agent.
    b. presence of ulcerations on the oropharynx.
    c. presence of exanthem on the hands and feet.
    d. length of treatment.

8. A 16-year-old male presents with mild sore throat, fever, fatigue, posterior cervical adenopathy, and palatine petechiae. Without a definitive diagnosis for this patient, what drug would be the *least* appropriate to prescribe?

    a. ibuprofen
    b. erythromycin
    c. amoxicillin
    d. acetaminophen

9. The nurse practitioner should instruct the mother of an infant with thrush to:

    a. take oral nystatin since she is breastfeeding.
    b. stop breastfeeding until the thrush has resolved.
    c. administer antifungal medication to the infant prior to feedings.
    d. sterilize pacifiers and bottle nipples.

5. *d*   It is unlikely that this child has respiratory syncytial virus (RSV) because of his age. Mononucleosis is rarely accompanied by respiratory distress. Asthma can cause rapid onset of respiratory distress, but it is not frequently accompanied by stridor and is usually accompanied by cough. With a 2-day history of pharyngitis and fever, it is more likely an infectious condition such as epiglottitis. Immediate referral to an emergency department is indicated.

6. *b*   Herpangina is a viral infection common in toddlers and young children caused by *Coxsackie virus*. The clinical findings of numerous, small (1 to 2 mm) ulcerations on the tonsils and uvula are typical of herpangina. The ulcerations can be very painful but usually resolve in 7 to 10 days. Treatment is symptomatic.

7. *c*   Although there are oropharyngeal ulcerations in both diseases, there are usually lesions on the palms of hands and soles of feet in hand-foot-and-mouth disease and the ulcerations are usually larger than 1 to 2 mm. Both diseases are caused by Coxsackie virus and are treated symptomatically.

8. *c*   Sore throat and fatigue are the most common features of infectious mononucleosis (IM). The presence of palatine petechiae and posterior cervical lymphadenopathy makes this highly likely. Hepatosplenomegaly is another associated physical finding. Administration of ampicillin derivatives in patients with IM results in a pruritic, maculopapular rash 90 to 100% of the time. If IM is suspected, ampicillin is inappropriate to prescribe.

9. *d*   Oral antifungals should be administered to the infant *after* feedings. If the mother were breastfeeding, she could also apply an oral antifungal to her nipples. Sterilization of pacifiers and bottle nipples decreases the incidence of reinfection. Cessation of breastfeeding is not necessary.

10. The nurse practitioner notices tooth decay on the lingual surfaces of the maxillary incisors in a 12 month old. The most likely cause is:

    a. nursing bottle syndrome.
    b. lack of fluoride in the diet.
    c. lack of calcium and vitamin D in the diet.
    d. high sugar snacks.

11. Which case of epistaxis should concern the nurse practitioner most?

    a. A child under 2 years-of-age
    b. A teenager with allergies
    c. A child with fresh clots in one naris
    d. A teenager using a nasal decongestant

12. Which of the following is appropriate prophylactic medication for a 12 year old with allergic rhinitis?

    a. An oral antihistamine
    b. cromolyn nasal spray
    c. A β-agonist inhaler
    d. An oral decongestant

13. When, in childhood, do the frontal sinuses usually present?

    a. Birth
    b. 2 to 3 years
    c. 4 to 6 years
    d. 10 to 11 years

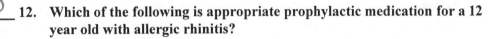

14. Which of the following factors would *not* place a child at increased risk for hearing loss?

    a. Allergic rhinitis
    b. Gestational age < 32 weeks
    c. Cleft palate
    d. Viral meningitis

15. Treatment of acute vertigo includes:

    a. bedrest and an antihistamine.
    b. fluids and a decongestant.
    c. a sedative and decongestant.
    d. rest and a low sodium diet.

10. *a*   Decay begins on the lingual surfaces of the teeth secondary to prolonged contact with milk, juice, or formula. These patients must be referred to a dentist. Parents should avoid putting a baby to bed with a bottle.

11. *a*   Allergies, decongestant use, chronic use of a nasal spray, mechanical trauma (e.g., nose picking), and viral or bacterial infection can all irritate mucosal membranes and cause bleeding. The finding of red irritated nares, with fresh blood or old crusts, is a typical finding. Epistaxis in a child under 2 years-of-age is unusual and warrants further investigation.

12. *b*   All the choices can be used to treat allergic rhinitis, but the only choice that helps to prevent symptoms before they begin is cromolyn nasal spray. This medication helps to prevent the release of mast cell contents which contain histamines and other chemical mediators responsible for allergy symptoms. Nasal steroids are the treatment of choice for allergic rhinitis.

13. *c*   Frontal sinuses usually appear as early as 5 to 6 years-of-age but they may be asymmetrical or absent. Infants are born with maxillary and ethmoid sinuses. Sphenoid sinuses may be identified radiographically by 9 years-of-age.

14. *a*   All the factors listed can place a child at increased risk for hearing loss except allergic rhinitis. Other factors include intrauterine infection, low birth weight (LBW, < 1500 grams), family history of hearing loss, use of a potentially ototoxic drug, head trauma, and hyperbilirubinemia.

15. *a*   Bedrest with vertigo is recommended for safety reasons. Antihistamines are vestibular suppressant drugs and help alleviate the symptoms. The vestibular system is one of 3 systems which helps to maintain spatial orientation and posture. The visual system gives clues to uprightness and the somatosensory system gives information from the muscles, joints, and skin about position. These systems work together to compensate when one system is deficient.

16. Risk factors for acute otitis media (AOM) include all of the following except:

    a. household cigarette smoke.
    b. group daycare attendance.
    c. sibling history of acute otitis media.
    d. African-American ethnicity.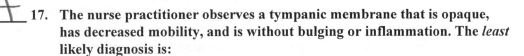

17. The nurse practitioner observes a tympanic membrane that is opaque, has decreased mobility, and is without bulging or inflammation. The *least* likely diagnosis is:

    a. acute otitis media (AOM).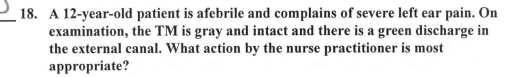
    b. otitis media with effusion.
    c. mucoid otitis media.
    d. serous otitis media.

18. A 12-year-old patient is afebrile and complains of severe left ear pain. On examination, the TM is gray and intact and there is a green discharge in the external canal. What action by the nurse practitioner is most appropriate?

    a. Irrigate the green discharge before examining the tympanic membrane.
    b. Prescribe an otic antibiotic/corticosteroid suspension.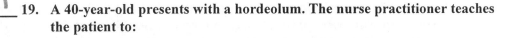
    c. Prescribe an oral antibiotic and analgesic for pain.
    d. Refer to an otolaryngologist for tympanocentesis.

19. A 40-year-old presents with a hordeolum. The nurse practitioner teaches the patient to:

    a. apply a topical antibiotic and warm compresses.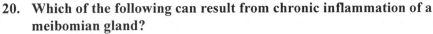
    b. apply cool compresses and avoid touching the hordeolum.
    c. use an oral antibiotic and eye flushes.
    d. apply light palpation to facilitate drainage.

20. Which of the following can result from chronic inflammation of a meibomian gland?

    a. A chalazion
    b. Uveitis
    c. Keratitis
    d. A pterygium

16. *d*   Bottle feeding, cleft palate, and Native-American or Eskimo heritage are also considered risk factors for acute otitis media. By 7 years-of-age, 90% of all children have had 1 occurrence of acute otitis media. Breastfeeding decreases the incidence.

17. *a*   Otitis media with effusion, mucoid otitis media, and serous otitis media all refer to the same condition. The classic finding is decreased mobility of the tympanic membrane. Patients may be asymptomatic except for reports of decreased hearing acuity. With acute otitis media, the membrane frequently is erythematous, and bulging with purulent fluid posteriorly.

18. *b*   The condition described is otitis externa, an infection of the external auditory canal. The most common pathogen is *Pseudomonas aeruginosa.* An otic antibiotic/corticosteroid combination is prescribed for the infection, inflammation, and pain. An oral analgesic is recommended as needed.

19. *a*   Treatment for a hordeolum (stye) consists of applying a topical antibiotic and warm compresses several times daily to facilitate pointing and drainage. If spontaneous drainage does not occur, incision and drainage may be required.

20. *a*   A chalazion results from chronic inflammation of a meibomian gland. It sometimes requires treatment by incision and drainage or excision. It can become secondarily infected resulting in an internal hordeolum.

_C_ 21. A patient presents with an inflamed upper eyelid margin. The conjunctiva is red and there is particulate matter along the upper eyelid. The patient complains of a sensation that "there is something in my eye." What is the diagnosis and how should it be treated?

a. Hordeolum; treat with a topical antibiotic and warm compresses
b. Conjunctivitis; treat with topical antibiotic and warm compresses
c. Blepharitis; treat with warm compresses and gentle debridement with a cotton swab
d. Chalazion; refer to an ophthalmologist for incision and drainage

_A_ 22. A patient presents with periorbital erythema and edema, fever, and nasal drainage. The nurse practitioner should:

a. start aggressive antibiotic therapy.
b. start treatment with a steroid.
c. recommend cool compresses and an oral antibiotic.
d. order sinus x-rays.

_C_ 23. A 21-year-old college student presents to the student health center with copious, markedly purulent discharge from her left eye. The nurse practitioner should suspect:

a. viral conjunctivitis.
b. common pink eye.
c. gonococcal conjunctivitis.
d. allergic conjunctivitis.

_A_ 24. A patient reports "something flew in my eye" about an hour ago while he was splitting logs. If there were a foreign body in his eye, the nurse practitioner would expect to find all *except*:

a. purulent drainage.
b. tearing.
c. photophobia.
d. a positive fluorescein stain.

_A_ 25. The following are all important tests of visual acuity in infants and children up to 3 years-of-age *except*:

a. the Hirschberg test.
b. the red reflex.
c. corneal and pupillary reflexes.
d. tracking of visual stimuli.

21. *c* Blepharitis is an inflammation of the eyelid and its margins and can be caused by bacteria or a seborrheic process. Treatment includes lid scrubs and a topical antibiotic if the cause is bacterial. Conjunctivitis presents in a similar fashion but does not involve eyelid margins.

22. *a* The condition described is periorbital cellulitis. This may be seen in children from ethmoid sinusitis. Periorbital cellulitis in children or adults, can lead to meningitis or cavernous sinus thrombosis. This patient should be aggressively treated with intramuscular or intravenous antibiotics and possible surgical consultation.

23. *c* A purulent and copious discharge should alert the nurse practitioner to the likely possibility of gonococcal or chlamydial conjunctivitis. Both require systemic antibiotic treatment and immediate referral to an ophthalmologist for evaluation.

24. *a* The nurse practitioner may observe all the findings listed except purulent drainage (which would indicate a bacterial infection). Although a bacterial infection is possible from a foreign object, it is unlikely that this would have occurred in the time frame reported by the patient.

25. *a* Visual acuity should be tested in children every time they present for a routine check-up and anytime there is eye trauma. The Hirschberg test evaluates ocular muscle coordination.

26. Which of the following is *most* likely to be the cause of ophthalmia neonatorum?

    a. *Neisseria gonorrhoeae*
    b. Silver nitrate
    c. *Chlamydia trachomatis*
    d. *Herpes simplex*

27. A 2 year old presents with a white pupillary reflex. What is the most likely cause of this finding?

    a. Viral conjunctivitis
    b. Glaucoma
    c. Corneal abrasion
    d. Retinoblastoma

28. Which of the following is *least* likely to cause cataract in a 4 year old child?

    a. Long term systemic steroid use
    b. Strabismus
    c. Trauma to the cornea
    d. Blepharitis

29. At what age should a patient with persistent dacryostenosis be referred to an ophthalmologist?

    a. 2 months-of-age
    b. 4 months-of-age
    c. 6 months-of-age
    d. 1 year-of-age

30. At what age does vision normally become approximately 20/20?

    a. 6 weeks
    b. 4 months
    c. 3 to 4 years
    d. 6 years

26. *a* Ophthalmia neonatorum is an acute inflammation of the conjunctiva most commonly caused by gonococcal infection in the mother. The neonate's eyes become infected during the birth process. Chlamydial conjunctivitis is more common in teens and young adults.

27. *d* Retinoblastoma is a rare retinal tumor with a familial tendency. The presenting age is about 2 years. Other causes of white pupillary reflex or leukocoria include cataract formation and certain retinal problems.

28. *d* Cataracts may be present at birth due to maternal prenatal infections or prematurity. Cataracts may be seen in some children with trisomy 21, diabetes mellitus, Marfan's syndrome, or different types of ocular abnormalities such as strabismus. A traumatic cataract may be formed within 24 hours of trauma or injury to the eye. Long term use of a systemic or oral corticosteroid may precipitate cataract formation.

29. *b* Dacryostenosis usually resolves spontaneously as the infant grows older and the ducts mature. It is important to distinguish dacryostenosis from dacryocystitis. Dacryocystitis is an infection of the tear duct. It usually results from dacryostenosis.

30. *d* At birth and at 6 weeks-of-age, an infant's vision is normally about 20/100. At 4 months-of-age, vision is about 20/80. At 3 to 4 years, vision is about 20/50. At 6 years-of-age, vision is normally 20/20 or 20/25.

Gastrointestinal Disorders

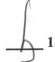 1. Appropriate therapy for peptic ulcer disease (PUD) is:

    a. primarily by eradication of infection.
    b. based on etiology.
    c. aimed at diminishing prostaglandin synthesis.
    d. dependent on cessation of (NSAID) use.

 2. A patient presents with classic symptoms of gastroesophageal reflux disease (GERD). He is instructed on life style modifications and drug therapy for 8 weeks. Three months later he returns, reporting that he was "fine" as long as he took the medicine. The most appropriate next step is:

    a. referral for surgical intervention such as partial or complete fundoplication.
    b. dependent upon how severe the practitioner believes the condition.
    c. to repeat the 8 week course of drug therapy while continuing lifestyle modifications.
    d. investigation with endoscopy, manometry, and/or pH testing.

 3. When a patient presents with symptoms of acute gallbladder disease, what is the appropriate nurse practitioner action?

    a. Order abdominal x-rays.
    b. Order an abdominal ultrasound.
    c. Refer the patient to a surgeon for evaluation.
    d. Prescribe pain medication.

 4. A 15 year old male presents with abdominal pain that began in the peri-umbilical area then localized to the right lower quadrant (RLQ). He complains of anorexia, and low grade fever. A complete blood count (CBC) reveals moderate leukocytosis. What is the most likely diagnosis?

    a. Acute gastroenteritis
    b. Recurrent abdominal pain
    c. Constipation
    d. Acute appendicitis

1. *b*   Peptic ulcer disease (PUD) is associated with *Helicobacter pylori* infection, NSAID use, and Zollinger-Ellison syndrome. Classification of ulcers into 1 of these 3 categories leads to appropriate therapy. The most appropriate management of PUD is based on etiology.

2. *d*   Indications for testing patients with suspected GERD include: incomplete response to treatment, recurrent disease, atypical symptoms, recurrent aspiration pneumonia, pulmonary fibrosis, or complications while receiving therapy. Diagnostic testing procedures should precede any surgical intervention. Complete relief of GERD symptoms does not exclude other more serious diseases.

3. *b*   The diagnosis of symptomatic cholelithiasis is made by clinical presentation and documentation of gallstones. Treatment is surgical. Plain x-rays demonstrate gallstones in only 20% of patients. Ultrasonography demonstrates gallstones in more than 95% of patients with cholelithiasis. Patient referral should take place when gallstones are identified or as patient condition dictates.

4. *d*   These are classic symptoms of acute appendicitis. The incidence is highest among adolescents and young adults and is most common among adolescent males.

5. How many kilocalories below one's requirement does it take to lose 1 pound?

   a. 3500
   b. 2500
   c. 2000
   d. 1000

6. A 70-year-old patient presents with left lower quadrant (LLQ) abdominal pain, a markedly tender palpable abdominal wall, fever, and leukocytosis. Of the following terms, which correctly describes the suspected condition?

   a. Diverticulosis
   b. Diverticula
   c. Diverticulitis
   d. Diverticulum

7. Before initiating an HMG CoA-reductase inhibitor for hyperlipidemia, the nurse practitioner orders liver function studies. The patient's aminotransferase (ALT) is elevated. What laboratory test(s) should be ordered?

   a. Serologic markers for hepatitis
   b. Serum bilirubin
   c. Serum cholesterol with HDL and LDL
   d. A liver biopsy

8. A patient has experienced nausea and vomiting, headache, malaise, low-grade fever, abdominal cramps, and watery diarrhea for 72 hours. His white count is elevated with a shift to the left. He is requesting medication for diarrhea. What is the most appropriate response?

   a. Prescribe loperamide (Imodium®) or atropine-diphenoxylate (Lomotil®) and a clear liquid diet for 24 hours.
   b. Prescribe a broad-spectrum antibiotic such as ciprofloxacin (Cipro®), and symptom management.
   c. Offer an anti-emetic medication such as prochlorperazine (Compazine®) and provide oral fluid and electrolyte replacement instruction.
   d. Order stool cultures.

5. *a*   A pound of body fat represents 3500 kilocalories. For every 3500 kcal decrease in the diet, 1 pound of body weight will be lost. The period of time over which the decreased intake occurs is not a factor.

6. *c*   Diverticula are outpouchings that occur along the wall of the alimentary tract. They are usually asymptomatic. Diverticulum is the singular form of diverticula. The presence of diverticula is referred to as diverticulosis. It is asymptomatic and requires no treatment. Clinical signs and symptoms of acute diverticulitis are LLQ abdominal pain, tenderness over the involved segment with or without a palpable mass, leukocytosis, and usually fever. Appropriate treatment is a course of oral antibiotics effective against both aerobic and anaerobic bacteria. A high fiber diet can help allay symptoms of irritable bowel that may accompany diverticulosis.

7. *a*   There is a correlation between serum ALT and abnormal antibodies to the hepatitis B virus. Patients with elevated ALT frequently have active hepatitis when assessed by liver biopsy. Bilirubin may be normal to slightly elevated.

8. *b*   The nurse practitioner's differential diagnoses should include infection with Salmonella, Shigella, and Campylobacter since all have similar signs and symptoms. Diagnosis can be confirmed only with stool or blood cultures. Most healthy adults have a course that is self-limiting to 72 hours and antibiotics may prolong excretion of the organism in the case of Salmonella. However, a course of ciprofloxacin after 72 hours is prudent if the patient's condition has not improved. Antidiarrheal agents potentially increase complications and predispose the patient to bacteremia.

9. After thorough history, physical examination, and laboratory tests, a patient is diagnosed with irritable bowel syndrome (IBS). Which of the following initial treatment plans is currently considered most effective?

   a. A low fat, tyramine-free, caffeine-free, high fiber diet, along with a daily diary, and attention to psychosocial factors
   b. Referral to a gastroenterologist for colonoscopy
   c. Treatment with a selective serotonin reuptake inhibitor (SSRI) such as fluoxetine (Prozac®) or sertraline (Zoloft®)
   d. Antibiotics, nutritional support, and high fiber diet

10. Which of the following are classic features of ulcerative colitis?

   a. Right lower quadrant pain, frequently accompanied by a palpable mass, fever, and leukocytosis
   b. Painful hematemesis, occasionally accompanied by melena
   c. Rapidly progressive dysphagia with ingestion of solid foods, anorexia, and weight loss out of proportion to the dysphagia
   d. Remissions and exacerbations of bloody diarrhea, tenesmus, fecal incontinence, abdominal pain, and weight loss

11. Of the following, the patient who should be referred for periodic colonoscopy is the patient with:

   a. diverticulitis resistant to traditional medical management.
   b. extensive ulcerative colitis of long duration.
   c. irritable bowel syndrome (IBS) complicated by psychiatric illness.
   d. history of severe Crohn's disease.

12. Diagnosis of Crohn's disease is made considering signs, symptoms and:

   a. a lesion identified by endoscopy.
   b. biopsy of bowel mucosa to rule out other causes.
   c. intestinal obstruction demonstrated by plain x-ray of the abdomen.
   d. the presence or absence of bloody diarrhea.

9. *a*   Irritable bowel syndrome (IBS) may be diagnosed with careful history and physical examination, along with complete blood count (CBC) to assess for anemia, and a biochemical profile and urinalysis for general information. Invasive procedures should be avoided unless age or family history indicates risk. A low fat, tyramine-free, caffeine-free diet, along with a daily diary and stress reduction are mainstays of therapy. Unresponsive patients should be referred to a gastroenterologist. Selective serotonin reuptake inhibitors (SSRI) may improve symptoms secondary to their anti-anxiety effect, but should not be considered initially. In some patients, SSRIs worsen symptoms via their excitatory effect on the bowel.

10. *d*   Ulcerative colitis is diffuse superficial inflammation of the colonic mucosa and submucosa. It almost always involves the rectum, and tends to extend throughout the entire colon. Etiology is unknown. Disabling features include exacerbations of bloody diarrhea, fecal incontinence, and tenesmus, resulting in weight loss.

11. *b*   Patients with extensive ulcerative colitis of long duration are at risk for colorectal cancer. Colonoscopic surveillance for these patients is recommended.

12. *a*   The diagnostic test most specific for Crohn's disease is colonoscopy with ileoscopy. Biopsies of the bowel mucosa are not diagnostic, but help rule out other causes. Plain x-rays will reveal intestinal obstruction but are not specific. Bloody diarrhea is commonly observed in Crohn's disease and other colonic diseases.

13. A 47 year old male patient presents to the clinic with a single episode of a moderate amount of bright red rectal bleeding. On examination, external hemorrhoids are noted. How should the nurse practitioner proceed?

    a. Instruct the patient on measures to prevent hemorrhoids such as bowel habits and diet.
    b. Order a topical hemorrhoid cream along with a stool softener.
    c. Refer the patient for a barium enema and sigmoidoscopy.
    d. Refer the patient for a surgical hemorrhoidectomy.

14. A patient with a diagnosis of giardiasis is being treated with metronidazole (Flagyl®). What information is important to obtain before prescribing this medication?

    a. Is the patient allergic to sulfa?
    b. Does the patient have peptic ulcer disease?
    c. Is the patient at least 18 years-of-age?
    d. Does the patient drink alcohol?

15. A 3-day-old infant is brought into the clinic with a history of failure to pass meconium, poor feeding, vomiting, and excessive flatus. The infant was diagnosed in the nursery with trisomy 21. Which of the following should be included in the differential diagnosis?

    a. Omphalocele
    b. Hirschsprung's disease
    c. Duodenal atresia
    d. Esophageal atresia

16. A 1-year-old presents with recurrent diarrhea and drawing up of the legs followed by periods of lethargy. On physical examination, a "sausage-like" mass is palpated in the upper right quadrant of the distended abdomen. Which of the following is the most likely diagnosis?

    a. Intussusception
    b. Volvulus
    c. Abdominal hernia
    d. Foreign body in the GI tract

13. *c*   Sigmoidoscopy is indicated in all instances of rectal bleeding. While hemorrhoids are common, they must be considered only a tentative source of bleeding. Colonic neoplasms may also present with rectal bleeding and can usually be diagnosed with barium enema and sigmoidoscopic biopsy.

14. *d*   Alcoholic beverages must be avoided during and 3 days after taking metronidazole due to potential for a disulfiram-like reaction.

15. *b*   Hirschsprung's disease (congenital aganglionic megacolon) is absence of ganglion cells in a portion of the intestinal wall, resulting in a lack of peristalsis in that portion of the bowel. It accounts for 33% of all obstructions. The disease is familial and is common with trisomy 21.

16. *a*   Intussusception, invagination (or "telescoping") of the bowel, is the most common cause of intestinal obstruction in the first 2 years of life. Barium enema is diagnostic and often also therapeutic. Volvulus is a twisting of the bowel on itself producing obstruction, but a mass is not palpable. Recurrent abdominal pain, foreign bodies, and an abdominal hernia do not cause diarrhea.

D   17. A 2-week-old infant presents with projectile vomiting, weight loss, dehydration, constipation, and history of insatiable appetite. An olive-shaped mass is palpable to the right of the epigastrium. The nurse practitioner, suspecting pyloric stenosis, refers the infant for an upper GI series. The expected finding is:

     a. double bubble pattern, secondary to air in the stomach, and a distended duodenum.
     b. dilated loops of bowel.
     c. bowel loops of varying width, with a grainy appearance.
     d. the "string sign," indicating a narrow and elongated pyloric canal.

C   18. After a thorough examination, a 2-month-old infant is diagnosed with infantile colic. What should be included in the initial education of the mother about this condition?

     a. Introduce solid foods into the diet, beginning with bananas and applesauce.
     b. Set strict limits on holding the infant to avoid manipulative infant behavior.
     c. Instruct the mother on appropriate feeding techniques. Then reinforce efforts to calm and comfort the infant.
     d. Restrict breast and bottle feeding to every 3 hours in frequency and 15 minutes in duration.

D   19. A patient is diagnosed with *Enterobius vermicularis* (pinworms) infection. He is treated with mebendazole (Vermox®) 100 mg today, to be repeated in 2 weeks. Who else should be treated?

     a. All household members, regardless of age
     b. All household members, as well as close friends
     c. All household members under 12 years-of-age
     d. Only infected or symptomatic household members

B   20. The most effective treatment of primary and secondary encopresis focuses on:

     a. psychotherapy for the entire family.
     b. establishment of a regular bowel routine.
     c. a daily laxative or enema.
     d. loss of privileges as a consequence for soiling.

17. *d*   Pyloric stenosis is due to a hypertrophied pyloric muscle. It is diagnosed by clinical signs and symptoms along with narrowing and elongation of the pyloric canal (evidenced by upper GI series as the classic "string sign"). Intervention is correction of fluid and electrolyte imbalance followed by surgical repair.

18. *c*   There is no "cure" for infantile colic. The situation can only be managed until it resolves on its own. Effective management includes appropriate feeding technique, calming strategies, and parental support. Dicyclomine (Antispas®), hyoscyamine (Levsin®), and simethicone (Mylicon®) have indications for treatment of infantile colic.

19. *d*   Examination of all household members may be advised in situations of recurrent infection. Diagnosis is established by sighting the eggs and/or worms. It is appropriate to recommend treatment for all infected and symptomatic contacts.

20. *b*   Treatment for encopresis differs depending on whether it is related to constipation, impaction, or simply inappropriately placed bowel movements. In all cases, the primary treatment involves establishment of a bowel routine. Medication and counseling may be involved. Incentives and rewards may be helpful. Punishment is ineffective and inappropriate.

21. After being thoroughly examined, a child is diagnosed with recurrent abdominal pain. Patient and parent counseling should include:

    a. acknowledgment that the pain is real, although there is no known physical cause.
    b. extensive education about inflammatory bowel diseases and the appropriate medication treatment.
    c. a list of foods to be avoided in the child's diet.
    d. necessary lifestyle changes to accommodate the child during episodes of abdominal pain.

22. An adult female patient is seeking information about her ideal weight. She is 5 feet 7 inches tall. Using the "height-weight formula," what is her ideal body weight (IBW)?

    a. 130 lbs
    b. 135 lbs
    c. 140 lbs
    d. 145 lbs

23. Which of the following is *not* a symptom of irritable bowel syndrome?

    a. Painful diarrhea
    b. Painful constipation
    c. Cramping and abdominal pain
    d. Weight loss

24. A patient reports to the nurse practitioner that he was diagnosed with hepatitis B a year ago and has not seen a health care provider since then. What information should this patient be given?

    a. Hepatitis B is enterically transmitted and does not cause chronic disease.
    b. About 10% of affected persons become carriers and are at increased risk for hepatocellular carcinoma.
    c. Hepatitis B vaccine is recommended to prevent the damaging effects of chronic infection.
    d. There is no known treatment that will normalize liver functions and improve liver histology.

21. *a* Recurrent abdominal pain is real pain with no known physical cause. High-fiber food may be helpful. Normalization of lifestyle and behavioral therapy for pain relief during pain episodes should be encouraged.

22. *b* The height-weight formula is a quick method for determining ideal weight. Females allow 100 pounds for the first 5 feet of height plus 5 pounds for each additional inch. Males allow 106 pounds for the first 5 feet of height plus 6 pounds for each additional inch. This method can only be used as an estimate because it does not account for body composition or age.

23. *d* Irritable bowel syndrome (IBS) is characterized by cramping abdominal pain with painful constipation and/or diarrhea. Bleeding, fever, weight loss, and persistent severe pain are indicative of other problems.

24. *b* Of the 6 identified hepatitis viruses, the following 4 are associated with chronic disease: hepatitis B, C, D, and G. Hepatitis A and E do not cause chronic disease. Hepatitis B is responsible for 43% of cases of viral hepatitis in the United States. Up to 10% of these cases become carriers. The carrier state is clearly associated with hepatocellular carcinoma. The hepatitis B series is recommended to prevent initial infection. There are successful treatments available for chronic hepatitis.

25. A 3-month-old infant is diagnosed with gastroesophageal reflux (GER). Initial interventions for this condition include:

    a. changing the infant's formula.
    b. adding 1 tablespoon of rice cereal to each ounce of formula.
    c. positioning the infant on his left side after feedings.
    d. offering large less frequent feedings.

26. An employee picnic menu includes grilled hamburgers, potato salad, and homemade ice cream sundaes. Within an hour after the meal, several children and parents begin to have nausea, vomiting and stomach cramps. None of those effected have fever. What is the most likely etiologic agent?

    a. *Salmonella*
    b. *Clostridium perfringens*
    c. *Staphylococcus aureus*
    d. *Escherichia coli*

27. Which intervention listed below is safe for long term use by an adult with constipation?

    a. Bulk-forming agents
    b. Stool softeners
    c. Laxatives
    d. Osmotic agents

28. The nurse practitioner is reviewing a patient's lab report who completed the hepatitis B series 3 months ago. Which of the following lab results reflects this?

    a. Positive hepatitis B surface antigen
    b. Positive hepatitis B surface antibody and negative core antibody
    c. Positive hepatitis B surface antibody and positive core antibody
    d. Positive core antibody only

25. *b* Small, frequent feedings with frequent burping, continued breastfeeding, addition of cereal, elevating the head of the bed, and positioning the infant on his right side are all treatments helpful in GER. Formula changes are generally not helpful and should be avoided. If nonpharmacological treatments are not sufficient, ranitidine (Zantac®), or cimetidine (Tagamet®) may be prescribed.

26. *c* "*Staph*" has a very short incubation period of 30 minutes to 6 hours. Fever is uncommon, but nausea, vomiting, and abdominal cramping are usual. *Clostridium* has an incubation period of 8 to 12 hours and produces the same symptoms, but is usually accompanied by fever. *Salmonella* has an incubation period of 6 to 72 hours, but usually less than 24 hours and the same abdominal symptoms present with the addition of fever. *E. coli* requires 10 hours to several days for incubation and produces only abdominal cramping and watery diarrhea.

27. *a* Bulk-forming agents, such as psyllium and methylcellulose, may be used safely and are often required long term. Stool softeners, osmotic agents, and laxatives, if used more regularly will lead to dependence for routine bowel movements. Patients should be encouraged to increase fiber intake gradually to prevent abdominal cramping that is frequently associated with high fiber intake. Adequate hydration should also be encouraged.

28. *b* Positive surface antibody and negative core antibody is indicative of immunity derived from the hepatitis vaccine. Immunity as a result of having had hepatitis B is reflected as positive surface antibody and positive core antibody. Positive surface antigen always reflects current hepatitis B infection.

Health Promotion and Disease Prevention

B 1. A hoarse cry in a newborn may indicate:

    a. problems with feeding.
    b. hypothyroidism.
    c. hearing impairment.
    d. cri du chat.

C 2. A first time mother asks how she should place her 3 month old during playtime. The nurse practitioner replies:

    a. always place him supine because this encourages kicking and leg muscle development.
    b. always place him prone because this helps development of chest and arm muscles.
    c. place him in a variety of positions to develop anterior and posterior muscles.
    d. it does not matter how the infant is placed because he will find the most comfortable position.

B 3. If a child receives his 1st dose of IPV at 2 months, how soon may he receive the 2nd dose?

    a. 2 weeks
    b. 1 month
    c. 6 weeks
    d. 2 months

D 4. What is the earliest age that MMR immunization can be administered?

    a. 2 months
    b. 4 months
    c. 6 months
    d. 1 year

C 5. Which behavior would *not* be expected of a 2 year old?

    a. Kicking a ball
    b. Running around a corner without falling down
    c. Riding a tricycle
    d. Climbing on a chair and standing up to reach an object

1. *b*   It is important to assess an infant's cry. A hoarse cry is associated with hypothyroidism (cretinism). A high-pitched cry is associated with cri du chat.

2. *c*   Infants should not be placed consistently in the same position while awake because this slows development and strengthening of the muscles which are least used in that position. Infants should always be positioned supine or side-lying for sleep.

3. *b*   The minimal period of time recommended between the 1st and 2nd doses of IPV is 4 weeks. The 2nd dose is usually scheduled 8 weeks after the 1st dose and the 3rd dose is usually scheduled 6 months after the 2nd dose.

4. *d*   MMR vaccine should not be administered before 12 months-of-age. If measles vaccination is indicated because of an outbreak, monovalent measles vaccine may be administered prior to 12 months-of-age. After this time, vaccination at 12 months with MMR may be initiated. The usual age for the 2nd dose is 4 to 6 years.

5. *c*   A 2 year old should be able to do all except choice *c.* Riding a tricycle is an expected skill for a 3 year old.

6. All of the following are typical of toddlers *except*:

a. increased appetite.
b. gender identity.
c. ritualistic behavior.
d. toilet training.

 7. Which activities are *not* characteristic of preschool children?

a. Social, cooperative, and shared play
b. Independent toileting with occasional accidents
c. Always follow rules during playground games
d. Use of security objects

 8. Which of the following would *not* be considered a developmental red flag to a nurse practitioner assessing a 4 year old?

a. Persistent fear of going to sleep
b. Missing speech sounds
c. Fire-setting
d. An imaginary friend

 9. When examining a 5 year old, the nurse practitioner knows that this is an appropriate age to teach the child about:

a. washing his hands before eating.
b. not allowing anyone to touch his private parts without permission.
c. the importance of balanced meals so that he can grow tall and strong.
d. getting his preschool immunizations.

 10. What is the recommendation of the U.S. Preventive Services Task Force concerning vision screening of the school-aged child?

a. School-age children should be screened for vision impairment every 3 years.
b. There is no recommendation for or against vision screening of asymptomatic school-age children.
c. School-age children should be screened for vision impairment on entry into kindergarten and annually thereafter.
d. Screening with the Snellen visual acuity test is recommended but frequency is left to clinical discretion.

6. *a*   Toddlers are classified as 1 to 3 year olds. They generally exhibit a *decreased* appetite as their growth slows and they are more easily distracted by their environment. They generally request or refuse the same foods repeatedly. They rarely use eating utensils and prefer finger foods.

7. *c*   Since preschoolers are just beginning to learn moral behaviors, they often cheat to win. While most preschoolers toilet independently, accidents occasionally occur and bed-wetting is not unusual. The use of a security item, such as a blanket, is common.

8. *d*   Imaginary play, typical of 4 year olds, is demonstrated by frequent make-believe, magical thinking, and fantasy. While many children are afraid of "the dark," persistent fear of going to sleep may indicate other problems that should be explored.

9. *b*   Anticipatory guidance by the nurse practitioner should include an explanation about not allowing anyone to touch his private parts without permission. This is the age of sexual exploration for the child.

10. *b*   The U.S. Preventive Services Task Force has not yet gathered sufficient evidence to support routine screening of asymptomatic school-age children for vision impairment. However, health care providers often incorporate vision screening into routine exams.

D _____ 11. Which of the following descriptions of the Denver II Developmental Screening Test is most accurate?

    a. Applicable to children from birth to 2 years; evaluates 4 major categories of development: motor, intellectual, emotional, and language to determine whether a child is within normal range for various behaviors or is developmentally delayed

    b. Applicable to children from birth to 5 years; evaluates 4 major categories of development: motor, vision, hearing, and psychosocial to determine whether a child is normal or developmentally compromised

    c. Applicable to children from age 6 months to 6 years; evaluates 4 major categories of development: intellectual, verbal, social, and memory to determine IQ and aptitude

    d. Applicable to children from birth to 6 years; evaluates 4 major categories of development: gross motor, fine motor-adaptive, language, and personal-social to determine whether a child is within normal range for various behaviors or is developmentally delayed

B 12. Anticipatory guidance with the most potential to benefit the adolescent mortality rate should be directed toward:

    a. prevention of sexually transmitted diseases, upper respiratory infections, and other infectious diseases.

    b. prevention of accidents, homicide, and suicide.

    c. prevention of lung cancer, breast cancer, and testicular cancer.

    d. increased physical fitness, low fat diet, and smoking cessation.

B 13. Which group is considered to be at high risk for development of testicular tumor?

    a. Pre-adolescence

    b. Late adolescence through early adulthood

    c. Mid-life, 40 to 60 years-of-age

    d. 65 years-of-age and older

11. *d* The Denver II relies on children's play behavior for developmental assessment data and is a good general assessment tool for anticipatory guidance and early intervention.

12. *b* Accidents, homicide, and suicide account for 75% of deaths among teenagers and young adults 15 to 24 years-of-age.

13. *b* The peak incidence of tumors of the testes is in late adolescence and early adulthood; therefore, palpation of the testes is most likely to yield valuable information at this age.

A

14. Healthy People 2010 published by the U.S. Department of Health and Human Services:

a. is a set of national health objectives designed to improve the overall health of people and communities.
b. provides guidelines for adolescent preventive services.
c. reviews evidence for 169 interventions to prevent 60 illnesses across the life span.
d. removes barriers to prenatal and infant health care to narrow the gap between services provided to African-American and Caucasian mothers and infants.

D

15. A 23-year-old female college student is being evaluated by the nurse practitioner for immunization status. She has documentation of completion of the IPV, DTaP, and MMR series only. She states "I got a shot when I was 12 years old, but I don't know what it was." Which vaccine(s) should she receive today?

a. Td
b. HBV and Hib
c. Hib and Td
d. Td and HBV

C

16. The nurse practitioner is counseling a 24-year-old sexually active male patient about male condom use. Which of the following statements is *incorrect*?

a. Adequate lubrication is needed to prevent damage to the condom.
b. Unroll the condom over an erect penis before any sexual contact.
c. Make sure the condom is tight against the head of the penis.
d. Withdraw while the penis is erect so that the condom stays in place.

B

17. A 26-year-old male patient in good health has a blood pressure of 135/80. How soon should his blood pressure be re-assessed?

a. 1 day
b. 2 months
c. 1 year
d. 2 years

14. *a* Healthy People 2010 is a report released by the U.S. Department of Health and Human Services. It contains goals to be met by the year 2010. The 2 main goals are to increase quality and years of healthy life and to eliminate health disparities. It is designed to identify common preventable health threats and to establish national goals to help reduce these threats.

15. *d* It is recommended that adolescents and young adults not previously immunized against hepatitis B receive the HBV series. A tetanus and diphtheria (Td) booster is recommended every 10 years. Hib is not recommended after 5 years of age.

16. *c* A space should be left at the tip of the condom to prevent breakage and to serve as a reservoir.

17. *b* U.S. Preventive Services Task Force strongly recommends screening adults aged 18 and older for high blood pressure. An elevated reading (135/80) should be confirmed on at least 2 visits over a period of 1 to several weeks. There is insufficient evidence at this time to recommend an optimal interval. Therefore, the best choice in this question is response "b". JNC VII characterizes a blood pressure of 135/80 as "pre-hypertension."

A

18. Colorectal cancer screening recommendations for a 50-year-old male include annual:

    a. fecal occult blood testing.
    b. colposcopy.
    c. barium enema.

C

    d. digital rectal exam.

19. The most accepted recommendation regarding skin cancer prevention is:

    a. monthly skin self-examination.
    b. use of sunscreen at all times.
    c. avoidance of excessive sun exposure.

B

    d. avoidance of tanning devices.

20. During a routine pre-employment screen, a patient is noted to have a positive hepatitis B surface antigen. This finding indicates he:

    a. has received the hepatitis B immunization.
    b. has an active infection with hepatitis B.
    c. has recovered from a hepatitis B infection.
    d. requires re-immunization for protection from hepatitis B.

B

21. What is the leading cause of death and unintentional injury in the elder population?

    a. Motor vehicle accident (MVA)
    b. Fall
    c. Asphyxiation from choking
    d. House fire

R

22. Which statement is true regarding dental health?

    a. A diet high in sugar has no effect on dental caries.
    b. Individuals with dentures should visit the dentist every 2 years.
    c. About one inch of toothpaste on a brush is appropriate for 2 to 5 year olds.
    d. Swishing with water after eating does not help to reduce tooth decay.

18. *a*   Colorectal cancer screening is recommended for all persons 50 years-of-age and older with annual fecal occult blood testing, or sigmoidoscopy, or both. Many learned authorities believe a colonoscopy is superior to a sigmoidoscopy for detection of colon abnormalities because more of the colon can be visualized.

19. *c*   Avoidance of excessive sun exposure is the most accepted recommendation for prevention of skin cancer. All the other items are recommended by particular groups, but are not as widely accepted. Clinicians should remain alert for suspicious lesions in fair-skinned men and women > 65 years, those with atypical moles, those with > 50 moles. These groups have a substantially increased risk for melanoma.

20. *b*   A positive surface antigen means that the patient is currently infected with hepatitis B. From the information given, it is not known whether he has acute hepatitis B or chronic hepatitis B. In order to determine this, an anti-HBc IgM (antibody to the core hepatitis B virus) should be measured. If it is positive, the patient has acute hepatitis B. If it is negative, the patient has chronic hepatitis B.

21. *b*   In the United States, fall is the leading cause of nonfatal injury and death from accidental injury among older persons.

22. *b*   Patients with dentures should be evaluated by a dentist every 2 years to assess gum health and denture fit. Diets high in sugar increase the likelihood of dental caries because sugar adheres to the dental enamel and provides an excellent medium for bacterial growth. Swishing the mouth with water after eating reduces the amount of sugar remaining in the mouth. "Pea-size" most accurately describes the amount of toothpaste that 2 to 5 year olds should use for brushing.

C 23. Previously immunized elderly patients should receive a tetanus and diphtheria (Td) booster every:

    a. 2 to 3 years.
    b. 5 years.
    c. 10 years.
    d. 15 years.

C 24. Which of the following is an example of Piaget's concrete logical operations?

    a. A 4-year-old child insists that a ball of clay "has more" once it is shaped into a snake.
    b. A 5-year-old child demonstrates the ability to read a paragraph to decode the words.
    c. A 7-year-old child maintains that a ball of clay weighs the same amount after it has been shaped into a snake.
    d. An 8-year-old child must re-calculate basic mathematics facts each time he attempts to solve a word problem.

B 25. The first sign of puberty in girls is:

    a. enlargement of the ovaries, uterus, and clitoris.
    b. development of breast buds.
    c. the occurrence of menarche.
    d. acne resulting from stimulation of the sebaceous glands.

C 26. The CDC recommends the pneumococcal polysaccharide vaccine for:

    1. all adults > 60 years-of-age.
    2. asplenic persons ≥ 2 years-of-age.
    3. HIV positive individuals and diabetic adults.
    4. patients with CHF or chronic liver disease.

    a. 1, 2
    b. 3, 4
    c. 2, 3, 4
    d. All of the above

23. *c*   The standard practice is to get a tetanus and diphtheria (Td) booster at least once every 10 years.

24. *c*   The shift from pre-operational to concrete logical operations is exemplified by the child's ability to determine that since nothing was added to the ball of clay, it must weigh the same when reshaped. This cognitive reorganization occurs generally in the early school-age period.

25. *b*   The first sign of puberty in girls is the development of breast buds, at the average age of 10 years. The first sign of puberty in boys is testicular enlargement, which usually occurs at about 10 years-of-age.

26. *c*   The CDC recommends that all adults 65 years-of-age and older receive the pneumococcal vaccine. In addition to the other groups listed, individuals with a chronic cardiovascular or pulmonary disorder, chronic liver disease, alcoholism, COPD, or renal failure. Alaskan natives and certain American Indian populations should also receive the pneumococcal immunization.

27. A 37-year-old female is found to have a negative rubella titer. How long after immunization should she avoid pregnancy?

    a. 28 days
    b. 60 days
    c. 90 days
    d. 120 days

28. Which immunization(s) is(are) contraindicated in an immunodeficient individual?

    1. Varicella
    2. IPV
    3. MMR
    4. HBV

    a. 4
    b. 1, 3
    c. 1, 3, 4
    d. All of the above

29. Which of the following is a function of aging?

    a. Loss of adipose tissue
    b. Increased oxygen demand and consumption
    c. Increased total body water
    d. Decreased absorption of iron, folic acid, and vitamin B-12

27. *a* Women should be asked if they are pregnant prior to administration of the rubella vaccine. The CDC advises waiting 28 days before attempting pregnancy. Traditionally, women were asked to avoid pregnancy for 3 months.

28. *b* IPV is an inactivated form ("dead") virus and therefore is not contraindicated for the immunodeficient individual. The varicella and MMR are attenuated or weakened viruses with potential to cause disease in an immunodeficient individual. IPV is only contraindicated for individuals who have had anaphylactic reactions to a previous dose or to streptomycin, polymyxin B, or neomycin. The Hepatitis B vaccine (HBV) is only contraindicated in patients with history of anaphylactic reaction to yeast.

29. *d* Iron, folic acid, and vitamin B-12 require an acidic environment to be absorbed. After age 80, there is decreased absorption of these nutrients because the stomach secretes less acid. Loss of muscle mass occurs in both genders (more commonly in men). There is an increase in truncal adipose tissue. Total body water decreases (increasing risk of dehydration) and metabolism and oxygen consumption decreases (decreasing oxygen demand).

Hematological Disorders

1. The nurse practitioner is caring for a 19 year old female college student with moderate iron deficiency anemia secondary to heavy menstrual bleeding. The appropriate initial treatment for this patient is:

   a. intramuscular iron dextran.
   b. a daily oral multivitamin with iron.
   c. oral ferrous sulfate.
   d. increased intake of dietary iron.

2. Thalassemia should be included in the differential diagnosis of an infant with microcytic anemia when the infant's parents are of what ethnicity?

   a. Italian
   b. Swedish
   c. Irish
   d. Japanese

3. The most appropriate therapy for an elderly patient with pernicious anemia is:

   a. increased dietary intake of vitamin B-12.
   b. oral vitamin B-12 supplementation.
   c. intramuscular injections of vitamin B-12.
   d. oral multivitamin supplementation.

4. A 23-year-old male patient presents with a hemoglobin 10 g/dL, and mean corpuscular volume (MCV) 115 fl. These laboratory values are most consistent with which of the following?

   a. Thalassemia major
   b. Anemia of chronic disease
   c. Iron deficiency anemia
   d. Folic acid deficiency anemia

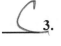

5. The most effective treatment for anemia of chronic disease is:

   a. iron replacement therapy.
   b. treatment of the underlying disease.
   c. an oral folate supplement.
   d. corticosteroid therapy.

1. *c*   With iron deficiency anemia, iron stores of the body must be replenished as well as the underlying cause corrected. A daily iron supplement is used initially and will provide more iron than the iron contained in a multivitamin. The most common form is ferrous sulfate. Intramuscular iron dextran is usually not needed, but may be required in the presence of a malabsorption disorder, inflammatory bowel disease, intolerance to oral iron, or blood loss too great to be compensated adequately with oral iron.

2. *a* β-thalassemia is most common in people of Mediterranean descent and α-thalassemia is more common in African-Americans. There are no known connections between thalassemias and persons of Swedish, Irish, or Japanese descent.

3. *c*   The most effective therapy for pernicious anemia is intramuscular injections of vitamin B-12. Oral B-12 is usually not absorbed efficiently enough for effective treatment; however, more recent studies have shown that this may be effective in younger patients. Oral multivitamin therapy and increased dietary intake of vitamin B-12 are probably NOT adequate for treatment in the elderly.

4. *d*   Folic acid deficiency anemia is a macrocytic anemia commonly seen with alcoholism. MCV 80-100 fl is considered normal; > 100 fl is macrocytic; < 80 fl is microcytic. Thalassemia major and iron deficiency anemia are microcytic anemias. Anemia of chronic disease is usually normocytic.

5. *b*   Anemia of chronic disease is best treated with control of the underlying problem. Since the underlying problem is not iron or folate deficiency, replacement of either of these is of no benefit. Corticosteroid treatment may be used to treat a patient with idiopathic thrombocytopenia (ITP).

C

6. A 2-year-old African-American child is being evaluated by the nurse practitioner. His clinical appearance and history are consistent with sickle cell anemia. What is the appropriate laboratory test to screen for sickle cell anemia?

   a. DNA analysis
   b. CBC with peripheral smear
   c. Sickledex®
   d. Serum haptoglobin level

C

7. A 23-year-old female patient of Italian descent has been diagnosed with anemia secondary to glucose-6-phosphate dehydrogenase (G-6-PD) deficiency. It is important to teach this patient to avoid which of the following?

   a. Organ meats
   b. Black beans
   c. Aspirin
   d. Milk and milk products

8. A 3-year-old male is being evaluated by the nurse practitioner for frequent respiratory infections and fatigue. His laboratory tests show thrombocytopenia, granulocytopenia, and anemia. Which of the following is consistent with these lab findings?

   a. Acute lymphocytic leukemia (ALL)
   b. Hodgkin's lymphoma
   c. Chronic myelocytic leukemia (CML)
   d. Multiple myeloma

9. A newborn infant develops jaundice at 12 hours-of-age. Which of the following causes of hyperbilirubinemia should be suspected?

   a. Breastfeeding jaundice
   b. Cephalhematoma
   c. Physiological hyperbilirubinemia
   d. ABO incompatibility

6. *c*   The Sickledex® is commonly used to screen for sickle cell anemia. Hemoglobin electrophoresis is used for the definitive diagnosis. Examination of peripheral smear and haptoglobin levels are useful as supportive evidence, but are not used for screening.

7. *c*   Hemolytic anemia occurs in persons with G-6-PD deficiency when they are exposed to certain substances that cause precipitation of hemoglobin, red cell injury, and hemolysis. Fava beans, aspirin, sulfonamides, and anti-malarials are examples of known precipitants of anemia in persons with G-6-PD deficiency.

8. *a*   Acute lymphocytic leukemia (ALL) is most common in children. It is characterized by immunosuppression, thrombocytopenia, granulocytopenia, and anemia. Fatigue is a prominent clinical feature.

9. *d*   Jaundice that develops within 24 hours of birth is not considered physiological. Jaundice secondary to cephalhematoma and breastfeeding jaundice usually develop 24 hours after birth. Hyperbilirubinemia caused by ABO incompatibility can, and usually does, occur within 24 hours of birth.

10. A 36-year-old patient is diagnosed with iron deficiency anemia and started on iron replacement therapy. To evaluate the patient's response, how soon should a reticulocyte count be ordered?

    a. 7 days
    b. 2 weeks
    c. 3 weeks
    d. 1 month

11. Acute idiopathic thrombocytopenia purpura (ITP) is most commonly seen in childhood following:

    a. trauma.
    b. glucocorticosteroid therapy.
    c. aspirin ingestion.
    d. acute infection.

12. All parents of a child newly diagnosed with hemophilia should be taught:

    a. to discourage the child from outdoor physical activity.
    b. to have the child vaccinated against the hepatitis B virus.
    c. encourage routine immunizations.
    d. to seek emergency care for any sign of bleeding.

13. A 76-year-old female patient with chronic atrial fibrillation is taking warfarin (Coumadin®) and being managed on an outpatient basis. What is the preferred laboratory test to evaluate this patient's coagulation status?

    a. Partial thromboplastin time (PTT)
    b. Prothrombin time (PT)
    c. International normalization ratio (INR)
    d. Clotting time

14. A 24-year-old male patient diagnosed with Hodgkin's lymphoma is concerned about long term survival. The most accurate response by the nurse practitioner is:

    a. "The 5-year survival rate is 75 to 80%."
    b. "Non-Hodgkin's lymphoma has a better prognosis."
    c. "With radiation and chemotherapy, there is almost a 100% cure rate."
    d. "With surgical treatment, there is a 95% cure rate."

10. *a* Response to iron therapy should be apparent within 7 to 10 days of beginning therapy. Reticulocytosis is the first indication of response followed by an increase in hemoglobin level. The reticulocyte count changes daily in response to bone marrow activity.

11. *d* Acute idiopathic thrombocytopenia purpura (ITP) is an illness of childhood, most frequently seen following an acute infection. Glucocorticosteroid therapy is the treatment of choice. There is no relationship between trauma and acute ITP. Aspirin ingestion may cause drug-induced thrombocytopenia, but not acute ITP.

12. *c* Routine childhood immunization should be encouraged because they will help prevent illnesses. Children with hemophilia should be allowed as much physical activity as appropriate for their factor deficiency. It is not necessary to seek emergency treatment for all bleeding; some may be treated at home or in an outpatient non-emergency setting.

13. *c* INR is the standard method for evaluating the coagulation status of patients taking warfarin (Coumadin®). PTT is be used to monitor heparin therapy. Clotting time is not useful for determining coagulation status.

14. *a* The 5-year overall survival rate for Hodgkin's lymphoma is 75 to 80%. Hodgkin's lymphoma carries a better prognosis than does non-Hodgkin's lymphoma. Surgical treatment is not indicated for Hodgkin's lymphoma.

15. An important measure to prevent complications in children with sickle cell anemia is:

    a. tight restriction of physical activity.
    b. trace mineral supplementation.
    c. staying well hydrated.
    d. home schooling for infection control.

16. A 76-year-old male patient with chronic renal failure is on renal dialysis. He has repeated problems with anemia. Which of the following therapies is indicated for this patient?

    a. An iron supplement
    b. Blood transfusions
    c. Erythropoietin replacement
    d. A folic acid supplement

17. Iron deficiency anemia in an elderly male patient is most commonly associated with:

    a. a malignant process.
    b. gastrointestinal bleeding.
    c. insufficient dietary iron.
    d. hypothyroidism.

18. A 61-year-old female presents with headaches, epistaxis, and plethora of the hands and face. On physical examination, the nurse practitioner notes splenomegaly. The patient's laboratory studies reveal increased red blood cells and increased platelet count. She is otherwise in good health. What is the most likely diagnosis?

    a. Hypersplenism
    b. Idiopathic thrombocytopenic purpura (ITP)
    c. Polycythemia vera
    d. Acute myelogenous leukemia (AML)

19. Which of the following ecchymotic lesions in a 4-year-old patient most likely represents a bleeding disorder?

    a. 4 cm on the right lateral thigh
    b. 7 cm on the abdomen
    c. 3 cm on the left upper arm
    d. 2 cm on the forehead

15. *c* Staying well hydrated is necessary for children with sickle cell anemia because dehydration triggers sickling. Physical activity should be limited during crises to maintain adequate tissue oxygenation, but not necessarily at other times. Home schooling, for reasons of infection control, is not necessary.

16. *c* Persons with chronic renal failure (CRF) develop erythropoietin deficiency. Recombinant erythropoietin injections are considered the therapy of choice in these patients.

17. *b* The most common cause of iron deficiency anemia is blood loss. In women, blood loss through menses is usually the underlying cause. In the elderly, gastrointestinal bleeding is the most common cause. A malignant process may be the cause of the anemia, but it is not the most likely cause.

18. *c* Splenomegaly, erythrocytosis, and thrombocytosis are characteristic of polycythemia vera. The cause is unknown and may be treated by therapeutic phlebotomy or cytotoxic agents.

19. *b* Ecchymotic lesions greater than 6 cm, without history of significant trauma, most likely indicate an underlying bleeding problem. This is especially true if they are located in an area not usually subject to trauma.

D

20. Persons with thalassemia should avoid which of the following?

    a. Iron chelation therapy
    b. Drinking tea
    c. Folic acid supplements
    d. Iron supplementation

A

_____ 21. A 17 year old has mononucleosis. His CBC is characterized by:

    a. increased lymphocytes and decreased total white count.
    b. increased neutrophils and increased total white count.
    c. decreased monocytes and decreased total white count.
    d. decreased lymphocytes and increased neutrophils.

C

_____ 22. The patient who has iron deficiency anemia should be educated that foods high in iron content include:

    a. bananas, apples, and oranges.
    b. yellow vegetables.
    c. organ meats and dark green leafy vegetables.
    d. milk and dairy products.

C

_____ 23. The client with iron deficiency anemia should be advised to take the iron supplement:

    a. with milk to avoid stomach upset.
    b. with milk of magnesia at bedtime to avoid constipation.
    c. on an empty stomach between meals.
    d. for 30 days to 6 weeks.

A

_____ 24. Which of the following postpartum mothers should receive RhoGAM® to prevent Rh isoimmunization?

    a. A G_1P_1 mother is Rh negative without Rh antibodies, the cord blood is Coombs negative, and her newborn is Rh positive.
    b. A G_2P_2 mother is Rh negative without Rh antibodies, the cord blood is Coombs negative, and her newborn is Rh negative.
    c. A G_2P_2 mother is Rh negative with Rh antibodies, the cord blood is Coombs negative, and her newborn is Rh negative.
    d. A G_1P_1 mother is Rh positive with Rh antibodies, the cord blood is Coombs positive, and her newborn is Rh negative.

20. *d* Persons with thalassemia should avoid iron replacement therapy due to the risk of iron overload.

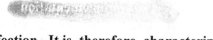

21. *a* Infectious mononucleosis is a viral infection. It is, therefore, characterized by an increased number of lymphocytes and a decreased number of neutrophils. Bacterial infection is characterized by an increased number neutrophils and a decreased number of lymphocytes. Early in the course of a bacterial infection the total WBC count may be within normal range.

22. *c* Examples of dietary sources of iron include red meat, organ meat (liver and kidney), dark green leafy vegetables, apricots, peaches, raisins, soybeans, dried peas and beans, clams and oysters, and oatmeal. Some cereals and bread products are fortified with iron. Dairy products are poor sources of iron.

23. *c* Iron is best absorbed when taken on an empty stomach or with a vitamin C-rich food or supplement. The best recommendation is to take it between meals. Milk and dairy products decrease iron absorption. Oral iron replacement therapy is usually required for at least 6 to 12 months. Constipation is avoided with a concomitant stool softener. Patients who have a malabsorption syndrome or who are unable to tolerate oral iron therapy may require parenteral therapy.

24. *a* When the mother is Rh negative without Rh antibodies, the cord blood is Coombs negative, and the newborn is Rh positive, the mother must receive Rh O (D) immunoglobulin (RhoGAM®) following delivery to prevent Rh isoimmunization.

25. A young couple presents for preconceptual counseling. Both carry the sickle cell trait. The nurse practitioner would be accurate to tell them that the baby:

a. will have normal hemoglobin.
b. might have the sickle cell trait.
c. will have the sickle cell trait, but not the disease.
d. will have sickle cell disease.

25. *b* When both parents carry the sickle cell trait, their offspring will have a 25% chance of a normal hemoglobin, a 50% chance of sickle cell trait, and a 25% chance of sickle cell disease.

Male and Female Disorders

1. A 20-year-old male patient complains of "scrotal swelling." He states his scrotum feels heavy, but denies pain. On examination, the nurse practitioner notes transillumination of the scrotum. What is the most likely diagnosis?

    a. Indirect inguinal hernia
    b. Hydrocele
    c. Orchitis
    d. Testicular torsion

2. A 45-year-old patient voices concern about her "hot flashes" and irregular menstrual periods. What diagnostic test would the nurse practitioner order to confirm the beginning of menopause?

    a. Serum follicular stimulating hormone (FSH)
    b. Serum prolactin level
    c. Pelvic ultrasound
    d. Thyroid stimulating hormone (TSH)

3. A 40-year-old female presents for a routine well woman exam. On examination, the nurse practitioner notes a scant nipple discharge, absence of a palpable mass, and absence of lymph node enlargement. Which of the following is the most likely diagnosis?

    a. Intraductal papilloma
    b. Breast cancer
    c. Chest wall syndrome
    d. Fibrocystic breast disease

4. A 22-year-old patient has a single, nontender, freely movable lump in her right breast. She denies any nipple discharge. Which of the following diagnoses is this clinical presentation most consistent with?

    a. Fibrocystic breast disease
    b. Breast cancer
    c. Fibroadenoma
    d. Intraductal papilloma

1. *b*   The clinical presentation of a hydrocele includes scrotal swelling, a feeling of heaviness in scrotum, and transillumination. The condition is usually painless. Indirect inguinal hernias are often associated with a communicating hydrocele. Hydrocele may also present secondary to injury, infection, or tumor.

2. *a*   In early menopause, follicle stimulating hormone (FSH) is > 30-40 mIU/ml, luteinizing hormone (LH) is > 30 mIU/ml, and the FSH:LH ratio is > 1. Pelvic ultrasound and prolactin level are not useful in determining onset of menopause. TSH may be considered for an atypical menopausal presentation or a very early presentation. FSH is not necessary to confirm diagnosis of menopause. It may be measured on any day if patient is not having menses. Measure on Day 3 in menstruating women.

3. *a*   Intraductal papilloma often presents as a nontender mass with serous or bloody nipple discharge. The lesion is located in the ductal system near the areola. Breast cancer, although usually nontender, may present with pain. Chest wall syndrome may present in some women as breast pain. Fibrocystic breast disease often presents with bilateral breast pain.

4. *c*   Fibroadenoma usually presents as a single, nontender, freely mobile mass in the breast and there is usually absence of nipple discharge. Fibrocystic breast disease is usually painful and there are multiple lumps present. Breast cancer is typically a fixed mass and nipple discharge may or may not be present. Intraductal papilloma is characterized by serous or bloody nipple discharge.

B

5.   The nurse practitioner diagnoses epididymitis in a 24-year-old sexually active male patient. The drug of choice for treatment of this patient is:

   a.   oral ciprofloxacin (Cipro®).
   b.   oral doxycycline (Vibramycin®) plus intramuscular ceftriaxone.
   c.   oral trimethoprim-sulfamethoxazole (Bactrim® DS).
   d.   intramuscular penicillin.

D

6.   Which of the following is *not* a common early sign of benign prostatic hyperplasia (BPH)?

   a.   Difficulty initiating a urine stream
   b.   Nocturia
   c.   Urinary retention
   d.   Increased force of urine flow

D

7.   Which of the following is *not* appropriate suppression therapy for chronic bacterial prostatitis?

   a.   doxycycline 100 mg qd
   b.   nitrofurantoin 100 mg qd
   c.   Bactrim® DS qd
   d.   erythromycin qd

C

8.   A 25-year-old overweight patient presents with a complaint of dull achiness in his groin and history of a palpable lump in his scrotum that "comes and goes." On physical examination, the nurse practitioner does not detect a scrotal mass. There is no tenderness, edema, or erythema of the scrotum, and the scrotum does not transilluminate. What is the most likely diagnosis?

   a.   Testicular torsion
   b.   Epididymitis
   c.   Inguinal hernia
   d.   Varicocele

D

9.   A nurse practitioner diagnoses a 60-year-old male with balanitis. Which disease is commonly associated with balanitis?

   a.   Congestive heart failure (CHF)
   b.   Dyslipidemia
   c.   Erectile dysfunction (ED)
   d.   Diabetes mellitus (DM)

5. *b*   Among men < 35 years-of-age, epididymitis is most commonly caused by *Neisseria gonorrhoeae* or *Chlamydia trachomatis*. Oral doxycycline plus intramuscular ceftriaxone should be administered to patients with epididymitis who are sexually active and < 35 years old. An alternative to doxycycline is azithromycin 1 gram.

6. *d*   Patients with early clinically significant urethral obstruction secondary to BPH typically present with decreased force of urine flow, hesitancy, frequency, nocturia, a sense of incomplete voiding, stream interruption, and dribbling. Other early signs may be prostatitis, urinary tract infection, and hematuria. Late manifestations are uremia, urinary retention, anorexia, anemia, and bleeding diathesis.

7. *d*   A daily dose of doxycycline, nitrofurantoin, or TMP/SMZ (Bactrim® DS) is recommended for chronic bacterial prostatitis (CBP) suppression therapy. These 3 antibiotics are effective against many Gram negative organisms, the likely causative agent. Erythromycin has poor Gram negative coverage.

8. *c*   The clinical manifestations associated with inguinal hernia are a dull ache in the groin and a mass in the scrotum that may or may not be reducible. An inguinal hernia that is not easily seen may be palpated when the examiner's finger is inserted through external inguinal canal as the patient forcefully coughs or bears down.

9. *d*   Balanitis is inflammation of the glans penis. It may be a complication of a sexually transmitted disease or from a noninfectious cause. Diabetes mellitus predisposes males to balanitis.

10. The most commonly recommended method for prostate cancer screening in a 55 year old male is:

    a. digital rectal examination (DRE) plus prostate specific antigen (PSA).
    b. prostate specific antigen (PSA) alone.
    c. transrectal ultrasound (TRUS) alone.
    d. prostate specific antigen (PSA) and transrectal ultrasound (TRUS).

11. A 35-year-old male presents with a complaint of low pelvic pain, dysuria, hesitancy, urgency, and reduced force of stream. The nurse practitioner suspects acute bacterial prostatitis. Which of the following specimens would be *least* helpful for diagnosis?

    a. Voided midstream bladder urine.
    b. Voided urethral urine.
    c. Voided post-prostate massage urine.
    d. Sterile in-and-out catheter urine specimen.

12. A 24-year-old female insists on having a screening mammogram. Upon further questioning, the nurse practitioner discovers the patient is concerned about breast cancer because her mother has fibrocystic breast disease. The nurse practitioner would be accurate if she tells the patient that a major risk factor for development of breast cancer in women is:

    a. benign breast disease in a first degree relative.
    b. late menarche (after age 15 years).
    c. first full term pregnancy after age 30 years.
    d. early menopause (before age 45 years).

13. A 60-year-old male patient with multiple health problems presents with a complaint of erectile dysfunction (ED). Of the following, which medication is most likely to be causing the problem?

    a. Thiazide diuretic
    b. Insulin
    c. Famotidine (Pepcid®)
    d. Albuterol

10. *a* Digital rectal examination (DRE), prostate specific antigen (PSA), and transrectal ultrasound (TRUS) are all methods of screening for prostate cancer. Any method used alone is not as effective as 2 used together. The American Cancer Society recommends annual DRE beginning at 40 years-of-age. Beginning at 50 years-of-age, annual DRE plus PSA is recommended.

11. *d* A sterile in-and-out catheter specimen would identify only organisms in the bladder and would not differentiate between bladder, kidney, or prostate site of infection. The sequence for obtaining specimens when prostate infection is suspected is: (1) voided urethral urine, (2) voided midstream bladder urine, and (3) voided post-prostate massage urine.

12. *c* Risk factors for development of breast cancer include first degree relative with breast cancer, early menarche (age 11 years or younger), late menopause (age 55 years or older), nulliparity, first full term pregnancy after age 30 years, and postmenopausal obesity.

13. *a* Diuretics and many other antihypertensive drugs are common causes of erectile dysfunction (ED) in men. The other drugs do not affect erectile function.

14. The treatment of choice for chronic bacterial prostatitis (CBP) is:

    a. erythromycin 4 times daily for 7 to 10 days.
    b. doxycycline twice daily for 7 to 10 days.
    c. a fluoroquinolone daily for 3 weeks to 4 months.
    d. Bactrim® DS daily for 4 to 16 weeks.

15. A 25 year old obese female has a history of frequent candidal vaginal infections in the past year. She is in a monogamous sexual relationship and uses an intrauterine device (IUD) for contraception. Of the following, which is the most likely underlying condition predisposing her to recurring candidal vaginitis?

    a. Tampon use
    b. Diabetes mellitus
    c. Trichomoniasis
    d. Pregnancy

16. It is imperative that the nurse practitioner teach patients taking an oral contraceptive to report any of the danger signs of complications. Which of the following, would be of *least* concern to the nurse practitioner?

    a. Lower leg pain
    b. Upper abdominal pain
    c. Chest pain
    d. Weight gain

17. The nurse practitioner is discussing contraception options to be used during lactation with a 24-year-old pregnant patient. Which of the following methods of contraception would *not* be appropriate for use while breastfeeding?

    a. levonorgestrel (Norplant®)
    b. A low dose oral contraceptive
    c. An intrauterine device
    d. A diaphragm and spermicide

14. *c*   The treatment of choice is a fluoroquinolone daily for 3 weeks to 4 months. The cure rate with Bactrim® DS is only about 30% to 40%.

15. *b*   A common underlying cause of frequent candidal infection is diabetes mellitus. Pregnancy increases the incidence of candidiasis, but is an unlikely factor in this patient.

16. *d*   The danger signs to teach patients who are taking oral contraceptives are: *A*-abdominal pain; *C*-chest pain; *H*-headache; *E*-eye problems; and *S*-severe leg pain. Weight gain may be a side effect, but is not associated with any known serious complication.

17. *b*   Combination oral contraceptives may cause decreased breast milk production in the lactating woman and should be avoided. Levonorgestrel (Norplant®), an intrauterine device, and the diaphragm with spermicide are all appropriate contraceptive choices for the breastfeeding woman.

18. A 19-year-old sexually active female is being counseled by the nurse practitioner about contraception. The nurse practitioner is accurate when she tells the patient that a diaphragm:

    a. with a flat spring is easier to use.
    b. increases the incidence of urinary tract infection.
    c. must be inserted immediately before intercourse.
    d. increases the risk of sexually transmitted diseases.

19. The side effect of medroxyprogesterone (Depo-Provera®) that often leads women to discontinue use is:

    a. pain at the injection site.
    b. weight gain.
    c. heavy menstrual bleeding.
    d. nausea and vomiting.

20. A 25-year-old married woman is being taught the natural family planning method (NFP) of contraception by the nurse practitioner. Which of the following statements by the patient demonstrates her understanding of NFP?

    a. "Abstinence is required during the 14th through 16th day of my cycle."
    b. "Coitus is 'safe' when my basal body temperature increases."
    c. "Cervical mucus is clear and thin during ovulation."
    d. "Douching does not affect my ability to effectively practice NFP."

21. A 16-year-old female is brought to the nurse practitioner by her mother. When counseling an adolescent about sexual activity and contraception, it is *not* appropriate to:

    a. ask the mother to leave the room for part of the interview.
    b. encourage condom use even if other contraceptive methods are utilized.
    c. include the intrauterine device as a contraceptive option to consider.
    d. discuss the adolescent's sexual experience with her privately.

18. *b* Use of a diaphragm for contraception is associated with an increased incidence of urinary tract infection. The arching spring type is easier to properly place than the flat spring type. The diaphragm can be inserted up to 6 hours before intercourse. The risk of contracting a sexually transmitted disease is decreased with diaphragm use.

19. *b* Weight gain is a common side effect of medroxyprogesterone (Depo-Provera®) which causes many women to discontinue the method. Menstrual bleeding is decreased but unpredictable, another major reason for discontinuation. Nausea and vomiting are not usually associated with medroxyprogesterone.

20. *c* Cervical mucus is abundant, clear, thin, wet, and elastic, before and during ovulation. Increase in basal body temperature indicates ovulation. Abstinence is required when basal body temperature and cervical mucus assessment indicate ovulation. Specific dates of the cycle cannot be used with confidence. Douching can interfere with the ability to accurately assess mucus changes.

21. *c* Intrauterine devices are not recommended for adolescents due to increased risk of pelvic inflammatory disease in this age group. Adolescents should be counseled without parents in the room for at least part of the session to assure confidentiality. Condoms should be used by adolescents even with other contraceptive methods to decrease the risk of contracting a sexually transmitted disease. All adolescents should be asked about their sexual experience in a matter-of-fact and non-judgmental manner to facilitate open and meaningful discussion.

C

_____ 22. The nurse practitioner is counseling a young woman who desires pregnancy. She discontinued her oral contraceptive 4 months ago. Her urine pregnancy test (UPT) is negative. She expresses concern that she might have an infertility problem. The nurse practitioner accurately tells her that a couple is not considered infertile until there has been unprotected intercourse without conception for what period of time?

    a. 4 months
    b. 8 months
    c. 1 year
    d. 1½ years

_____ 23. The treatment(s) with demonstrated effectiveness relieving symptoms of dysmenorrhea in women with premenstrual syndrome is(are):

    a. nutrition therapy with vitamin E.
    b. antipsychotic medication.
    c. antihypertensive agents.
    d. the NSAIDs.

_____ 24. The Papanicolaou (Pap) smear report on a 36-year-old female patient indicates atypical squamous cells of undetermined significance (ASCUS). Which of the following constitutes appropriate care for this patient?

    a. Repeat the Pap smear in 4 months.
    b. Prescribe estrogen cream.
    c. Perform a hysteroscopic examination.
    d. Refer the patient to a gynecologist.

_____ 25. A 38-year-old patient is being treated by the nurse practitioner for heavy vaginal bleeding secondary to multiple uterine leiomyomas. Her uterus is greater than 12 weeks gestational size, her hematocrit is 28%, and she has not responded to hormonal therapy. The most appropriate intervention at this time is to:

    a. start iron replacement therapy.
    b. obtain a gynecological consultation.
    c. order a urine pregnancy test.
    d. begin medroxyprogesterone (Depo-Provera®).

22. *c* By definition, infertility is when a couple has not conceived after a year of unprotected sexual intercourse or has not been able to carry a pregnancy to term after 1 year.

23. *d* Nonsteroidal anti-inflammatory drugs (NSAIDs) are often helpful in relieving pain associated with pre-menstrual syndrome (PMS, PMDS) due to the prostaglandin-inhibiting mechanism of action.

24. *a* If the Pap smear report shows ASCUS without neoplastic process suspected, the exam should be repeated every 4 to 6 months for 2 years. If a neoplastic process is favored as the underlying cause, colposcopy is recommended. Estrogen cream is used with this diagnosis when the patient is postmenopausal and not receiving hormone replacement therapy. Hysteroscopic examination is indicated for high-grade squamous intraepithelial lesions (HSIL), not for ASCUS. Referral to a gynecologist is not necessary at this time.

25. *b* Gynecological consultation is recommended for a patient with a uterus greater than 12 weeks gestational size, significant anemia (hematocrit < 30%), or a normal endometrial biopsy with failure to respond to hormonal therapy.

26. Which of the following does *not* increase a woman's risk for developing cervical cancer?

    a. A husband with penile cancer
    b. Multiple sexual partners
    c. History of tobacco abuse
    d. Nulliparity

27. A 50-year-old patient has abnormal vaginal bleeding with heavy periods and intermenstrual watery discharge with a small amount of blood. What is the most likely diagnosis?

    a. Uterine fibroids
    b. Normal perimenopause
    c. Endometrial cancer
    d. Cervical cancer

28. A 16-year-old high school student athlete is concerned that she has not had a menstrual period yet. On physical examination, the nurse practitioner finds normal growth and development including appropriate secondary sexual characteristics, and an otherwise normal exam. What is the most appropriate nurse practitioner action?

    a. Referral to another healthcare provider.
    b. Order a pregnancy test.
    c. Attempt a progesterone challenge.
    d. Prescribe an oral contraceptive.

29. A 6-month-old female is brought to the nurse practitioner by a child protection caseworker. On physical examination, the nurse practitioner notes a well developed, but undernourished, child. The examination is essentially negative except for the presence of labial adhesions. The nurse practitioner is concerned about urinary obstruction. The most appropriate intervention at this time is:

    a. labial separation under local anesthesia.
    b. local application of conjugate estrogen cream.
    c. instruction in perineal hygiene.
    d. referral to a physician.

26. *d* Risk factors for cervical disease are multiple and include partner with carcinoma in situ of the penis, high parity, multiple sexual partners (due to the risk of exposure to HPV), smoking, sexual intercourse prior to 18 years-of-age, first pregnancy before 18 years-of-age, low socioeconomic status, viral exposure, and immunodeficiency.

27. *c* Typically, endometrial cancer presents in women over 40 years-of-age who are postmenopausal, but 20% of women develop the disease while still menstruating. Bleeding is characterized by heavy menstrual periods and intermenstrual watery discharge with small amounts of blood, especially early in the disease process.

28. *a* Primary amenorrhea is defined as no menstrual bleeding by age 14 years and a lack of secondary sexual characteristic development *or* no menstrual bleeding by age 16 years with normal development of secondary sexual characteristics. All patients with primary amenorrhea should be referred to a physician or nurse practitioner familiar with the work-up.

29. *b* Labial adhesions may be secondary to poor hygiene. However, when there is a concern that labial adhesions are impeding vaginal or urinary drainage, topical conjugate estrogen cream twice a day for 14 to 21 days should be prescribed. This will usually thin the vulval tissue and induce separation. If there is no concern about urinary or vaginal discharge obstruction, the caregiver can be taught to use an ointment (e.g., A&D®) and apply pressure gently for several weeks to separate the adhesion. Separation under local anesthesia should be planned if therapy with conjugate estrogen cream fails. Referral to a physician is required if the adhesions are persistently thick, even after application of estrogen cream.

Neurological Disorders

1. The physiological explanation for syncope is:

   a. accelerated venous return and increased stroke volume resulting in deactivation of the parasympathetic nervous system.
   b. a cycle of inappropriate vasodilation, bradycardia, and hypotension.
   c. a sudden rise in blood pressure due to overly efficient vasoconstriction.
   d. emotional stress resulting in hypertension, tachycardia, and increased venous return.

2. The diagnosis which must be considered in a patient who presents with a severe headache of recent onset, with neck stiffness and fever, is:

   a. migraine headache.
   b. subarachnoid hemorrhage.
   c. glaucoma.
   d. meningitis.

3. An 65-year-old patient complains of recurrent bilateral temporal headaches, malaise, muscle aches, and low grade fever. The headache is described as superficial tenderness rather than deep pain. Giant cell arteritis is suspected. Appropriate treatment is:

   a. refer for temporal artery biopsy and initiation of oral prednisone.
   b. aspirin or acetaminophen every 4 hours as needed for pain and fever.
   c. a daily β-blocker such as propranolol (Inderal®).
   d. CT scan of the head and lumbar puncture for CSF evaluation.

4. The typical description of a tension headache is:

   a. periorbital pain, sudden onset, often explosive in quality, and associated with nasal stuffiness, lacrimation, red eye, and nausea.
   b. bilateral, occipital, or frontal tightness or fullness, with waves of aching pain.
   c. hemicranial pain that is accompanied by vomiting and photophobia.
   d. steadily worsening pain that interrupts sleep, is exacerbated by orthostatic changes, and may be preceded by nausea and vomiting.

1. *b*   Syncope occurs in the presence of diminished venous return and resulting decreased stroke volume. The reduction in stroke volume triggers a sympathetic reaction of cardiac contractility followed by sympathetic withdrawal. The parasympathetic nervous system is then activated, causing vasodilation, bradycardia, hypotension, and syncope.

2. *d*   Acute severe headache with nuchal rigidity and fever should lead the nurse practitioner to suspect meningitis. Positive Brudzinski's sign and positive Kernig's sign have > 80% association with bacterial meningitis. Lumbar puncture is mandatory for confirmation. Migraine, glaucoma, and subarachnoid hemorrhage are not usually associated with fever.

3. *a*   Temporal arteritis, or giant cell arteritis, is a common cause of headache among the elderly. Inflammation of the cranial arteries may lead to ischemic optic neuropathy and resulting blindness. Erythrocyte sedimentation rate (ESR) is often elevated. Temporal artery biopsy provides the definitive diagnosis and prednisone therapy is the recommended treatment.

4. *b*   Tension headache is usually bilateral and located in the occipital and/or frontal area. It is often described as constant fullness with waves of aching pain. Tension headaches may be triggered by emotional stress or worry. The recommended therapy is acetaminophen, aspirin, or NSAIDs.

5. The most effective intervention(s) to prevent stroke is (are):

    a. 81 mg of aspirin daily.
    b. carotid endarterectomy for patients with high-grade carotid lesions.
    c. routine screening for carotid artery stenosis with auscultation for bruits.
    d. smoking cessation and treatment of hypertension.

6. The most common symptoms of transient ischemic attack (TIA) include:

    a. nausea, vomiting, syncope, incontinence, dizziness, and seizure.
    b. weakness in an extremity, abruptly slurred speech or partial loss of vision, and sudden gait changes.
    c. headache and visual symptoms such as bright spots or sparkles crossing the visual field.
    d. gradual onset of ataxia, vertigo, generalized weakness, or lightheadedness.

7. A 60-year-old female patient complains of sudden onset unilateral, stabbing, surface pain in the lower part of her face lasting a few minutes, subsiding, and then returning. The pain is triggered by touch or temperature extremes. Physical examination is normal. Which of the following is the most likely diagnosis?

    a. Trigeminal neuralgia
    b. Temporal arteritis
    c. Parotiditis
    d. Bell's palsy

8. A 12 month old, who was premature at birth, has a history of prolonged febrile seizures on 2 occasions. The mother requests information about the prognosis. The nurse practitioner would be correct to tell the mother:

    a. the child has 2 risk factors for developing epilepsy.
    b. the child already has the diagnosis of epilepsy because he has a history of seizure.
    c. the child has no greater likelihood of developing a seizure disorder than the general population.
    d. children with febrile seizures are less likely than the general population to develop epilepsy.

5. *d*   According to the U.S. Preventive Services Task Force, the most important modifiable risk factors for stroke are hypertension and smoking. Improved treatment of hypertension has resulted in greater than 50% age-adjusted reduction in incidence of stroke.

6. *b*   Most symptoms of TIA are sudden and temporary. Slurred speech, diplopia, partial loss of vision, prickling, tingling, numbness, paresis, and sudden gait abnormalities are the most common symptoms of TIA. Symptoms typically last < 24 hours.

7. *a*   The typical clinical presentation of trigeminal neuralgia (tic douloureux) is sudden onset of sharp, stabbing, or shooting "electrical" facial pain that is triggered by touch, eating, speaking, or temperature extremes. It lasts seconds to minutes, subsides, then returns. Women over 50 years-of-age are affected most. The diagnosis is made by history after dental origin, sinus origin, cluster headache, structural lesion, and other related disorders have been ruled out. Physical exam, CT scan, and ESR are usually normal.

8. *a*   Risk factors for developing epilepsy include head trauma, CNS infection, febrile seizures (especially atypical seizures lasting > 3 minutes), and premature or low birth weight.

9. A 27-year-old female patient with epilepsy is well controlled with phenytoin (Dilantin®). She requests information about contraception. The nurse practitioner should instruct her that while taking phenytoin:

    a. the effectiveness of an oral contraceptive may be reduced.
    b. she should use a very low dose estrogen oral contraceptive.
    c. she should use another anticonvulsant along with the phenytoin.
    d. bilateral tubal ligation is recommended.

10. A 20-month-old child has been brought to the clinic after having a simple febrile seizure. The most appropriate intervention is to:

    a. recommend phenytoin (Dilantin®) therapy for 6 to 12 months.
    b. have an EKG performed.
    c. educate the parents about febrile seizures and first aid.
    d. refer the child for immediate lumbar puncture and blood work.

11. What is the most appropriate intervention for a 2-month-old febrile infant who appears ill but has no evidence of specific infection upon examination?

    a. Prescribe oral broad-spectrum antimicrobial therapy and recommend acetaminophen as needed.
    b. Hospitalization, and blood, urine and spinal fluid cultures, followed by antimicrobial therapy.
    c. Refer to a pediatric neurologist.
    d. Instruct the parent on the signs and symptoms of serious illness and recommend acetaminophen for fever.

12. A 2-year-old child is diagnosed with *Haemophilus influenza type b*. The child's parents will not allow any of his siblings to be immunized. There are 2 other children in the home, ages 1 year and 3 years. How should the nurse practitioner manage contacts?

    a. Only the 1-year-old child is at risk; therefore, only this child needs rifampin prophylaxis.
    b. Rifampin prophylaxis should be given to all household contacts, including the adults.
    c. Only the 2 children who are household contacts need rifampin prophylaxis.
    d. The 2 children who are household contacts should receive the Hib vaccine immediately.

9. *a*   Oral contraceptive effectiveness may be reduced when taken concomitantly with phenytoin, carbamazepine, phenobarbital, or primidone. A higher dose estrogen oral contraceptive may be more effective. The lowest effective dose of a single anticonvulsant is the most desirable medical treatment, especially when considering teratogenicity of this drug class. The patient should be educated about the increased incidence of congenital anomalies in infants born to mothers taking anticonvulsant medication.

10. *c*   The parents should be educated about febrile seizures and their management. Anticonvulsants are not necessary or appropriate for a first time febrile seizure. A lumbar puncture is recommended for children under 1 year of age experiencing a first seizure. The American Academy of Pediatrics does not recommend routine blood work, EEG, lumbar puncture, or neuroimaging for a first simple febrile seizure.

11. *b*   If the febrile infant under 3 months-of-age appears well, has been healthy, and a careful history and physical examination (including CBC and urinalysis) is negative for evidence of infection, the nurse practitioner can then be 95% confident that there is no serious bacterial infection. If the febrile infant < 3 months-of-age appears ill or toxic, that infant should be hospitalized promptly for cultures and parenteral antibiotics.

12. *b*   Rifampin prophylaxis should be given to all household contacts, including the adults. Children up to age 5 years may be immunized against Hib.

13. The 4 classic features of Parkinson's disease are:

    a. mask-like facies, dysarthria, excessive salivation, and dementia.
    b. tremor at rest, rigidity, bradykinesia, and postural disturbances.
    c. depression, cognitive impairment, constipation, and shuffling gait.
    d. tremor with movement, cogwheeling, repetitive movement, and multi-system atrophy.

14. Which of the following statements about multiple sclerosis (MS) is correct?

    a. MS is a chronic, untreatable illness that is almost always fatal.
    b. MS is a disease of steadily progressive and unrelenting neurologic deterioration.
    c. MS is a chronic, treatable illness with unknown cause and a variable course.
    d. Patients with MS who take active steps to improve their health have the best cure rate.

15. A 72-year-old patient exhibits sudden onset of fluctuating restlessness, agitation, confusion, and impaired attention. This is accompanied by visual hallucinations and sleep disturbance. What is the most likely cause of this behavior?

    a. Dementia
    b. Delirium
    c. Medication reaction
    d. Depression

16. Interventions that have proven most successful in the initial treatment of bulimia nervosa are:

    a. intensive individual and group psychotherapy.
    b. hospitalization followed by outpatient psychotherapy focusing on underlying issues.
    c. antidepressant medication and cognitive therapy that focuses on behavior.
    d. short-term use of a benzodiazepine and supportive group therapy to address underlying psychological issues.

13. *b* Tremor is the most frequent initial presenting feature of Parkinson's disease. It appears at rest and usually disappears with movement. Rigidity eventually presents in everyone with this illness. Bradykinesia refers to slow onset of movement and impaired ability to initiate movement. Postural disturbances tend to develop later in the illness.

14. *c* Multiple sclerosis (MS) is a chronic illness that is treatable and rarely fatal, but is not curable. It is a disease of remission and relapse in 90% of patients. There is no reliable predictor of who will have a benign course and who will become disabled.

15. *b* Sudden onset of these signs and symptoms is suspicious for delirium. Medication reaction is an example of delirium, but it is not the most likely cause of the behavior. Behavior changes in dementia are usually insidious, persistent, and stable. Visual hallucinations are frequently part of the delirium syndrome. Any cognitive disorder may present with confusion.

16. *c* Antidepressants, especially selective serotonin reuptake inhibitors (SSRIs), have been found to have an anti-bulimic effect. Eating behavior is best stabilized with individual or group cognitive therapy that focuses on the bingeing and purging behavior rather than on underlying issues.

17. What is the most frequent cause of death in patients with anorexia nervosa?

    a. Renal failure
    b. Suicide
    c. Hepatic failure
    d. Cardiac arrest

18. Successful management of a patient with attention deficit hyperactivity disorder (ADHD) may be best achieved with:

    a. stimulant medication along with behavioral and family intervention.
    b. methylphenidate (Ritalin®) in conjunction with diet changes.
    c. treatment by a pediatric psychiatrist.
    d. discipline and removal of offending foods from the diet.

19. The child at high risk for developing hydrocephaly often has a history of:

    a. Down syndrome, *cri du chat*, or other genetic abnormality.
    b. prematurity, meningitis, or intrauterine infection.
    c. microcephaly with head circumference below the 5th percentile.
    d. fetal alcohol syndrome (FAS) with growth restriction.

20. Advances in obstetric and neonatal care have:

    a. helped to identify the cause of cerebral palsy.
    b. demonstrated that cerebral palsy is a direct result of birth asphyxia.
    c. had no effect on the incidence of cerebral palsy.
    d. resulted in a dramatic decrease in the incidence of cerebral palsy.

21. Which of the following set of symptoms should raise suspicion of a brain tumor?

    a. Recurrent, severe headaches that awaken the patient and are accompanied by visual disturbances
    b. Vague, dull headaches that are accompanied by a reported sense of impending doom
    c. Periorbital headaches occurring primarily in the evening and accompanied by pupillary dilation and photophobia
    d. Holocranial headaches present in the morning and accompanied by projectile vomiting without nausea

17. *d* The most frequent cause of death associated with anorexia nervosa is cardiac arrest. Suicide is the second most frequent cause of death.

18. *a* Stimulant medication, family education, and behavioral intervention have been successful for about 70% of children diagnosed with ADHD. Children taking methylphenidate (Ritalin®) should avoid over-the-counter antihistamines. A multidisciplinary approach involving medical, psychological, educational, and social intervention is preferred. Diet modification has not proven effective.

19. *b* Obstructive hydrocephalus usually develops as a result of an abnormality or lesion in the 4th ventricle or aqueduct of Sylvius. Neonatal meningitis, subarachnoid hemorrhage in a premature infant, or intrauterine viral infection may result in obstruction of CSF flow. Down syndrome, *cri du chat*, and fetal alcohol syndrome (FAS) are all causes of microcephaly.

20. *c* Cerebral palsy is a common, non-progressive, encephalopathy that is believed to be due to a defect in the developing brain. Improvements in perinatal care have not affected the incidence.

21. *d* Brain tumor size (mass) increases intracranial pressure which manifests as a holocranial headache on morning awakening, often accompanied by projectile vomiting. Personality changes and focal neurological deficits are other frequently associated clinical findings.

22. The nurse practitioner performs a routine physical examination of a 3-year-old child. A hard, painless mass is palpated in the abdomen, along with lymph node enlargement and lower limb paresis. Blood and imaging studies provide markers for neuroblastoma. What information is correct to give to the parents?

    a. The diagnosis must be confirmed by tissue biopsy or by bone marrow aspiration plus urine or serum catecholamine levels.
    b. Neuroblastoma is the final diagnosis based on physical examination and blood and imaging markers.
    c. Signs and symptoms, along with blood imaging markers, define the tumor as stage D, metastasis beyond lymph nodes.
    d. Prognosis is poor, based on the likelihood that there is metastasis to the bone.

23. The hallmark of neurofibromatosis (von Recklinghausen's disease) present in almost 100% of patients is:

    a. acoustic neuroma.
    b. astrocytoma of the retina.
    c. distinctive osseous lesions.
    d. *cafe au lait* spots.

24. Initial treatment of a child presenting with a severe head injury is:

    a. aimed at the prevention of seizure activity with prophylactic anticonvulsant medication.
    b. prevention of coma, which is the most important determinant of neurological recovery.
    c. aimed at resuscitation, then maintenance of oxygenation and blood flow.
    d. normalization of intracranial pressure, followed by intracranial pressure monitoring.

25. The routine primary poliovirus vaccination regimen for adults is:

    a. 3 doses of live oral trivalent polio vaccine (OPV), each 2 months apart.
    b. 3 doses of inactivated trivalent polio vaccine (IPV), each 2 months apart.
    c. recommended only for persons with compromised immunity.
    d. not routinely recommended in non-immunized adults.

22. *a*   A definitive diagnosis of neuroblastoma requires tissue biopsy or documentation of bone marrow involvement plus increases in levels of urine or serum catecholamines.

23. *d*   *Cafe au lait* spots, a clinical finding in almost 100% of patients with neurofibromatosis, are present at birth and gradually increase in size, number, and degree of pigmentation. Approximately 40% of patients are reported to have osseous lesions and skeletal abnormalities. Acoustic neuromas are present in most cases of neurofibromatosis-2, which accounts for 10% of all cases. Astrocytoma of the retina is a lesion often associated with tuberous sclerosis.

24. *c*   A head injured patient requires that all related injuries be identified and treated, but the most immediate need is airway resuscitation, maintenance of oxygenation, and maintenance of blood flow. Cerebral edema, a major complication of head injury, is managed with adequate oxygenation, elevation of the head and trunk to facilitate venous return from the head, isotonic intravenous fluid administration maintaining low central venous pressure, and maintenance of normal body temperature.

25. *d*   Adults at risk for exposure to poliovirus should receive IPV. However, routine administration of polio vaccine to non-immunized adults is not recommended.

Orthopedic Disorders

1. A 72-year-old female patient reports a 6-month history of gradually progressive swollen and painful distal interphalangeal (DIP) joints of one hand. She has no systemic symptoms but the erythrocyte sedimentation rate (ESR), antinuclear antibody (ANA), and rheumatoid factor (RF) are all minimally elevated. What is the most likely diagnosis?

   a. Rheumatoid arthritis (RA)
   b. Osteoarthritis (OA)
   c. Lupus
   d. Peripheral neuropathy

2. What intervention does the American College of Rheumatology recommend as first-line therapy for osteoarthritis?

   a. Extensive diagnostic work-up
   b. NSAIDs at therapeutic doses
   c. Early joint replacement
   d. Exercise and weight loss

3. Which of the following physical modalities recommended for treatment of rheumatoid arthritis provides the most effective long term pain relief?

   a. Superficial and deep heat
   b. Application of cold
   c. Transcutaneous electrical nerve stimulation (TENS)
   d. Exercise

4. The nurse practitioner is following a child with juvenile rheumatoid arthritis (JRA) who has been previously diagnosed and is being managed for the disease by a pediatric rheumatologist. The mother asks for information about the child's long term prognosis. What is the most appropriate reply?

   a. Since her child is under the care of a rheumatologist, she should direct questions concerning the JRA to him.
   b. JRA is a childhood form of rheumatoid arthritis and her child will have the illness for a lifetime.
   c. Most children with JRA achieve complete remission by adulthood, but the effects may cause lifelong limitations.
   d. Most children with JRA do not live to adulthood.

1. *b*   When osteoarthritis affects the hands, the distal interphalangeal (DIP) joints are usually involved. Rheumatoid arthritis is usually symmetrical, and the proximal interphalangeal (PIP) joints are more often affected. Inflammation develops quickly, not gradually. This patient is elderly; therefore, it is expected that the ESR, ANA, and RF will be only somewhat elevated. Over-interpretation of laboratory tests without evidence of systemic inflammation can lead to misdiagnosis.

2. *d*   Exercise, weight loss, and rest are recommended by the American College of Rheumatology guidelines for initial management of osteoarthritis (OA). Given the adverse effects of medications indicated for the treatment of OA, it is best to minimize dosage and delay use as long as possible. An extensive diagnostic work-up is not recommended unless the presentation is in question. Patients who have severe degenerative joint disease (DJD), joint fusion, or whose pain severity is not relieved by more conservative therapies may be candidates for joint replacement.

3. *d*   Exercise is most consistently effective in reducing the pain associated with rheumatoid arthritis. Exercise improves blood flow, cartilage health, range of motion, and muscle strength. Exercise can also improve self-efficacy. Patients with RA should be cautioned to limit joint range of motion, and/or splint affected joints, during acute flare-ups to preserve joint integrity. Heat, cold, and TENS application also have a role in pain relief.

4. *c*   Although the active disease process does not continue into adulthood, contractures, growth retardation, bone deformities, and visual impairment associated with (JRA) may lead to lifelong functional impairments. A comprehensive treatment program involving physical therapy, occupational therapy, nutrition, education, and regular ophthalmologic care can limit residual functional disability.

5. The most reliable diagnostic indicator of gout is:

 a. monosodium urate (MSU) crystals in the synovial fluid.
 b. tophi visible over joints or in connective tissue.
 c. elevated serum uric acid level.
 d. abrupt onset of single joint inflammation and pain.

6. A 14-year-old female cheerleader reports gradual and progressive dull anterior knee pain, exacerbated by kneeling. The nurse practitioner notes swelling and point tenderness at the tibial tuberosity. X-ray is negative. What is the most likely diagnosis?

 a. Patellar fasciitis
 b. Cruciate ligament tear
 c. Osgood-Schlatter disease
 d. Patellar fracture

7. The most reliable indicator(s) of neurological deficit when assessing a patient with acute low back pain is(are):

 a. patient report of bladder dysfunction, saddle anesthesia, and motor weakness of limbs.
 b. history of significant trauma relative to the patient's age.
 c. decreased reflexes, strength, and sensation in the lower extremities.
 d. patient report of pain with the crossed straight leg raise test.

8. The most commonly recommended pharmacological treatment regimen for low back pain (LBP) is:

 a. acetaminophen or an NSAID.
 b. a muscle relaxant as an adjunct to an NSAID.
 c. an oral corticosteroid and diazepam (Valium®).
 d. colchicine and an opioid analgesic.

9. Diagnostic radiological studies are indicated for low back pain:

 a. routinely after 3 weeks of low back pain symptoms.
 b. to screen for spondylolithiasis in patients less than 20 years-of-age with 2 weeks or more of low back pain.
 c. when there is suspicion of a space-occupying lesion, fracture, cauda equina, or infection.
 d. as part of a pre-employment physical when heavy lifting is included in the job description.

5. *a* Demonstration of monosodium urate (MSU) crystals is the most reliable sign for establishing the diagnosis of gout. Serum uric acid levels are unreliable for diagnosis but play a role in management.

6. *c* Osgood-Schlatter disease, a common cause of knee pain in adolescents, is a periostitis caused by repetitive traction of the patellar tendon over the tibial tuberosity. Rest, analgesics, and quadriceps strengthening exercises are recommended for treatment.

7. *c* Research has shown that report of dysfunction or pain with crossed straight leg raises is a significant indicator of neurological impairment. However, compromised reflexes, sensation, and strength are more reliable. History of significant trauma increases the likelihood of fracture. Choice *a* describes cauda equina syndrome.

8. *a* Acetaminophen and NSAIDs have been found through research to be reasonably safe and effective for treating low back pain. Muscle relaxants have not been shown to be significantly beneficial when combined with NSAIDs unless the injury is recent and there is evidence of muscle spasm. Oral steroid treatment and diazepam are not recommended. A short-term opioid analgesic may be an option early in severe cases, but colchicine is not indicated.

9. *c* Lumbar x-rays rarely detect changes that are unexpected. X-ray, CT, MRI, and myelography are recommended only in the presence of red flags from history and physical exam, or after 1 month of symptoms without relief. Imaging studies should be ordered in consultation with a surgeon since findings may call for prompt surgical intervention.

10. The most effective treatment for noninfectious bursitis includes:

    a. systemic antibiotic therapy effective against penicillin resistant *Staphylococcus aureus*.
    b. rest, an intra-articular corticosteroid injection, and a concomitant oral NSAID.
    c. a tapering regimen of oral corticosteroid therapy.
    d. frequent active range of joint motion.

11. A 26-year-old female presents with elbow pain that is described as aching and burning. There is point tenderness along the lateral aspect of the elbow and painful passive flexion and extension. She reports she has been playing tennis almost daily for the past month. The most likely diagnosis is:

    a. radial tunnel syndrome.
    b. ulnar collateral ligament sprain.
    c. olecranon bursitis.
    d. lateral epicondylitis.

12. Phalen's test, 90° wrist flexion for 60 seconds, reproduces symptoms of:

    a. ulnar tunnel syndrome.
    b. carpal tunnel syndrome.
    c. tarsal tunnel syndrome.
    d. myofascial pain syndrome.

13. A positive drawer sign supports a diagnosis of:

    a. sciatica.
    b. cruciate ligament injury.
    c. meniscal injury.
    d. patellar ligament injury.

14. The correct treatment for ankle sprain during the first 48 hours after injury includes:

    a. alternating heat and ice, and ankle exercises.
    b. resistive ankle exercises, ankle support, and pain relief.
    c. rest, elevation, compression, ice, and pain relief.
    d. referral to an orthopedist after x-rays to rule out fracture.

10. *b*   The affected joint should be rested. A sling, cane, or splint may be helpful.
A long-acting corticosteroid injected into the bursa along with an oral NSAID
should be effective in relieving the inflammation and pain of bursitis.

11. *d*   Lateral epicondylitis (also called tennis elbow) is associated with aching,
burning, sharp pain along the lateral aspect of the elbow. It usually follows
repetitive overuse or a single traumatic event. All other choices are associated
with medial elbow pain.

12. *b*   Carpal tunnel syndrome occurs with median nerve compression at the wrist,
resulting in dysesthesia of the palmar surface of the thumb, index finger, 3rd
finger, and radial side of the 4th finger.

13. *b*   A positive drawer sign indicates cruciate ligament pathology. Position the
patient supine with the hip flexed 45°, the knee flexed 90°, and the foot flat on
the exam table. While stabilizing the distal femur with one hand, the examiner
applies anterior force and applies posterior force with the opposite hand.
Increased forward and backward motion is a positive anterior drawer sign.

14. *c*   Approximately 85% of ankle injuries are sprains. X-ray is recommended with
history of severe trauma or if the swelling is inconsistent with the reported
injury. Immediate intervention can be remembered by the acronym RICE:
Rest, and avoidance of weight-bearing; Ice applied as often as possible for 20
minutes at a time; Compression, with an elastic wrap; and Elevation of the
affected limb. Acetaminophen or ibuprofen is recommended as needed for
pain. Gentle ROM should be initiated after fracture is ruled out.

15. Radiographic evaluation of talipes equinovarus must be performed:

    a. while weightbearing.
    b. after 4 years-of-age.
    c. with oblique views.
    d. while non weightbearing.

16. A 6-month-old patient with type III metatarsus adductus (i.e., rigid and does not correct to neutral) should be treated with:

    a. stimulation of the perineal musculature by stroking the lateral border of the foot.
    b. straight or corrective shoes.
    c. serial plaster casts.
    d. surgical intervention.

17. The infant 1 to 6 months-of-age with a diagnosis of developmental hip dysplasia is correctly treated with:

    a. closed reduction of the hips.
    b. surgical open reduction followed by pelvic and/or femoral osteotomy.
    c. a variety of adduction orthoses.
    d. the Pavlik harness.

18. A 7-year-old presents with a painless limp, antalgic gait, muscle spasm, mildly restricted hip abduction and internal rotation and proximal thigh atrophy. The most likely diagnosis is:

    a. transient monoarticular synovitis.
    b. slipped capital femoral epiphysis.
    c. congenital dysplasia of the hip.
    d. Legg-Calve-Perthes disease.

19. A 6-year-old presents with acute onset of ipsilateral hip pain, limp, and limited abduction. He was seen in the clinic ten days ago with an upper respiratory infection. He complains of pain in the groin and anterior thigh. He is afebrile. Laboratory values are all within normal limits. AP and lateral x-rays of the pelvis are normal. The most likely diagnosis is:

    a. transient monoarticular synovitis.
    b. septic arthritis.
    c. osteomyelitis of the hip.
    d. Legg-Calve-Perthes disease.

15. *a*   AP and lateral, standing or simulated weightbearing x-rays are used to diagnose talipes equinovarus (club-foot). Recently, ultrasound (US) has gained acceptance and confidence because many positions can be noted during the US; compared to the x-ray where a single position is viewed. Non-surgical correction should be achieved by 3 months-of-age. If this is unsuccessful, surgical treatment is indicated between 6 months and 1 year-of-age.

16. *c*   Type I and II metatarsus adductus feet are flexible and usually require corrective shoes or no treatment. Between 85% to 90% resolve spontaneously. Type III feet are rigid and corrected with serial plaster casting followed by orthosis. Metatarsus adductus deformities in children 4 years-of-age or older require surgery, usually followed by serial casting.

17. *d*   The objective of treatment for hip dysplasia is to enlarge and deepen the hip socket by applying constant pressure on the head of the femur into the acetabulum. The Pavlik harness and the von Rosen splint maintains this position. Surgical correction may be required for infants older than 6 months-of-age.

18. *d*   These are the classic signs and symptoms of Legg-Calve-Perthes disease, a local, self-healing disorder. It is characterized by loss of circulation to the femoral head resulting in avascular necrosis. The mean age of presentation is 7 years. Justification for treatment is prevention of secondary osteoarthritis and femoral head deformity.

19. *a*   The average age of onset of transient monoarticular synovitis is 7 years. About 70% of patients will have a history of upper respiratory infection 7 to 14 days prior to the onset of symptoms. The diagnosis is one of exclusion. Septic arthritis and osteomyelitis must be ruled out before a diagnosis of transient monoarticular synovitis can be made.

20. Establishment of a definitive diagnosis of osteomyelitis requires:

    a. a known causative injury such as a puncture wound, bite, or decubitus ulcer.
    b. biopsy or culture of the pathogen from blood or bone aspirate.
    c. visualization of purulent material draining into soft tissue.
    d. lucent areas identified on plain x-ray.

21. At what age is screening most likely to detect scoliosis?

    a. 4 to 6 years
    b. 8 to 10 years
    c. 12 to 14 years
    d. 18 to 20 years

22. The obligatory criteria for diagnosis of muscular dystrophy (MD) are:

    a. progressive, genetic myopathy with degeneration and death of muscle fibers.
    b. asymmetric overgrowth of extremities, angiomas, thickening of bones, and excessive muscle growth.
    c. hypotonia that persists into adulthood, and recurrent joint dislocation.
    d. hypotonicity, developmental delay, and symmetric congenital absence of individual muscles.

23. A 2-week-old infant, with a history of a difficult delivery, is brought to the nurse practitioner clinic. The mother says the infant fusses when handled or picked up. On physical examination, the nurse practitioner notes decreased movement of the right arm during the Moro reflex, and crepitus on palpation of the right clavicle. The diagnosis is fracture of the clavicle and recommended management is:

    a. a "figure-8" clavicle brace.
    b. a shoulder/trunk spica cast to immobilize the fracture for 6 weeks.
    c. instructions to the parents to handle the neonate gently.
    d. referral to an orthopedic surgeon.

20. *b*   The definitive diagnosis of osteomyelitis is made with culture of blood, bone aspirate, or biopsy.

21. *c*   Screening tests should be performed at the age in which manifestation of the condition is most prevalent. Starting at 8 years, parents should watch for uneven shoulders, uneven hips or waist, prominent shoulder blades, and leaning to one side. Scoliosis manifests itself during the time of peak growth which is age 12 in females and age 14 in males.

22. *a*   There are 4 obligatory criteria which distinguish muscular dystrophy from other neuromuscular diseases: primary myopathy with a genetic basis, progressive nature, muscle degeneration, and death of muscle fibers. The muscular dystrophies are a group of related diseases with different clinical courses and genetic traits.

23. *c*   A frequent complication of a difficult birth is fracture of the clavicle. Neonates generally require only gentle handling of the arm and shoulder for 3 to 5 weeks. If severe, safety pin the infant's sleeve to his shirt. Older children may require a sling. X-ray is not usually necessary for diagnosis.

_____ 24. The cornerstone of treatment for stress fracture of the femur or metatarsal stress fracture is:

    a. rest from activities which may further stress the bone.
    b. daily passive range of motion exercises.
    c. continuation of the patient's routine physical activities.
    d. application of ice after activity.

24. *a*   Absolute rest from aggravating activities is essential until healing has occurred. The patient should engage in pain free activity for 4 to 8 weeks while the fracture heals. An alternate activity referred to as cross-training is recommended.

Pregnancy and Lactation

1. Which of the following should the nurse practitioner encourage preconceptually to decrease the risk of neural tube defect in the fetus?

   a. Maternal α-fetoprotein level
   b. Folic acid 0.4 mg daily
   c. Rubella vaccine today
   d. Vitamin E 400 IU daily

2. A 28-year-old pregnant patient, at 18 weeks gestation, complains of feeling light-headed when standing. Which of the following is an appropriate response by the nurse practitioner?

   a. Blood pressure normally decreases during pregnancy and can cause this symptom.
   b. The lightheadedness is a concern. A CBC should be ordered to check for anemia.
   c. Lightheadedness may be caused by an abnormal elevation in blood pressure during pregnancy.
   d. Low blood sugar may be causing this problem. An oral glucose tolerance test is indicated.

3. Which of the following is the current recommendation for human immunodeficiency virus (HIV) screening during pregnancy?

   a. All pregnant women should be counseled and encouraged to be tested.
   b. No screening is necessary once a woman becomes pregnant.
   c. Women who have risk factors should be tested in early pregnancy.
   d. Use polymerase chain reaction (PCR) testing in pregnancy.

4. RhoGAM® is indicated for an Rh-negative mother:

   a. routinely at 28 to 30 weeks gestation.
   b. before amniocentesis.
   c. within 72 hours of birth of an Rh-positive infant.
   d. after a vaginal ultrasound.

1. *b*   Supplemental folic acid, 0.4 mg/day, has been shown to decrease the incidence of neural tube defects when taken prior to and during pregnancy. Pregnancy should be avoided for 28 days after receiving the rubella vaccine. Vitamin E has no known role in prevention of neural tube defects. Maternal α-fetoprotein level may detect neural tube defect, but it has no role in prevention.

2. *a*   Blood pressure normally decreases during pregnancy, reaching the lowest point during the 2nd or early 3rd trimester and rising thereafter. Patient education to rise slowly from sitting or lying is important. Low blood glucose may be the etiology, but an oral glucose tolerance test at this point is not indicated. A fasting blood glucose could be ordered, however. A CBC could be ordered, but it is unlikely that anemia is the problem unless it has suddenly become severe.

3. *a*   There is varied opinion about screening for HIV in pregnancy. Early treatment during pregnancy has been shown to reduce the incidence of perinatal transmission; therefore, the CDC recommends all pregnant women be counseled about testing and encouraged to do so. Screening is by enzyme linked immunosorbent assay (ELISA).

4. *c*   RhoGAM® is indicated after amniocentesis, within 72 hours after delivery of an Rh positive infant, after uterine evacuation (miscarriage, molar pregnancy), but not after a vaginal ultrasound. No sensitization takes place in the Rh-negative mother when she is pregnant with an Rh-negative infant.

D

_____ 5.   A 19-year-old pregnant patient, at 20 weeks gestation, complains of pain in the right lower quadrant. She is afebrile and denies nausea and vomiting. The most likely diagnosis is:

   a.   appendicitis.
   b.   urinary tract infection.
   c.   muscle strain.
   d.   round ligament pain.

A

_____ 6.   Which of the following is *not* a component of the fetal biophysical profile?

   a.   Gestational age estimate
   b.   Fetal breathing
   c.   Amniotic fluid volume
   d.   Fetal movement

C

_____ 7.   A 28-year-old pregnant patient gives a history of smoking 1 pack of cigarettes per day (1 PPD). The nurse practitioner is accurate when she tells the patient that cigarette smoking is associated with:

   a.   microcephaly.
   b.   fetal hypoglycemia in the first 24 hours of life.
   c.   intra uterine growth restriction.
   d.   increased incidence of fetal cardiac anomalies.

C

_____ 8.   A 20-year-old female patient presents to the emergency department with lower abdominal pain, moderate vaginal bleeding, and right shoulder pain. Her blood pressure is 85/50 mmHg, pulse 140, respirations 28, and temperature 98°F (36.6°C). She has a history of pelvic inflammatory disease (PID). Her urine pregnancy test is positive. Which of the following is the most likely diagnosis?

   a.   Threatened spontaneous abortion
   b.   Abruptio placenta
   c.   Ectopic pregnancy
   d.   Placenta previa

A

_____ 9.   Which of the following laboratory tests is useful in the diagnosis of spontaneous abortion?

   a.   Serial quantitative β-human chorionic gonadotropin levels
   b.   Qualitative plasma estradiol levels
   c.   Plasma dehydroepiandrosterone sulfate (DHEA-S®) levels
   d.   Qualitative plasma human chorionic gonadotropin levels

5. *d*   As the fetus grows and the uterus rises out of the pelvis, strain is placed on the uterine round ligaments causing lower abdominal pain. This common discomfort in pregnancy is not associated with any other systemic symptoms. The pain is often relieved by left side-lying while bringing both knees closer to the chest.

6. *a*   There are 5 components in the fetal biophysical profile: fetal heart rate acceleration, fetal breathing, fetal movements, fetal tone, and amnionic fluid volume measurement.

7. *c*   Due to a variety of reasons, smoking during pregnancy causes small for gestational age fetuses, and increased incidence of prematurity and perinatal death.

8. *c*   The classic presentation of ectopic pregnancy with a ruptured fallopian tube is vaginal bleeding, sudden severe lower abdominal pain, neck or shoulder pain, and hypotension. The neck and shoulder pain is secondary to diaphragmatic irritation from blood. Women with pelvic inflammatory disease (PID) frequently have an elevated temperature as well as increased incidence of ectopic pregnancy due to scarring.

9. *a*   Serial quantitative β-human chorionic gonadotropin levels are the most useful for diagnosing spontaneous abortion. The levels progressively decline over several days. During early pregnancy, the levels double every 2 to 3 days.

C 10. A 30-year-old female patient is seeking advice from the nurse practitioner about becoming pregnant. She is currently taking an oral contraceptive. She gives a history of having a hydatidiform molar pregnancy 2 years ago. The appropriate plan of care for this patient should include:

    a. delaying pregnancy for 1 more year.
    b. measuring serum chorionic gonadotropin level.
    c. discontinuing the oral contraceptive.
    d. recommending hysterectomy.

B 11. An autosomal recessive disorder such as cystic fibrosis is expressed in the offspring when:

    a. neither parent carry the gene.
    b. both parents carry the gene.
    c. 1 parent has the disease.
    d. 1 parent carries the gene.

C 12. Children born with Down syndrome often have other anomalies. They require specific evaluation of what body system?

    a. Respiratory
    b. Gastrointestinal
    c. Cardiac
    d. Endocrine

B 13. Turner's syndrome presents exclusively in:

    a. male infants.
    b. female infants.
    c. Jewish infants.
    d. Asian infants.

C 14. The best way for a pregnant woman to avoid injury to herself and her fetus in the event of a motor vehicle accident (MVA) is to:

    a. use the lap restraint only.
    b. avoid exposure to air bag deployment.
    c. use both the lap restraint and shoulder restraint.
    d. use the shoulder restraint only.

10. *c* Women who have a hydatidiform molar pregnancy should delay pregnancy for 1 year and be followed with serum chorionic gonadotropin levels. After 1 year of normal levels, follow up may be discontinued and pregnancy permitted. She may discontinue the oral contraceptive and begin attempting pregnancy.

11. *b* An autosomal recessive disorder is expressed when the child inherits an affected gene from each parent. Because the parents have only 1 affected gene each, they do not have expression of the disease.

12. *c* Approximately 50% of children born with Down syndrome have congenital heart disease. It is imperative that the infant be evaluated for cardiac anomalies.

13. *b* Turner syndrome is a sex-linked abnormality occurring only in female offspring. Eastern European Jewish infants may be at higher risk of Tay-Sachs disease, a progressive, destructive central nervous system disease.

14. *c* No evidence has been found to indicate that lap and shoulder seat restraints increase risk of fetal injury. The leading cause of fetal death in motor vehicle accidents is death of the mother; therefore, use of properly positioned lap and shoulder restraints should be encouraged. The lap restraint should be placed under the abdomen and across the upper thighs.

B 15. When counseling a woman who is breastfeeding her 6-month-old infant, the nurse practitioner should recommend a caloric intake over her pre-pregnancy requirements of:

a. 200 kcal/day.
b. 500 kcal/day.
c. 900 kcal/day.
d. 1000 kcal/day.

A 16. To prevent breast trauma during breastfeeding, the nurse practitioner should stress the importance of:

a. positioning of the infant.
b. prenatal breast care.
c. keeping the nipples dry.
d. using breast shields.

B 17. A 26-year-old female patient presents with cracked and sore nipples. She is breastfeeding her first child who is 4 weeks old. The nurse practitioner would be accurate to advise the patient to:

a. stop breastfeeding until the nipples have healed.
b. apply a vitamin E moisturizing cream after each feeding and continue to breast-feed.
c. use a breast shield with each feeding.
d. apply an antibiotic cream after each feeding.

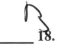 18. An 18-year-old mother who is breastfeeding her 2-week-old infant, expresses concern about how much milk the baby is getting. Which of the following parameters is reassuring to the nurse practitioner that the infant is receiving adequate nutrition?

a. The infant is nursing 6 times per day.
b. The infant has at least 6 wet diapers per day.
c. The infant has a formed stool twice daily.
d. Weight loss is 10% of the infant's birth weight.

D 19. A 23-year-old pregnant patient who works as a secretary in a large law firm is seeing the nurse practitioner for early pregnancy evaluation and education. It would be very important to teach this patient about:

a. the dangers of standing too much during pregnancy.
b. the need for rest periods during the day.
c. avoidance of heavy lifting.
d. proper hand positioning when typing.

15. *b* Although the caloric cost of producing 1 liter of breast milk is 940 kcal, only 500 kcal/day is necessary for lactation because of pregnancy stores. The only exception is women with known high metabolic rates.

16. *a* In the first few days of breastfeeding, positioning is the most common cause of painful nipples. Correct positioning of the infant is essential to prevent sore nipples.

17. *b* Rarely is discontinuation of breastfeeding necessary because of cracked or sore nipples. Breast shields have no role in the care of cracked nipples. Antibiotic cream is not indicated unless there is a secondary infection present. Application of a moisturizing cream after each feeding, which contains vitamin E or aloe, will aid healing and relieve the discomfort.

18. *b* Signs of adequate intake of breast milk include: alert and healthy appearance; good muscle tone and skin turgor; at least 6 wet diapers per day; pale dilute urine; frequent, seedy stools; nursing 8 or more times per day for 15 to 20 minutes; adequate let down reflex; consistent weight gain.

19. *d* Carpal tunnel syndrome is more common during pregnancy. It would be very important to teach this patient about appropriate hand positioning when typing to decrease the risk of developing this syndrome.

D   20. A 15-year-old pregnant patient presents for her first prenatal visit. On
physical examination, her uterus is approximately 24-week gestational
size. She does not know when her last menstrual period was or when she
might have conceived. Gestational age for this patient can most accurately
be assessed by:

    a. Naegele's rule.
    b. biophysical profile.
    c. measurement of fundal height.
    d. ultrasonography.

C   21. A nurse practitioner is holding a prenatal nutrition class for a group of
patients. Considering cultural variations, which of the following women
may be at increased risk for inadequate intake of calcium?

    a. A 30-year-old orthodox Jew
    b. A 35-year-old Caucasian
    c. A 27-year-old Native-American
    d. A 24-year-old Hispanic

B   22. During pregnancy, it is important to be physically active. The nurse
practitioner should encourage her pregnant patient who has a very
sedentary lifestyle to:

    a. begin an aerobics class for maximum benefit.
    b. begin any exercise program that she might enjoy.
    c. start walking daily and slowly build up distance.
    d. avoid beginning any new exercises until after delivery.

23. What is the recommended timing for gestational diabetes screening?

    a. 12-16 weeks gestation
    b. 24-28 weeks gestation
    c. 30-34 weeks gestation
    d. 34-38 weeks gestation

C   24. Which of the following diseases is *not* acquired transplacentally?

    a. Rubeola
    b. Toxoplasmosis
    c. Tuberculosis
    d. Varicella

20. *d* Prior to the 26th week of pregnancy, ultrasound will accurately estimate gestational age within days. Between the 18th and 30th week of pregnancy, measurement of fundal height is accurate within 2 weeks of the estimated gestational age. Naegele's rule would not be accurate due to the lack of this patient's inability to report her last menstrual period. Gestational age estimation is not a component of the biophysical profile.

21. *c* Native-Americans have a high incidence of lactose intolerance. They are often unable to meet daily dietary calcium requirements during pregnancy.

22. *c* Women who are accustomed to exercise before pregnancy can safely continue, if there are no complications of the pregnancy which would be a contraindication. Beginning an aerobic exercise program or intensifying training is not recommended. For women who have not previously exercised, a walking regimen is recommended.

23. *b* All women not previously known to have diabetes should be screened at 24 to 28 weeks gestation. The recommended test is a blood glucose level checked 1 hour after a 50-gram oral glucose challenge. If it is abnormal, a 3-hour glucose tolerance test should follow. If 2 of the 3 values are abnormal, immediate interventions should follow to treat gestational diabetes. If one value is abnormal, manage with diet and exercise and retest at 32 to 34 weeks.

24. *c* Tuberculosis is not transmitted transplacentally, but may be transmitted in the early newborn period if the mother has active untreated disease. Rubeola, toxoplasmosis, and varicella are all transmitted transplacentally and have teratogenic potential.

25. Which of the following maternal situations is considered an absolute contraindication to breastfeeding?

    a. Early HIV infection
    b. History of breast cancer
    c. Taking tuberculosis medication
    d. Hepatitis C infection

25. *a* There are few absolute contraindications to breastfeeding. HIV infection and intravenous drug abuse are 2 contraindications. Recent studies have raised the possibility that HIV-positive mothers may safely breast-feed if the babies are being treated for HIV. This study has not been recommended or adopted by any US agency.

Professional Issues

A 1. Nurse practitioner services are filed with Medicare for reimbursement:

   a. and paid by Medicare Part B.
   b. using special procedure codes specific to nurse practitioner services.
   c. only as incident to the services of the physician.
   d. by the patient, using the nurse practitioner's UPIN.

B 2. An example of an indirect role of the nurse practitioner is:

   a. response to illness and assessment of health status and health risks.
   b. educator, administrator, or researcher, influencing the delivery of direct care.
   c. diagnosing actual or potential health problems based on analysis of the data collected.
   d. evaluating the effectiveness of an intervention with the client.

C 3. Certification for nurse practitioners is offered through:

   a. the American Nurses Association.
   b. individual state boards of nursing.
   c. national certifying organizations.
   d. universities providing graduate education.

C 4. The mechanism for handling first contact into the health care system and providing a continuum of care, evaluation and management of symptoms, maintenance of health, and appropriate referrals is called:

   a. administrative service.
   b. flexible care.
   c. case management.
   d. care planning.

B 5. The requirement that a nurse practitioner practice under the direct supervision of a physician is:

   a. not a requirement in any state.
   b. dependent on state regulations.
   c. illegal, according to standards of nursing care.
   d. a standard national requirement.

1. *a*   There are no special procedure codes specific to nurse practitioner services. Nurse practitioners or their employers should file with Medicare Part B for reimbursement. The patient cannot file the claim, and the nurse practitioner cannot charge the patient for completion of any paperwork involved.

2. *b*   Nurse practitioners have traditionally delivered direct patient care. Since there are increasing numbers of nurse practitioners who are prepared at the graduate level of education, there is increasing need for indirect roles such as educator, administrator, consultant, and researcher.

3. *c*   Nurse practitioners are individually certified, making them accountable for their own practice, and helping to legitimize specialty nursing practice. National certifying agencies, such as the American Nurses Credentialing Center (ANCC) and American Academy of Nurse Practitioners (AANP), offer certification.

4. *c*   Case management is a major shift from the traditional medical model to one that coordinates and integrates services within the constraints of reimbursement.

5. *b*   The requirement for a nurse practitioner to practice under "the medical direction of a physician" is dependent on the state in which the nurse practitioner practices. Most states describe nurse practitioners' practice as "in collaboration with" a physician. Some states allow the nurse practitioner to practice independently, while other states require a collaborative or supervisory physician.

d 6. The authority for nurse practitioners to practice as primary care providers is extended through:

  a. educational programs.
  b. national nursing organizations.
  c. national certifying bodies.
  d. state legislatures.

C 7. Advance directives are:

  a. documents specifying who the patient has designated, or assigned, the legal authority to make health care decisions for him or her.
  b. documents which establish the patient's wish not to receive life-prolonging medical treatment.
  c. documents that guide medical decision making in the event an individual becomes incompetent or unable to convey his wishes.
  d. legally binding in all 50 states in the United States.

d 8. Standards of practice are:

  a. treatment protocols.
  b. a means to identify providers who can be reimbursed for services.
  c. a process by which a state board of nursing grants individuals permission to engage in practice.
  d. minimum levels of acceptable performance.

 9. What is the exception to the graduate level preparation requirement for advanced practice registered nurse (APRN) certification?

  a. Advanced practice registered nurses who have completed an approved educational program prior to implementation of graduate level education are considered to have met the requirements for advanced practice registered nursing.
  b. Advanced practice registered nurses who plan to practice in a hospital or other controlled setting are not required to have graduate education.
  c. Advanced practice registered nurses who pass both the American Nurses Credentialing Center (ANCC) and the American Academy of Nurse Practitioners (AANP) certification examinations are allowed to practice without graduate level education.
  d. There are no exceptions to the rule requiring graduate education to practice as an advanced practice registered nurse.

6. *d*   Legislative activity at the state level is necessary to permit nurse practitioners to practice as primary care providers.

7. *c*   A document which designates authority to make health care decisions is a health care proxy or durable power of attorney, which is only one example of an advance directive. Another type of advance directive is a living will, which usually states the patient's wishes not to receive life-prolonging treatment. Advance directives refer to several different kinds of documents that guide medical decision making. They are recognized in some, but not all states.

8. *d*   Standards of practice describe a minimal competency level.

9. *a*   Some advanced practice registered nurses in current practice have not been educated at the graduate level. Advanced practice registered nurses who have completed an accredited or approved educational program prior to implementation of the graduate level education requirement are considered to have met the educational requirements for advanced practice registered nurse (APRN) certification.

_C_ 10. Which of the following factors created an opportunity for the
development of the nurse practitioner movement?

a. Oversupply of registered nurses in traditional roles
b. Increased need for specially trained cardiovascular nurses
c. Shortage of primary care physicians
d. Hospital-based nurse practitioner programs

_D_ 11. A nurse practitioner has just diagnosed a patient as having acute
hepatitis B. The principle which prohibits the nurse practitioner from
notifying the patient's spouse without permission is:

a. breach of contract.
b. malpractice.
c. ethics.
d. confidentiality.

_B_ 12. A nurse practitioner plans to open a private clinic. Each patient will be
expected to pay $45 immediately following the visit. This is an example of:

a. utilitarianism.
b. fee-for-service.
c. contracted services.
d. case management.

_B_ 13. A nurse practitioner has recently been hired to work in a fast track
facility. The nurse practitioner's employer asks if she has "a problem
prescribing medication for emergency contraception." The NP replies
affirmatively. This is:

a. grounds for dismissal.
b. an ethical dilemma for the NP.
c. illegal according to the standards of nursing.
d. patient abandonment.

_B_ 14. Nurse practitioners are permitted to perform male circumcisions in some
states but not in others. This is related to:

a. standards of practice.
b. scope of practice.
c. prescriptive authority.
d. reimbursement.

10. *c*   The first nurse practitioner program was started in the late 1960's by Loretta Ford, RN, EdD and Henry Silver, MD in Colorado. The first program was designed to increase access to care for children. The shortage of primary care physicians was an opportunity for nursing to develop the nurse practitioner role.

11. *d*   Confidentiality refers to the privileged information that a health care provider obtains about the patient. It cannot be disclosed to a third party without specific consent from the patient or legal guardian. In some circumstances related to protection of public health, it may be illegal not to disclose the information (e.g. in the case of an infectious condition).

12. *b*   Fee-for-service refers to that amount of money collected (as in this case) by a nurse practitioner for providing a specific service. Fee for services rendered may be paid directly by a patient or paid directly by an insurance company.

13. *b*   In this instance, the nurse practitioner has a difference of opinion with her employer based on her religious or moral beliefs about providing emergency contraception. This situation is an example of an ethical dilemma. Failure to participate in the provision of care to the patient based on the nurse practitioner's beliefs is neither against the law nor a violation of the standards of practice.

14. *b*   Scope of practice for nurse practitioners varies from state to state and is dictated by each individual state. In order to ascertain whether a particular procedure is permitted, the nurse practitioner should consult with the board which governs the practice of nursing in the state where he/she practices. In most instances, this is the state board of nursing.

15. A nurse practitioner has been sued by a patient for malpractice. The nurse practitioner is considered to be a:

    a. defendant.
    b. plaintiff.
    c. judicial claimant.
    d. litigator.

16. Which is true about nurse practitioner practice in all 50 states?

    a. Nurse practitioners must function in collaboration with a physician.
    b. Reimbursement is consistent for nurse practitioner services from state to state.
    c. Certification is not required by all states to practice as a nurse practitioner.
    d. Practice is governed jointly by State Boards of Medicine and Nursing.

17. Subsequent to successful completion of the nurse practitioner certification exam, the candidate is considered which of the following?

    a. Licensed
    b. Certified
    c. Credentialed
    d. "Incident to"

18. An example of primary prevention is:

    a. routine immunizations for healthy children.
    b. screening for hypertension.
    c. cholesterol reduction in a patient with CAD.
    d. an annual PAP smear.

19. Prescriptive authority:

    a. requires successful completion of the NP certification exam as a prerequisite.
    b. occurs independent of physician collaboration or supervision.
    c. may be exercised by giving a verbal medication order to a pharmacist.
    d. is a legal right granted to all nurse practitioners.

15. *a* In a civil court of law, the plaintiff is the party seeking remedy for damages. The defendant is the party who allegedly caused the damages.

16. *c* Most states do require certification by AANP or ANCC for nurse practitioner practice, but certification is not mandatory in all 50 states. Some states allow practice after completion of an accredited graduate program.

17. *b* ANCC and AANP confer certification when the candidate successfully completes the certification exam. Licensure is determined by individual states.

18. *a* The goal of primary prevention is to prevent the development of a targeted problem. Screening for high blood pressure and PAP smear are examples of secondary prevention. These measures detect an already existing condition in an asymptomatic patient. Cholesterol reduction in a patient with CHF is an example of tertiary prevention. That is, it is a measure to help treat the patient with an existing disease which may help prevent complications.

19. *c* An example of exercising prescriptive authority is giving a verbal order to a pharmacist or writing an order for a prescription medication. Prescriptive authority rules and regulations vary from state to state. Prescriptive authority is granted only to those APRNs who meet the requirements of the governing body for the state in which the APRN practices.

A

20. In comparing sensitivity to specificity, sensitivity refers to a:

    a. true positive.
    b. false positive.
    c. false negative.
    d. true negative.

B

21. A nurse practitioner performs an in office procedure that is considered outside his scope of practice. The patient suffers a bad outcome. This is an example of which of the following?

    a. Negligence
    b. Malpractice
    c. Incompetence
    d. Beneficence

C

22. A professional liability insurance policy that provides coverage for injuries arising out of incidents occurring during the period the policy was in effect, even if the policy subsequently expires, or is not renewed by the policy-holder, is termed a(an):

    a. claims-made policy.
    b. individual policy.
    c. occurrence-based policy.
    d. supplemental policy.

20. *a* Sensitivity refers to the proportion of individuals who test positive for a disease or condition when the disease or condition is actually present. Specificity refers to the proportion of individuals who test negative when no disease/condition is present.

21. *b* Malpractice is professional misconduct or unreasonable lack of skill. Performing a procedure outside the scope of this nurse practitioner's practice constitutes malpractice for which he could be held liable.

22. *c* An "occurrence-based" policy provides coverage for injuries arising out of incidents occurring during the period the policy was in effect, even if the policy subsequently expires or is not renewed by the policy-holder. A "claims-made" professional liability insurance policy provides coverage only if an injury occurs, and the claim is reported to the insurance company, during the active policy period or during an uninterrupted extension of the policy ("policy tail").

Psychosocial Disorders and Mental Health

_____ 1. An elderly patient is taking an effective dose of doxepin (Sinequan®) for treatment of agitated depression with insomnia. Constipation has become a significant problem, even though the patient has been vigilant about maintaining adequate hydration and uses bulk laxatives frequently. Which of the following is the course of action most likely to be successful?

    a. Stop the doxepin (Sinequan®) and initiate fluoxetine (Prozac®).
    b. Suggest the addition of a daily hypertonic enema.
    c. Remind the patient that constipation is a common symptom of depression.
    d. Stop the doxepin and initiate trazodone (Desyrel®).

_____ 2. A patient has been taking fluoxetine (Prozac®) since being diagnosed with major depression, first episode, 2 months ago. She reports considerable improvement in her symptoms and her intention to discontinue the medication. What should be the nurse practitioner's recommendation?

    a. Advise the patient to stop the antidepressant medication.
    b. Question the patient to determine if the self-assessment is correct before advising her to discontinue the medication.
    c. Recommend that the patient continue the antidepressant medication for at least 4 more months.
    d. Discuss with the patient the need to take the antidepressant medication indefinitely.

_____ 3. The intervention known to be most effective in the treatment of severe depression, with or without psychosis, is:

    a. psychotherapy.
    b. electroconvulsive therapy (ECT).
    c. a selective serotonin reuptake inhibitors (SSRIs).
    d. a tricyclic antidepressant (TCA).

_____ 4. A patient has been diagnosed with generalized anxiety disorder (GAD). Which of the following medications may be used to treat generalized anxiety disorder (GAD)?

    a. alprazolam (Xanax®) or diazepam (Valium®)
    b. venlafaxine (Effexor®) or buspirone (BuSpar®)
    c. trazodone (Desyrel®) or sertraline (Zoloft®)
    d. venlafaxine (Effexor®) or hydroxyzine pamoate (Vistaril®)

1. *d*   Fluoxetine tends to contribute to constipation. A daily enema may cause fluid and electrolyte imbalance. Trazodone is a good alternative. It is a sedating antidepressant with properties similar to doxepin, but without anticholinergic effects. Constipation often accompanies depression and should be treated.

2. *c*   A patient being treated for a first episode of major depression should continue the full therapeutic dose of antidepressant medication for at least 6 months after remission is achieved. The first 2 months after remission of symptoms is a time of particular vulnerability to relapse.

3. *b*   Electroconvulsive therapy (ECT) is generally the most effective and most rapid treatment for severely depressed or acutely suicidal patients. ECT is the treatment of choice for psychotic depression and is also useful for the patient with poor response to medication.

4. *b*   Effexor®, BuSpar®, and Paxil® are approved by the FDA for the treatment of generalized anxiety disorder (GAD). Other medications listed may be used off-label for anxiety symptoms.

C   5.   The primary goals of treatment for patients with alcohol abuse disorder are:

a.   reduction in withdrawal symptoms and reduction in desire for alcohol.
b.   psychotherapeutic and pharmacological interventions to decrease desire for and effects of alcohol.
c.   abstinence or reduction in use, relapse prevention, and rehabilitation.
d.   marital satisfaction, improvement in family functioning, and reduction in psychiatric impairment.

a   6.   The AUDIT questionnaire is useful to assess:

a.   alcohol use disorders.
b.   types of headaches.
c.   dementia as differentiated from depression.
d.   cognitive dysfunction.

C   7.   What is the most commonly abused substance?

a.   Heroin
b.   Cocaine
c.   Alcohol
d.   Marijuana

d   8.   All of the following are medical emergencies which may be attributed to acute cocaine intoxication *except*:

a.   hyperthermia leading to extreme rhabdomyolysis.
b.   hypertension with or without vasculitis causing cerebrovascular accident (CVA).
c.   depression of cardiac conduction and contractility resulting in arrhythmias and myocardial infarction (MI).
d.   decreased heart rate and vasodilation leading to hypersomnia.

a   9.   A patient has smoked for 10 years. What statement should guide the nurse practitioner's intervention with this patient?

a.   Encourage the use of nicotine replacement except in the presence of medical contraindications.
b.   Offer nicotine replacement only to those smokers who are unsuccessful after 3 attempts to stop smoking.
c.   Discourage the use of nicotine replacement.
d.   Offer nicotine replacement only to select populations of heavy smokers with a long history of smoking.

5. *c*   It is controversial whether abstinence or reduction in alcohol use should be the goal of treatment. Relapse is expected, but gradual reduction in occurrence is a goal. A comprehensive treatment plan should address social, vocational, educational, and psychiatric aspects of this disorder.

6. *a*   AUDIT is an acronym for Alcohol Use Disorders Identification Test designed by the World Health Organization. It is a 10-item questionnaire that screens for harmful alcohol use in primary care settings.

7. *c*   Alcohol accounts for 50% of known cases of substance abuse. Cocaine, heroin, benzodiazepines, hallucinogens, and inhalants constitute the majority of the other 50% of known cases of substance abuse. Polypharmacy use is very common.

8. *d*   The toxidrome of cocaine use is created by its blocking effect on the re-uptake of dopamine, norepinephrine, and serotonin. Phase 1 of intoxication causes euphoria and hyper-alertness. The second phase of the toxidrome, after large doses, poses high risk for a medical emergency such as cardiac arrhythmias, myocardial infarction, cerebral vascular accident (CVA), seizure, and hyperthermia.

9. *a*   Except in special circumstances such as pregnancy and recent myocardial infarction, every smoker should be offered nicotine replacement therapy. Six month abstinence rates are 2 to 3 times higher for patients who use nicotine replacement as compared to placebo.

_b_ 10. Once a competent adult patient is identified as a victim of domestic abuse, the best plan is to:

a. recommend joint counseling sessions for the pair.
b. suggest resources that will help the victim to develop survival skills.
c. refer the abuser for individual psychological counseling.
d. insist that the victim leave the abusive environment immediately.

_a_ 11. Which of the following behaviors should the nurse practitioner recognize as most typical of the adolescent female who has been sexually abused?

a. Runaway attempts, substance abuse, hysterical seizures, and indiscriminate sexual activity
b. Anorexia or bulimia, difficult mother-daughter relationship, and violence toward siblings
c. Academic over-achievement, social isolation, and lack of religious affiliation
d. Frequent clinic visits for insignificant medical problems and apathetic or bored affect

_d_ 12. What is the most common method of suicide?

a. Hanging
b. Drug overdose
c. Poisoning
d. A firearm

_a_ 13. Which of the following adolescents has the strongest potential for substance abuse?

a. The adolescent with a family history of alcohol or drug dependence.
b. The adolescent who feels alienated from peers.
c. The adolescent whose parents are inconsistent with parental discipline.
d. The adolescent with a history of early sexual activity.

_b_ 14. The CAGE, MAST, and AUDIT questionnaires to detect problem drinking should be used:

a. to detect early problems and hazardous drinking.
b. as supplements to the standard patient history.
c. as diagnostic tools for the early detection of problem drinking.
d. to determine the degree and pattern of alcohol use.

10. *b*   If violence exists between 2 competent adults, the best plan of action is to help the victim to develop survival skills. Recommending joint counseling sessions runs the risk that the abuser will punish the victim for speaking out. Leaving may also be risky. Emergency shelter may be recommended in a life-threatening situation. Otherwise, suggest development of a safety plan.

11. *a*   In the adolescent population, the most common signs and symptoms of sexual abuse are drug and alcohol abuse, indiscriminate sexual activity, early pregnancy, hysterical seizures, and runaway attempts.

12. *d*   Firearms are used in 60% of all suicides and account for almost all of the increase in suicides during the last decade. The risk of suicide is about 5 times greater for persons living in a household where a firearm is kept. Men commit suicide four times more often than women.

13. *a*   Although all of these factors influence substance abuse in adolescents, the strongest predisposing risk factor is family history of alcohol or drug dependence.

14. *b*   Standard screening instruments such as CAGE, AUDIT, and MAST should be used only as supplements to the standard patient history as they may not detect early signs of problem development.

C 15. Which of the following is the best response to a woman who has just admitted she is a victim of spousal abuse?

  a. "What was it you did to make him angry?"
  b. "You must seek refuge immediately."
  c. "I am concerned about your safety."
  d. "I am going to call a shelter for you."

d 16. The daughter of a 75-year-old patient reports that her mother roams the house at night saying she cannot fall asleep. She has fallen twice. Of the following choices, which would be the most appropriate to treat her insomnia?

  a. doxepin (Sinequan®)
  b. trazodone (Desyrel®)
  c. diazepam (Valium®)
  d. zolpidem (Ambien®)

a 17. Which of the following drugs is *not* appropriate for the patient with comorbid anxiety and depression?

  a. buspirone (BuSpar®)
  b. A selective serotonin reuptake inhibitor (SSRI)
  c. A tricyclic antidepressant (TCA)
  d. bupropion (Wellbutrin®)

b 18. Which commonly used herbal remedy is *not* associated with anxiety and/or depressive symptom relief?

  a. Valerian root
  b. Ginkgo biloba
  c. Kava kava
  d. St. John's wort

d 19. The family of a 78-year-old man has moved him into an assisted living center because he can no longer be left at home alone. On examination, he is pleasant but mildly confused and having incontinent episodes. Which of his medications is *least* likely contributing to his behavior?

  a. imipramine (Tofranil®)
  b. hydrochlorothiazide
  c. cimetidine (Tagamet®)
  d. ramipril (Altace®)

15. *c* The nurse practitioner cannot make decisions for a competent adult. It is inappropriate to insinuate that the victim was somehow responsible for the violence. The patient should be treated as a responsible adult and reminded that the nurse practitioner is a patient advocate.

16. *d* Since this patient is having difficulty falling asleep, she needs a drug which will produce drowsiness at bedtime. Because of her age and risk for falling, she requires a drug with a short half-life so she will not have continued sedative effects the next day. Although the other choices would provide sedation, they have longer half-lives and would likely cause drowsiness the next morning/day. Additionally, use of the other drugs listed for primary treatment of insomnia would be off-label. Zolpidem should be used cautiously in older adults.

17. *a* Buspirone (BuSpar®) is only indicated for the treatment of anxiety. In general, anxiolytics have demonstrated little efficacy in the treatment of depression. However, antidepressants have a long history of use in the treatment of anxiety disorders. Bupropion (Wellbutrin®, Zyban®) has demonstrated efficacy in efforts at smoking cessation.

18. *b* Ginkgo biloba is a common herbal remedy associated with enhancement of vascular and cerebral perfusion and memory. The nurse practitioner should be aware when the patient is taking any herbal supplement to avoid risk of drug interactions.

19. *d* Tricyclic antidepressants, such as imipramine, have anticholinergic side effects which are especially problematic in the elderly because they contribute to urinary retention. Hydrochlorothiazide (HCTZ) is a diuretic and may contribute to his incontinence. Cimetidine is well known to produce adverse reactions, such as confusion, in elders. Ramipril, an ACE inhibitor, is unlikely to contribute to this patient's incontinence or confusion. Toileting may be complicated by the anticholinergic medication and/or the diuretic causing diuresis, urge incontinence, or inability to void at will.

Respiratory Disorders

_____ 1. Which of the following is the most important diagnosis to rule out in the adult patient with acute bronchitis?

    a. Pneumonia
    b. Asthma
    c. Sinusitis
    d. Pertussis

_____ 2. Antibiotic administration has been demonstrated to be of little benefit in the treatment of which of the following disease processes?

    a. Chronic sinusitis
    b. Acute bronchitis
    c. Bacterial pneumonia
    d. Acute exacerbation of chronic bronchitis

_____ 3. Which antibiotic would be the most effective in treating community acquired pneumonia (CAP) in a young adult without any comorbid conditions?

    a. erythromycin
    b. clarithromycin (Biaxin®)
    c. doxycycline (Vibramycin®)
    d. penicillin

_____ 4. A 20-year-old is diagnosed with mild persistent asthma. What drug combination would be most effective in keeping him symptom-free?

    a. A long-acting bronchodilator
    b. An inhaled corticosteroid and cromolyn (Intal®)
    c. Theophylline and a short-acting bronchodilator
    d. A bronchodilator PRN and inhaled corticosteroid

_____ 5. The purpose of a spacer for inhaled asthma medications is to:

    a. allow a longer period of time for inhalation.
    b. eliminate cough associated with drug inhalation.
    c. prevent oral fungal infection when using an inhaled steroid.
    d. reduce the dose of medication delivered per spray

1. *a* The hallmark of acute bronchitis is a productive cough. There is no gold standard for diagnosing acute bronchitis. In pneumonia, 80% of patients present with fever, 80% have crackles on auscultation, and the majority have a respiratory rate greater than 20 breaths per minute. Chest x-ray is considered the gold standard for a pneumonia diagnosis.

2. *b* Although frequently prescribed for acute bronchitis, studies have failed to demonstrate that antibiotic administration shortens duration of the illness. This is probably due to the fact that viral infections cause about 90% of acute bronchitis.

3. *b* Clarithromycin is an antibiotic recommended by the American Thoracic Society for treatment of community acquired pneumonia (CAP) in young adults without comorbid conditions. Clarithromycin provides antimicrobial activity against *Streptococcus pneumoniae*, the most common causative organism in CAP, and provides coverage for other less common pathogens, including *Mycoplasma pneumoniae*, *Chlamydia pneumoniae*, and *Legionella pneumophila*. Erythromycin is less well tolerated.

4. *d* A patient with mild persistent asthma has symptoms > 2 times per week but < 1 time per day. Daily medications should include an inhaled corticosteroid or cromolyn and an inhaled bronchodilator as needed for symptoms.

5. *a* The same amount of medication is delivered per spray, but the spacer allows a longer time interval between breaths for the patient to inhale it. A deep breath often triggers asthma patients to cough. Smaller breaths mediate the cough reflex.

6. A 65-year-old presents with past medical history of coronary artery disease, temperature 101°F (38.3°C) and tachypnea at 24 breaths per minute. Chest x-ray confirms left lower lobe pneumonia. What antimicrobial agent(s) should the nurse practitioner prescribe?

    a. amoxicillin-clavulanic acid (Augmentin®)
    b. **levofloxacin (Levaquin®)**
    c. erythromycin
    d. erythromycin and doxycycline

7. Salmeterol (Serevent®) is prescribed for a patient with asthma. What is the most important teaching point about this medication?

    a. It is not effective during an acute asthma attack.
    b. It may take 2 to 3 days to begin working.
    c. This drug works within 10 minutes.
    d. This drug may be used by patients 6 years and older.

8. What condition is associated with mucus production greater than 3 months per year for at least 2 consecutive years?

    a. Asthma
    b. Emphysema
    c. Chronic obstructive lung disease
    d. Chronic bronchitis

9. The most common correlate(s) with chronic bronchitis and emphysema is(are):

    a. familial and genetic factors.
    b. cigarette smoking.
    c. air pollution.
    d. occupational environment.

10. Which of the following patient characteristics are associated with chronic bronchitis?

    a. Overweight, cyanosis, and normal or slightly increased respiratory rate
    b. Underweight, pink skin, and increased respiratory rate
    c. Overweight, pink skin, and normal or slightly increased respiratory rate
    d. Normal weight, cyanosis, and greatly increased respiratory rate

6. *b*   The American Thoracic Society's recommendation for treatment of community acquired pneumonia (CAP) in the adult patient with cardiopulmonary disease (or other "modifying factors") is a fluoroquinolone with anti-pneumococcal activity or a beta-lactam, plus a macrolide or doxycycline. The most common etiologic agents in CAP are *Streptococcus pneumoniae*, *Mycoplasma* (or other atypicals like *Legionella* or *Chlamydia trachomatis*), and drug resistant *S. pneumoniae*. A third or fourth generation quinolone will provide coverage against all these organisms.

7. *a*   This drug is a long-acting (12 hour) β-agonist. It does not provide the immediate relief from bronchospasm that a short-acting inhaled bronchodilator does. For this reason, it should never be used during an acute attack. This drug is best for the patient who requires regular daily treatment with a short-acting inhaled bronchodilator for asthma symptom control.

8. *d*   Chronic bronchitis is the condition associated with mucus production greater than 3 months duration per year for at least 2 consecutive years. There are other classifications such as asthmatic bronchitis. Chronic obstructive lung disease is a disease classification of chronic obstruction due to either chronic bronchitis or emphysema or a combination of both.

9. *b*   Although all of these factors contribute to the development of chronic bronchitis and emphysema, cigarette smoking causes impaired ciliary function, inhibited alveolar macrophage function, and hyperplasia and hypertrophy of the mucus-secreting cells in the lungs.

10. *a*   Patients with classic chronic bronchitis ("blue bloaters") resemble the description in choice *a*. Typical emphysema patients ("pink puffers") more closely resemble the description in choice *b*.

D

11. Which of the following is *not* a goal of treatment for the patient with cystic fibrosis?

   a. Prevent intestinal obstruction
   b. Provide adequate nutrition
   c. Promote clearance of secretions
   d. Replace water-soluble vitamins

C

12. Which type of lung cancer has the poorest prognosis?

   a. Adenocarcinoma
   b. Epidermoid carcinoma
   c. Small cell carcinoma
   d. Large cell carcinoma

D

13. In order to decrease deaths from lung cancer:

   a. all smokers should be screened annually.
   b. all patients should be screened annually.
   c. only high risk patients should be screened routinely.
   d. patients should be counseled to quit smoking.

D

14. What prophylactic medication is commonly recommended for the patient under 35 years-of-age with a positive PPD?

   a. ethambutol
   b. streptomycin
   c. pyrazinamide
   d. isoniazid (INH)

D

15. The most appropriate treatment for a child with mild croup is:

   a. a bronchodilator.
   b. an antibiotic.
   c. a decongestant.
   d. a cool mist vaporizer.

A

16. Which statement below is *correct* about pertussis?

   a. It is also called whooping cough.
   b. It begins with symptoms like strep throat.
   c. It lasts about 3 weeks.
   d. It occurs most commonly in toddlers and young children.

11. *d*   Most patients with cystic fibrosis have insufficient release of pancreatic enzymes. This results in malabsorption of the fat-soluble vitamins: A, D, E, and K. Intestinal obstruction, termed meconium ileus, resembles appendicitis in these patients.

12. *c*   Small cell carcinoma, also called oat cell carcinoma, has a 5-year survival rate of less than 1%. Epidermoid carcinoma has the best 5-year survival rate of 37%. Adenocarcinoma is the type of lung tumor most frequently found in nonsmokers.

13. *d*   The risk of lung cancer for a man who smokes 2 packs of cigarettes per day for 20 years is 60 to 70 times greater than the risk for nonsmokers. The proportion is similar in women. Multidimensional studies have failed to demonstrate that screening decreases deaths from lung cancer. The most effective means of decreasing deaths from lung cancer is cigarette smoking prevention.

14. *d*   The CDC (Centers for Disease Control and Prevention) recommends administration of isoniazid (INH) to persons under 35 years-of-age with a positive PPD. The goal of this treatment is to prevent progression from latent infection to active infection. The other medications are used to treat active tuberculosis, but not for prophylaxis.

15. *d*   Mild croup usually does not need treatment. However, a cool mist vaporizer may be of benefit because it moistens the upper airway. Croup is characterized by a barking cough and inspiratory stridor. A child with inspiratory stridor at rest probably needs hospitalization. Emergency treatment of croup consists of dexamethasone and aerosolized epinephrine bronchodilator.

16. *a*   Pertussis typically presents in 3 phases. The first phase begins with symptoms like the common cold and lasts about 1 week. The second phase presents with paroxysmal coughing spells and can last several weeks (the Chinese word for pertussis means 100 days of cough). In the third phase, the cough gradually subsides. It is more likely in unimmunized populations like infants < 3 months of age.

C

_____ 17. What is the most common causative agent of bronchiolitis in infants and children?

    a. *Staphylococcus aureus*
    b. *Haemophilus influenza (H. flu)*
    c. Respiratory syncytial virus (RSV)
    d. Adenovirus

B

_____ 18. A 2-year-old presents with sudden onset of respiratory distress with unilateral wheezing. What is the likely cause?

    a. Pneumonia
    b. Foreign body aspiration
    c. Asthma exacerbation
    d. Epiglottitis

C

_____ 19. Which statement about bronchopulmonary dysplasia (BPD) is *false*?

    a. This disease is a sequela of mechanical ventilation in the neonatal period.
    b. It is characterized by tachypnea, wheezing, and increased respiratory effort.
    c. Clinical symptoms of BPD usually resolve after the first 6 months of life.
    d. Exacerbation of BPD is treated with a bronchodilator and corticosteroid.

C

_____ 20. Which of the following is a risk factor for sudden infant death syndrome (SIDS)?

    a. Maternal age > 19 years
    b. Summer months
    c. Low birth weight
    d. Female gender

17. *c*   Respiratory syncytial virus (RSV) is responsible for more than 50% of bronchiolitis in infants and children. Other common causative agents include parainfluenza, influenza, and adenovirus. This can be devastating to infants because their airways are smaller and they are less able to accommodate swelling and edema than older children and adults.

18. *b*   Unilateral wheezing in a child should always be considered abnormal. Taking into account the child's age, strong consideration should be given to the presence of a foreign body. Other causes of unilateral wheezing are infection, asthma, and lung mass. Asthma is overwhelmingly bilateral, but it can be unilateral depending on the cause.

19. *c*   Clinical symptoms of bronchopulmonary dysplasia (BPD) usually resolve after 3 years-of-age. BPD is diagnosed on the basis of history and radiological findings. These children are particularly susceptible to viral infections.

20. *c*   Males are at highest risk for sudden infant death syndrome (SIDS). There is no known cause, but several interventions may decrease risk: positioning the infant in a lateral or supine position for sleep, breastfeeding, and parental smoking cessation. Risk factors are maternal age < 19 years, male gender, and history of SIDS in a sibling. More infants die from SIDS in winter months.

C

21. Of the following choices, the *least* likely cause of cough is:

    a. asthma.
    b. gastroesophageal reflux (GER).
    c. acute pharyngitis.
    d. allergic rhinitis.

B

22. Which of the following medication classes should be avoided in patients with acute or chronic bronchitis because it will contribute to ventilation-perfusion mismatch in the patient?

    a. Xanthines
    b. Antihistamines
    c. Steroids
    d. Anticholinergics

A

23. Which of the following statements about tuberculosis (TB) testing is accurate?

    a. A positive skin test (PPD) reaction indicates exposure to tuberculosis, but follow up confirmatory cultures are required for a diagnosis.
    b. The tuberculosis bacillus is slow growing and a positive sputum culture requires at least 3 weeks.
    c. Frequent serial x-rays are required to monitor progression of tuberculosis lesions in the lungs.
    d. If the smear is positive, the culture will be positive.

D

24. Expected spirometry readings when the patient has chronic emphysema include:

    a. decreased residual volume (RV).
    b. increased vital capacity (VC).
    c. increased forced expiratory volume (FEV-1).
    d. increased total lung capacity (TLC).

B

25. A patient complains of "an aggravating cough for the past 6 weeks." There is no physiological cause for the cough. Which medication is most likely causing the cough?

    a. methyldopa (Aldomet®)
    b. enalapril (Vasotec®)
    c. amlodipine (Norvasc®)
    d. hydrochlorothiazide (HCTZ)

21. *c*   Acute pharyngitis is not associated with throat clearing or cough. If the patient with acute pharyngitis has a cough, it is due to a comorbid condition.

22. *b*   Antihistamines cause thickening and increased tenaciousness of secretions, contributing to increased airway obstruction and subsequent ventilation-perfusion mismatch. Xanthines and anticholinergics increase airway diameter. Steroids decrease edema and inflammation, thereby increasing airway diameter. Increased fluid intake and mucolytics contribute to thinning and expectoration of secretions, thus increasing airway diameter. Increasing the airway diameter facilitates ventilation and perfusion.

23. *a*   A positive PPD only indicates exposure to tuberculosis (TB) and does not necessarily indicate active disease process. A smear may be positive and cultures negative if the patient has been taking anti-tuberculosis medications. Even very small TB lesions can be visualized on chest x-ray in contrast to air in the lungs; therefore, frequent chest x-rays are not necessary. The causative organism requires 4 to 6 weeks to grow in culture medium.

24. *d*   RV is increased, VC is decreased, FEV-1 is decreased, and TLC is increased with emphysema. RV, VC, and FEV-1 spirometry readings are the same whether the COPD is due to chronic emphysema or chronic bronchitis; however, TLC is normal or only slightly increased with chronic bronchitis.

25. *b*   The ACE inhibitors are long known to produce nonproductive persistent cough in some patients. Reports demonstrate that cough related to ACE inhibitor use varies from < 1% to 25%. ACE inhibitors interfere with metabolism of bradykinin and the cough is related to rising bradykinin levels. Once the ACE inhibitor is discontinued, the cough abates.

Sexually Transmitted Diseases and Urological Disorders

C

1. The sexual partner of a symptomatic male patient with gonorrhea should be empirically treated:

   a. if symptoms are present.
   b. with ceftriaxone (Rocephin®) 1 gram intramuscularly.
   c. with ceftriaxone and doxycycline (Vibramycin®).
   d. only if exposed within 2 weeks of diagnosis.

B

2. The preferred therapeutic regimen for an 18-year-old pregnant patient diagnosed with *Chlamydia trachomatis* infection is:

   a. doxycycline 100 mg orally twice a day for 7 days.
   b. erythromycin base 500 mg orally 4 times a day for 7 days.
   c. a single IM dose of ceftriaxone (Rocephin®) 500 mg.
   d. a single dose of azithromycin (Zithromax®) 250 mg.

C

3. With a diagnosis of syphilis, which of the following tests remains positive for the patient's lifetime?

   a. VDRL
   b. RPR
   c. FTA-ABS or MHA-TP
   d. Darkfield examination

D

4. A 25-year-old patient presents with complaints of pain and burning in the vulvar area. Upon examination, the nurse practitioner notes 4 vesicles with an erythematous base arranged in a group on the patient's labia majora. The most likely diagnosis is:

   a. human papilloma virus (HPV).
   b. syphilis.
   c. chancroid lesions.
   d. *herpes simplex II.*

A

5. The diagnosis of human papilloma virus (HPV) infection in males is usually made by:

   a. clinical appearance.
   b. viral culture.
   c. Tzanck smear.
   d. KOH prep.

1. *c* The sexual partner(s) of a symptomatic patient who has gonorrhea should be evaluated and treated for gonorrhea and chlamydia (because both commonly present together) if sexual contact was within 30 days of onset of the patient's symptoms. The treatment of choice is a single dose of ceftriaxone 1 g IM (treatment for *N. gonorrhoeae*) and doxycycline 100 mg PO twice a day for 7 days (treatment for *C. trachomatis*). A single dose of one gram azithromycin may be substituted for doxycycline.

2. *b* The treatment of choice for *Chlamydia trachomatis* infection is doxycycline or azithromycin. Doxycycline should be avoided in pregnancy. An alternate regimen in pregnancy is 1gm azithromycin. According to the 2002 CDC STD Guidelines, the recommended treatment for Chlamydia during pregnancy is erythromycin base 500mg orally 4 times daily for 7 days. Clinical data and experience suggest that azithromycin is safe and effective during pregnancy.

3. *c* A patient who has a reactive treponemal test (i.e., FTA-ABS or MHA-TP) usually will have a reactive test for a lifetime, regardless of treatment or disease activity. VDRL and RPR are non-treponemal tests and their titers correlate with current disease activity. Darkfield examination of lesion exudate or tissue is the definitive method for diagnosing early syphilis and is only positive in the presence of active disease.

4. *d* *Herpes simplex II* (genital herpes) is characterized by painful vesicular lesions usually grouped together on an erythematous base. Human papilloma lesions are painless, flesh-colored papules. Syphilis lesions are painless ulcerations. Chancroid lesions are painful ulcerations.

5. *a* Appearance of human papilloma virus is usually sufficient for diagnosis in males or females. The presence of cervical HPV is diagnosed via Pap smear. Viral culture is not useful for diagnosing HPV. Tzanck smear is used to diagnose herpes infection. Application of potassium hydroxide (KOH) to a lesion is used to diagnose a fungal infection.

6. Which of the following diagnoses has a high comorbid association with HIV infection?

   a. Chancroid
   b. Secondary syphilis
   c. Chlamydia
   d. Lymphogranuloma venereum

7. An appropriate initial treatment for external genital warts caused by human papilloma virus (HPV) in a non-pregnant patient is:

   a. topical trichloroacetic acid (TCA).
   b. 5-fluorouracil cream.
   c. topical acyclovir (Zovirax®).
   d. intralesional interferon.

8. A 15-year-old patient has a complaint of vaginal discharge. She is sexually active with multiple partners. Which of the following would be most likely to lead the nurse practitioner to suspect pelvic inflammatory disease (PID)?

   a. Cervical motion tenderness (CMT)
   b. A report of dyspareunia
   c. A complaint of low back pain
   d. A yellow vaginal discharge

9. Which of the following must be present for the diagnosis of bacterial vaginosis?

   a. Presence of clue cells
   b. Vaginal pH < 4.0
   c. Presence of pseudohyphae on HPF
   d. Negative amine test

10. Which of the following is the most appropriate treatment for trichomoniasis in a non-pregnant woman?

    a. metronidazole (Flagyl®)
    b. doxycycline (Vibramycin®)
    c. clindamycin (Cleocin®)
    d. cephtriaxone (Rocephin®)

6. *a* Chancroid is a cofactor for HIV transmission. A high rate of HIV infection among persons with chancroid has been reported in the United States and other countries.

7. *a* Appropriate initial treatment of external genital warts caused by HPV includes cryotherapy with liquid nitrogen or cryoprobe, self-treatment with podofilox 0.5% solution, podophyllin 10%-25%, trichloroacetic acid (TCA), or electrodesiccation or electrocautery. 5-fluorouracil cream has not been evaluated in controlled studies and is not recommended for treatment of genital warts. Intralesional interferon is used for treatment of persistent and recurrent genital warts, but is not recommended by the CDC. Topical acyclovir is not indicated for treatment of genital warts.

8. *a* The CDC minimum criteria for clinical diagnosis of acute pelvic inflammatory disease (PID): lower abdominal tenderness, cervical motion tenderness, adnexal tenderness. The clinical diagnosis of PID is imprecise. No single clinical or historical finding is indicative of PID. Symptomatology varies among women.

9. *a* For a diagnosis of bacterial vaginosis, 3 of the following 4 criteria must be present: thin gray-white vaginal discharge, clue cells on microscopic examination, vaginal pH > 4.5, and positive 10% potassium hydroxide (KOH) "whiff" test.

10. *a* Metronidazole is the most commonly used medication in the United States for treatment of trichomoniasis. According to the 2002 CDC STD guidelines, the recommended treatment for trichomoniasis in pregnancy is a single dose of oral metronidazole 2 g.

11. A 3-year-old female with a palpable right upper quadrant abdominal mass, anemia, and fever is being evaluated for Wilms' tumor. Which of the following diagnostic tests would be most useful?

    a. Intravenous pyelogram (IVP)
    b. Flat and erect x-rays of the abdomen
    c. Abdominal ultrasound
    d. Voiding cystourethrogram (VCU)

12. A 32-year-old male patient complains of urinary frequency and burning on urination for 3 days. Urinalysis reveals bacteriuria. He denies any past history of urinary tract infection. The initial treatment should be:

    a. trimethoprim-sulfamethoxazole (Bactrim®) for 3 days.
    b. ciprofloxacin (Cipro®) for 7-10 days.
    c. trimethoprim-sulfamethoxazole for 14 days.
    d. ciprofloxacin for 3 days.

13. A 32-year-old female patient presents with fever, chills, right flank pain, right costovertebral angle tenderness, and hematuria. Her urinalysis is positive for leukocytes and red blood cells. The nurse practitioner diagnoses pyelonephritis. The most appropriate management is:

    a. to consult with a physician.
    b. a 14-day course of ciprofloxacin (Cipro®).
    c. to obtain blood cultures from separate sites.
    d. obtain urine cultures, a CBC, and initiate antibiotic therapy.

14. The mother of a new born infant with hypospadias requests circumcision for her infant. The nurse practitioner's best response to this mother should be to:

    a. wait until the infant is 6 weeks old.
    b. explain why an infant with hypospadias should not be circumcised.
    c. explain the benefits and risks of infant circumcision.
    d. have the mother sign a consent form for the procedure.

11. *c*   Abdominal ultrasound gives the best information about extensiveness of the tumor. Flat and erect x-rays of the abdomen may show linear calcifications, but are not as helpful as ultrasound. Intravenous pyelogram is rarely useful and voiding cystourethrogram is not indicated in the evaluation of Wilms' tumor.

12. *b*   This patient has a urinary tract infection. Ciprofloxacin for 7 to 10 days is an acceptable treatment for first time urinary tract infection in men. Trimethoprim-sulfamethoxazole (TMPS) may be used initially for 7 to10 days if the rate of TMPS resistance for the locale is <30%. Three days is usually adequate for women, but men require a longer course of treatment.

13. *d*   Choice *d* represents the most appropriate management. However, physician consultation should be considered in patients with pyelonephritis. Ciprofloxacin is a drug of choice for pyelonephritis and a 14-day course is probably needed. It is not usually necessary to order blood cultures unless sepsis is suspected.

14. *b*   Circumcision is contraindicated for newborns with hypospadias. The foreskin is needed for later repair of the defect. This child should be referred to urology for management.

_C_   15. A 10-year-old presents with hematuria, periorbital edema, and elevated blood pressure. He has a history of streptococcal pharyngitis 2 weeks earlier. What is the most likely diagnosis?

   a. Pyelonephritis
   b. Hydronephrosis
   c. Acute glomerulonephritis
   d. Kawasaki syndrome

_d_   16. Desmopressin acetate (DDAVP®) nasal spray has been found to be useful in the management of enuresis in children. In which of the following situations is the drug especially beneficial?

   a. Daytime incontinence
   b. Hypertensive children with enuresis
   c. Secondary enuresis
   d. Sleep overs

_C_   17.   Which of the following is an appropriate medication for a 64-year-old woman with stress incontinence (sphincter incompetence)?

   a. prazosin (Minipress®)
   b. bethanechol (Urecholine®)
   c. pseudoephedrine (Sudafed®)
   d. tolterodine tartrate (Detrol® LA)

_b_   18. A 78-year-old male patient has early chronic renal failure (CRF). The nurse practitioner is counseling him about his dietary requirements. Which of the following elements is most important to emphasize regarding his diet?

   a. Sodium restriction is essential.
   b. Protein intake must be limited.
   c. Fat calories must be restricted.
   d. Liberal intake of fluids is beneficial.

_b_   19. Which of the following patients requires radiological evaluation of a first incidence of urinary tract infection?

   a. A 9-year-old female
   b. An 11-year-old male
   c. A 13-year-old female
   d. An 18-year-old female

15. *c*   Hematuria, periorbital edema, and hypertension are all signs of acute glomerulonephritis. Acute glomerulonephritis most commonly follows a streptococcal infection, either pharyngeal or skin. It must be managed by treating the strep infection, correction of hypertension, and correction of fluid and electrolyte imbalances.

16. *d*   Desmopressin mimics the actions of vasopressin or antidiuretic hormone by reducing the amount of urine produced at nighttime. Desmopressin acetate is particularly useful for sleep overs, avoiding embarrassment until spontaneous resolution occurs. DDAVP is contraindicated in hypertension.

17. *c*   Pseudoephedrine is useful for patients with stress incontinence due to sphincter incompetence. Prazosin and bethanechol are indicated for patients with overflow incontinence. Detrol® LA is indicated for patients with detrusor instability (urge incontinence).

18. *b*   Protein intake is usually limited in patients with chronic renal failure who do not yet require dialysis treatment. Generally 0.5 grams/kg/day is prescribed with adjustments according to creatinine clearance. Sodium intake should not be either excessive or severely restricted. Fat and carbohydrate calories are needed to make up for the lack of calories from protein, and should not be restricted. Fluid intake should only be a quantity sufficient to maintain adequate urine volume.

19. *b*   The criteria for radiological work-up of children with UTI is: infants or any child < 3 years old; any child < 8 years old with acute symptoms; any child with pyelonephritis; male children with a first infection; females with a second infection; any child with suspicious factors; adolescents with pyelonephritis or after a second urinary tract infection.

_d_ 20. A 62-year-old with type 2 diabetes mellitus complains of increased nocturia, fatigue, and weakness. His fasting blood glucose is 110 mg/dL, he is slightly anemic, and his serum creatinine level is slightly elevated. All other laboratory tests and physical examination findings are within normal limits. What is the most likely diagnosis?

    a. Acute renal failure (ARF)
    b. Congestive heart failure (CHF)
    c. Insulin insensitivity
    d. Renal insufficiency

_c_ 21. When educating parents of children with enuresis, it is imperative that the nurse practitioner explain that:

    a. most children with enuresis have spontaneous resolution by 5 years-of-age.
    b. bedwetting alarms are of no value and may complicate the problem.
    c. nighttime enuresis is completely involuntary and the child cannot learn control.
    d. enuresis often indicates a disease process and the child should have a urological work-up.

_a_ 22. The nurse practitioner suspects early renal failure in a patient who presents with:

    a. polyuria, polydipsia, and low urine specific gravity.
    b. anuria and weight gain.
    c. oliguria and high urine specific gravity.
    d. hematuria and proteinuria.

_d_ 23. A 55-year-old male patient complains of blood in his urine for the past 2 weeks. He denies dysuria. Urinalysis is positive for red blood cells and negative for leukocytes and nitrites. The initial evaluation of this patient should include:

    a. magnetic resonance imaging (MRI).
    b. cystoscopy.
    c. bladder biopsy.
    d. renal ultrasonography and IVP.

20. *d*   Nocturia is a sign of moderate renal insufficiency due to impaired ability to concentrate urine. Prevention of renal failure involves good control of blood pressure, blood glucose, and lipid levels. A number of studies have demonstrated a relationship between hyperlipidemia and progressive renal dysfunction.

21. *c*   Emphasis should be placed on the involuntary nature of enuresis. When educating parents, it is important to stress that the child is not to blame for lack of control. The rate of spontaneous resolution is 15% per year after age 5 years. Bedwetting alarms are among the most effective management therapy for enuresis. Enuresis rarely indicates a disease process and the only initial evaluation needed is urinalysis and urine culture if indicated.

22. *a*   Renal tubular concentration of urine is decreased in early renal failure causing polyuria, low urine specific gravity, and thirst. This phase is transient and may not be noticed by the patient.

23. *d*   Intravenous pyelogram (IVP) and renal ultrasonography are usually recommended for evaluation of hematuria in the absence of urinary tract infection. Magnetic resonance imaging (MRI), cystoscopy, and bladder biopsy are not usually included in the initial work-up.

24. The nurse practitioner is conducting a routine health assessment of a 28-year-old patient. He states he is very "health conscious" and that he runs 6 miles daily. He denies current health problems and his past medical history is unremarkable. Routine urinalysis reveals proteinuria. What is the most likely cause of the proteinuria?

   a. Fever
   b. Exercise
   c. Urinary tract infection UTI)
   d. Trauma

25. Which of the following physical findings in a newborn would warrant an evaluation for genitourinary anomalies?

   a. Congenital cataracts
   b. Low set ears
   c. Hydrocele
   d. Polydactyly

26. The mother of a 2-year-old uncircumcised male patient is concerned that she cannot retract the foreskin over the glans penis. The appropriate response by the nurse practitioner is to:

   a. refer the patient to a urologist.
   b. forcibly retract the foreskin.
   c. treat the child for possible infection.
   d. reassure the mother that this is normal.

27. A 49-year-old male patient presents with sudden onset of severe left flank pain and hematuria. The nurse practitioner immediately suspects renal calculi. To verify this suspicion, the initial work-up should include:

   a. renal ultrasound.
   b. serum calcium and phosphorus.
   c. helical CT.
   d. an intravenous pyelogram (IVP).

24. *b*   Asymptomatic proteinuria is often seen in patients who participate in strenuous exercise programs or who do heavy physical labor. This patient is otherwise asymptomatic with a negative history; therefore, the other causes can probably be ruled out. Patients who do strenuous physical labor and exercise may also exhibit microscopic hematuria, but other causes must be ruled out before this can be attributed to physical exertion.

25. *b*   True low set ears are often associated with genitourinary anomalies and the patient should be evaluated. During fetal development, the pinna develops at the same time as the kidneys. A problem with ear development might indicate renal abnormalities.

26. *d*   Phimosis refers to foreskin that cannot be retracted over the glans penis. This is a normal finding in uncircumcised male children and usually resolves by age 5 years. Circumcision is not indicated unless there is urinary obstruction. The foreskin should never be forcibly retracted.

27. *c*   Intravenous pyelogram (IVP) was the diagnostic study of choice to differentiate details of any renal abnormality prior to helical CT. This method has superior sensitivity and specificity compared to an IVP. The disadvantage of CT is that it provides no information on renal function or degree of obstruction. Renal ultrasound is useful for detecting hydronephrosis, but cannot substitute for an IVP.

C 28. The history of a 3½-year-old healthy male reveals continuous failed attempts at toilet training. He is incontinent of urine at least once daily and wears "pull up" diapers. He is incontinent of urine nightly. He has used a toddler toilet chair successfully for bowel movements for the past 6 months. Urine dipstick is negative. The nurse practitioner correctly records a diagnosis of:

    a. secondary enuresis and provides the mother with more toilet training education.
    b. secondary enuresis and prescribes DDAVP.
    c. primary enuresis, provides the mother with more toilet training education, and considers referral to a urologist.
    d. primary enuresis, provides the mother with more toilet training education, and advises the mother to purchase regular boy's underwear and not to worry.

d 29. A 25-year-old sexually active single female is being seen for follow up of pelvic inflammatory disease (PID). As the nurse practitioner is leaving the examination room, the patient requests information on intrauterine device (IUD) contraception. Which of the following responses by the nurse practitioner would be most appropriate?

    a. "The IUD would be an appropriate method for you."
    b. "Because of your recent infection, abstinence is the best method for now."
    c. "You need to make another appointment for us to discuss contraception."
    d. "An IUD would not be a good choice for you right now, but we can discuss other methods."

28. *c* Enuresis is involuntary urination beyond age 5 years in girls and age 6 years in boys. Primary enuresis is defined as the absence of voluntary control of urination without a previous period of voluntary control. When enuresis presents after a period of at least 6 to 12 months of voluntary control, the condition is correctly referred to as secondary enuresis.

29. *d* An active pelvic infection is an absolute contraindication for use of an IUD. History of PID is a relative contraindication.

PRACTICE EXAMS

Practice Exam I

C 1. A 35-year-old man who has a history of intravenous drug abuse is diagnosed with *herpes zoster*. Which of the following diagnostic tests should the nurse practitioner now consider?

    a. Varicella titer
    b. Rapid plasma reagin (RPR)
    c. ELISA for HIV
    d. Viral culture

D 2. Which of the following is *not* consistent with the presentation of stress incontinence in women?

    a. Leaking of urine with exercise
    b. Perineal irritation
    c. History of multiparity
    d. Lower abdominal pain

A 3. Inclusion of CAGE questions in the patient interview may yield information about:

    a. problems related to alcohol use.
    b. the likelihood of domestic violence.
    c. symptoms of depression and suicidal ideation.
    d. motivating factors for smoking cessation.

 4. A 65-year-old man has a recent 5 pound weight gain, S3 heart sound, and bibasilar crackles on auscultation of the chest and thorax. What is the most likely diagnosis?

    a. Chronic renal failure
    b. Lobar pneumonia
    c. Secondary hypertension
    d. Congestive heart failure

B 5. Which of the following is *not* covered by Medicare Part B?

    a. Outpatient services
    b. Services in short-stay skilled nursing care facilities
    c. Physician and/or APRN provider services
    d. Lab and x-ray services

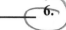

6. A 2-year-old has been diagnosed with bronchiolitis. Before leaving the nurse practitioner's office, the child's mother should know:

   a. how to assess the child's pulse.
   b. to take the child into a warm steam-filled bathroom for treatment of wheezing.
   c. that symptoms usually resolve in 1 to 3 days.
   d. to alternate acetaminophen and ibuprofen for fever.

7. A 23-year-old female is in the emergency room subsequent to a cocaine overdose. She is awake and alert. Her blood pressure is 160/104 mmHg, pulse 180 and regular, and respirations 28 and unlabored. Which of the following medications is indicated?

   a. Sublingual nifedipine (Procardia®)
   b. Oral lanoxin (Digoxin®)
   c. Intravenous propranolol (Inderal®)
   d. Intravenous morphine sulfate

8. An overweight male complains of low back pain after helping to move a refrigerator 2 days ago. To avoid future problems, the nurse practitioner should teach him:

   a. exercises to strengthen his lower back.
   b. to rest his back until he is pain free.
   c. to seek early medical attention after a back injury.
   d. to take his pain medication as prescribed.

9. What problem would be *least* expected in a pregnancy complicated by gestational diabetes?

   a. Cephalopelvic disproportion
   b. Placenta previa
   c. Neonatal hypoglycemia
   d. A macrosomic infant

10. A 48-year-old premenopausal patient was treated for a vaginal yeast infection (confirmed by microscopy) with a course of terconazole (Terazol®) 0.4% cream for seven days. The patient returned in 10 days with the same symptoms. The nurse practitioner re-examined the discharge and once again found budding yeast. The patient was treated with a course of miconazole (Monistat®) 2% cream. She continues to complain of itching and discharge after 5 days. What should the nurse practitioner do?

    a. Perform CBC, chemistry profile, HIV and re-examine the patient's medical history.
    b. Reculture the discharge and try a third antifungal agent.
    c. Perform another vaginal exam with cultures and sensitivity.
    d. Refer now.

11. Capillary blood glucose levels remain elevated in a patient with type 2 diabetes mellitus. The patient is currently taking a sulfonylurea medication. Which of the following drugs should be added next to the medication treatment regimen?

    a. glipizide (Glucotrol®)
    b. NPH insulin
    c. Regular insulin
    d. metformin (Glucophage®-XR)

12. Heberden's nodes are most commonly associated with what disease?

    a. Osteoarthritis (OA)
    b. Rheumatoid arthritis (RA)
    c. Psoriatic arthritis
    d. Bacterial arthritis

13. An 18-year-old college student lives in the dormitory. He was treated for scabies infestation with permethrin (Nix®). The burrows cleared and he was asymptomatic for 6 weeks. Now he is home for the weekend and complains again of intense itching and skin burrows. How should the nurse practitioner proceed?

    a. Retreat him with a different scabicide.
    b. Refer him to a physician for treatment.
    c. Tell him that itching can last 2 to 4 weeks after the mite has been eradicated.
    d. Re-treat him with permethrin and have him launder all of the contaminated bedding and clothing both at home and at school.

14. A 35-year-old male reports recurrent, severe, unilateral, headache over his left eye. The headaches last approximately 2 hours and usually occur at bedtime. Physical examination is negative. What is the most likely diagnosis?

    a. Common migraine headache
    b. Tension headache
    c. Cluster headache
    d. Classic migraine headache

15. A 45-year-old diabetic patient has periorbital cellulitis secondary to a sinus infection. What course of action should the nurse practitioner take?

    a. Initiate penicillin 1000 mg orally 2 times daily for 10 to 14 days.
    b. Initiate erythromycin 250 mg orally 4 times daily for 10 to 14 days.
    c. Initiate amoxicillin-clavulanate (Augmentin®) 875 mg orally twice a day for 14 days.
    d. Consider referral to a physician for IV antibiotic treatment and hospitalization.

16. A patient presents to the nurse practitioner with complaints of diarrhea and malaise which started at 2:00 am the morning of the visit. After history and examination, the nurse practitioner advises the patient that the problem should be self-limiting. If the diarrhea does not resolve, when should the nurse practitioner advise the patient to return?

    a. 24 hours
    b. 2 days
    c. 3 days
    d. 4 days

17. Most children who have been sexually abused have:

    a. dilation of the vagina or rectum.
    b. no detectable genital injury.
    c. a sexually transmitted infection.
    d. bruising of the genital area.

18. A 4-year-old female complains of leg pain on most nights which resolves by morning. This has lasted for the past 4 months. The nurse practitioner should tell the patient's mother:

    a. these are growing pains that last from 1 to 2 years. This is a common complaint in this age group.
    b. this complaint is typical of Osgood-Schlatter disease. It will resolve spontaneously in 2 to 4 months.
    c. this pain is typical with juvenile arthritis. Blood work will confirm the diagnosis.
    d. this pain is typical of children who need more attention. Spend more individual time with her at bedtime.

19. Which of the following diagnoses usually warrants referral for urgent care?

    a. Essential hypertension
    b. Vasovagal syncope
    c. Arterial insufficiency
    d. Unstable angina

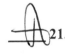

20. A 4 month old infant is not able to sit without support. The nurse practitioner should:

    a. refer the infant to a pediatrician.
    b. consider this normal and make sure other physical milestones are being achieved.
    c. give the infant another 4 weeks to achieve this milestone.
    d. wait until the infant is 6 months-of-age before referring to a pediatrician.

21. The nurse practitioner is evaluating a 35-year-old female nurse. She has a history of hospitalization for hepatitis B infection 2 years ago. Her laboratory tests demonstrate positive HBsAg. The nurse practitioner would correctly diagnose:

    a. chronic hepatitis B infection.
    b. acute hepatitis B infection.
    c. recovered hepatitis B infection.
    d. recent hepatitis B vaccination.

_____ 22. A 75-year-old patient is well controlled on timolol maleate (Timoptic®) for chronic open-angle glaucoma. Prescribing propranolol (Inderal®) for this patient may precipitate:

    a. hyperglycemia.
    b. elevated intraocular pressure.
    c. bradycardia.
    d. hypertension.

_____ 23. Koilonychia is indicative of what type of anemia?

    a. Pernicious
    b. Iron deficiency
    c. Sickle cell
    d. Folate deficiency

_____ 24. Adolescents need to be educated that human immunodeficiency virus (HIV) is transmitted by:

    a. homosexual intercourse, primarily.
    b. fecal-oral route.
    c. semen, vaginal secretions, and blood.
    d. saliva and tears.

_____ 25. Which of the following drugs is considered safest for use during pregnancy?

    a. clotrimazole (Gyne-Lotrimin®)
    b. isotretinoin (Accutane®)
    c. trimethoprim-sulfamethoxazole (Bactrim®)
    d. terconazole (Terazol®) vaginal cream

_____ 26. The most common cause of cerebral palsy is:

    a. unknown.
    b. intra-partal hypoxia.
    c. in utero infection.
    d. intra-ventricular hemorrhage.

_____ 27. The treatment of choice for recurrent *herpes simplex II* infection is:

    a. topical acyclovir.
    b. soaks with Burrow's solution.
    c. oral acyclovir.
    d. Nonsteroidal anti-inflammatory agents.

28. A 71-year-old male has recently lost his spouse of 49 years. He tells the nurse practitioner "I have nothing to live for." What essential question must the nurse practitioner ask him?

   a. "Have you told your family how you feel?"
   b. "Have you thought about killing yourself?"
   c. "What medication are you taking?"
   d. "Are you involved in any social activities?"

29. What kind of ophthalmology consultation should be planned for patients with diabetes mellitus (DM)?

   a. Dilated retinal examination should be performed by an ophthalmologist at the time of diagnosis of diabetes, then annually.
   b. A funduscopic exam should be included in every clinic visit, beginning at 65 years-of-age.
   c. Diabetic patients should have annual tonometry and cataract screening, beginning at 40 years-of-age.
   d. Beginning 5 years after diagnosis, patients with diabetes should have an annual dilated retinal examination.

30. A 72-year-old man has chronic prostatitis. What is the initial drug treatment of choice for this patient?

   a. ciprofloxacin (Cipro®)
   b. doxycycline (Vibramycin®)
   c. amoxicillin (Amoxil®)
   d. nitrofurantoin (Macrodantin®)

31. Enlargement of the scrotum and testes with little change in the size of the penis characterizes which Tanner stage of sexual development?

   a. Tanner 1
   b. Tanner 2
   c. Tanner 3
   d. Tanner 5

32. What is the most accurate comparison to use when evaluating peak expiratory flow rate (PEFR)?

   a. Predicted range for height
   b. Personal best
   c. Predicted range for weight
   d. Predicted range for age

D 33. A 59-year-old postmenopausal woman has atrophic vaginitis. She has a history of breast cancer at age 40 years. What is the appropriate initial treatment for this patient?

    a. Oral conjugated estrogens
    b. Oral medroxyprogesterone acetate
    c. Topical medroxyprogesterone acetate
    d. Topical conjugate estrogen cream

B 34. According to the current standard of care for obstetrical practice, women should be referred for amniocentesis who will be what age at the time of delivery?

    a. 30 years-of-age or older
    b. 33 years-of-age or older
    c. 35 years-of-age or older
    d. 40 years-of-age or older

B 35. On transillumination of the scrotum, the nurse practitioner identifies a hydrocele in a 3 month old infant. What course of action should be taken?

    a. Refer the patient to a urologist for surgical repair.
    b. Monitor the hydrocele until the infant is 6 months-of-age.
    c. Inspect the external genitalia for ambiguity.
    d. Inspect the penis for hypospadias.

A 36. Which of the following findings is usually associated with atopic dermatitis in infants?

    a. Positive family history
    b. Non-pruritic lesions
    c. Primary presentation in the diaper area
    d. Hyperpigmented areas of the skin

C 37. A prenatal patient is in the tenth week of pregnancy. Rubella titer was 1:18 on her first prenatal visit at 6 weeks gestation. She believes she was exposed to rubella yesterday and asks how this will affect her pregnancy. Which of the following responses by the nurse practitioner is appropriate?

    a. "The fetus could be affected. You may want to consider termination."
    b. "The outcome of the pregnancy depends on the closeness of proximity and length of time of exposure."
    c. "The pregnancy will be unaffected. You are immune to rubella."
    d. "A second rubella titer is needed to compare the results."

38. What diagnosis is associated with an elevated serum amylase?

    a. Cholecystitis
    b. Peptic ulcer disease (PUD)
    c. Pancreatitis
    d. Renal insufficiency

39. What is the most common cause of bronchopulmonary dysplasia (BPD) in infants?

    a. Perinatal infection
    b. Barotrauma
    c. Meconium aspiration
    d. A congenital anomaly

40. A 16-year-old patient with type 2 diabetes mellitus has sporadic blood glucose levels recorded in his glucose diary for the past 3 months. Every reading is between 100 and 140 mg/dL. A glycosylated hemoglobin of 12% for this patient would indicate:

    a. good overall glucose control.
    b. poor glucose control in the last 2 weeks.
    c. adequate glucose control in the last month only.
    d. poor glucose control for the last 1 to 3 months.

41. The process by which a professional association confers recognition that a licensed professional has demonstrated mastery of a specialized body of knowledge and skills is termed:

    a. licensure.
    b. quality assurance.
    c. certification.
    d. registration.

42. A common finding in patients with endometriosis is:

    a. dyspareunia.
    b. diarrhea.
    c. left upper quadrant abdominal pain.
    d. irregular menstrual cycles.

43. Which red blood cell (RBC) index is most useful for differentiating types of anemias?

   a. Mean corpuscular volume (MCV)
   b. Mean corpuscular hemoglobin concentration (MCHC)
   c. Hematocrit (HCT)
   d. Platelet count

44. At the end of the first year of therapy for type 2 diabetes mellitus, the patient asks, "How am I doing so far?" The best answer is provided by a review of the patient's:

   a. daily glucose diary for the past year.
   b. serial glycosylated hemoglobins for the past year.
   c. glucose diary for the last month compared to the first month.
   d. fasting serum glucose reports during the past year.

45. Which refractive error is commonly associated with the normal aging process?

   a. Myopia
   b. Anisometropia
   c. Presbyopia
   d. Hyperopia

46. A 13 month old presents with decreased mobility of the right tympanic membrane with pneumatic otoscopy. What office diagnostic test will help confirm the presence of fluid in the middle ear?

   a. Audiometry
   b. Tympanocentesis
   c. Tympanometry
   d. Swab of the external canal

47. What is the most sensitive and specific indicator of gonococcal infection in asymptomatic persons?

   a. DNA probe and enzyme immunoassay
   b. Urine dipstick for leukocyte esterase
   c. Detailed sexual history
   d. Direct culture from the site of exposure

48. Which of the following medications is useful in the treatment of patients with chronic emphysema?

    a. epinephrine
    b. ipratropium (Atrovent®)
    c. cromolyn sodium (Intal®)
    d. zafirlukast (Accolate®)

49. What is the leading cause of morbidity and mortality in postmenopausal American women?

    a. Alzheimer's Disease
    b. Osteoporosis
    c. Cancer
    d. Cardiovascular disease

50. The most appropriate premedication for treatment of exercise-induced asthma is a(n):

    a. inhaled corticosteroid.
    b. long-acting xanthine.
    c. inhaled β_2-agonist.
    d. leukotriene receptor antagonist.

51. An example of secondary prevention is:

    a. annual mammography for women age 40 years-of-age and older.
    b. educating parents about immunizations for children.
    c. introducing the subject of "safe sex" during an adolescent exam.
    d. annual influenza vaccination.

52. A critically ill patient states "my family is well provided for." This comment most likely means the patient:

    a. is suicidal.
    b. wishes to discuss the topic of death.
    c. is no longer interested in treatment.
    d. is in denial.

53. Education of women with fibrocystic breast disease should include which of the following statements?

    a. "Fibrocystic breast disease is often a precursor of breast cancer."
    b. "Annual mammography is recommended beginning at age 40."
    c. "Caffeine may trigger breast pain."
    d. "Oral contraceptives are not useful in the treatment of this disease."

54. On physical examination of a 3½-year-old child, the nurse practitioner auscultates a Grade II/VI heart murmur. Which statement about the murmur is *incorrect*?

    a. Functional or vibratory murmurs are innocent murmurs.
    b. There is a palpable thrill associated with this murmur.
    c. The murmur may become louder as the heart rate changes.
    d. This child does not need antibiotic prophylaxis prior to dental procedures.

55. Screening for anemia with hemoglobin and hematocrit is recommended for high risk infants between 6 and 12 months-of-age. Which group listed below is considered high risk?

    a. Caucasians
    b. Children in single parent households
    c. Low birth weight infants
    d. Children in daycare

56. A woman of childbearing age is contemplating pregnancy. By prescribing folic acid 1 mg daily, the nurse practitioner is practicing:

    a. primary prevention.
    b. secondary prevention.
    c. tertiary prevention.
    d. risk identification.

57. A 48-year-old normotensive male patient's total cholesterol is 250 mg/dL and low density lipoprotein is 140 mg/dL. He is a non-smoker. His father died of congestive heart failure at 80 years-of-age. What is the appropriate initial treatment for this patient's hyperlipidemia?

    a. Observe and re-assess in 6 months
    b. Start an HMG CoA-reductase inhibitor
    c. Diet and exercise
    d. Start daily niacin

58 . Evaluation for coarctation of the aorta is warranted in a 2 week old infant when there is unequal intensity of:

    a. brachial and radial pulses.
    b. brachial and femoral pulses.
    c. carotid and brachial pulses.
    d. radial and pedal pulses.

59. A 43-year-old female requests a nighttime sleep aid for insomnia. On further questioning, she reports feeling "hyper, uneasy, and nervous" during the daytime and "hot all of the time" for the past 3 or 4 months. Her appetite is "better than ever," yet she has lost 16 pounds in the past 2 months. What is the most likely diagnosis?

    a. Generalized anxiety disorder (GAD)
    b. Graves' disease
    c. Pheochromocytoma
    d. Menopause

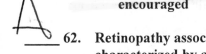

60. Which of the following is an appropriate drug for initial treatment of gastroesophageal reflux disease (GERD) in adults?

    a. famotidine (Pepcid®)
    b. sucralfate (Carafate®)
    c. metoclopramide (Reglan®)
    d. omeprazole (Prilosec®)

61. A 2-year-old female presents with a 3 day history of high fever, followed by abrupt resolution and development of a pink maculopapular rash today. What pharmacological intervention(s) should the nurse practitioner consider?

    a. amoxicillin (Amoxil®) 45 mg/kg/day for 10 days
    b. Calamine® lotion applied to the rash 4 times a day and as needed
    c. acetaminophen (dose by weight) and fluids
    d. No pharmacologic intervention is needed, but fluids should be encouraged

62. Retinopathy associated with poorly controlled or uncontrolled diabetes is characterized by all of the following *except*:

    a. papilledema.
    b. dot and blot hemorrhages.
    c. microaneurysms.
    d. cotton wool spots.

63. A 3 month old has diaper candidiasis. The nurse practitioner should advise the mother to apply nystatin (Mycostatin®) cream at each diaper change and:

    a. clean the skin with plain water prior to applying the medication.
    b. change diapers at least every 2 hours.
    c. return if there is no improvement in 24 hours.
    d. apply an absorbent powder to the diaper area.

64. An adult female presents with a hordeolum. A topical antibiotic is prescribed. Which of the following instructions is *not* appropriate for the nurse practitioner to give the patient?

    a. "Apply warm, moist compresses several times per day."
    b. "Do not use soap near the affected eyelid."
    c. "Do not wear eye makeup and discard all used eye makeup."
    d. "Do not rub your eyes."

65. Instructing caregivers and mothers of low birth weight (LBW) infants in a hospital nursery about sensory stimulation is likely to result in:

    a. children with higher intelligence quotient scores.
    b. no difference in outcomes.
    c. interruption of the infant's sleep cycle.
    d. a lower incidence of upper respiratory infection.

66. Of the following, which medication is the most effective treatment for acute anxiety?

    a. buspirone (BuSpar®)
    b. alprazolam (Xanax®)
    c. paroxetine (Paxil®)
    d. imipramine (Tofranil®)

67. A 50-year-old, non-smoker, without comorbidity, presents to the clinic and is diagnosed with pneumonia. His vital signs are normal except for temperature 101.6°F (38.6°C). A sputum specimen is collected and sent for culture and sensitivity. What action should the nurse practitioner take today?

    a. Wait for the culture report before starting antibiotic therapy.
    b. Start 2 tablets clarithromycin (Biaxin® XL) 500 mg daily.
    c. Start penicillin V 500 mg 4 times a day.
    d. Start ciprofloxacin (Cipro®) 500 mg twice a day.

68. Which of the following medications is indicated for prevention of febrile seizures?

    a. phenobarbital
    b. acetaminophen (Tylenol®)
    c. aspirin
    d. phenytoin (Dilantin®)

69. A 70-year-old female presents to the clinic with complaints of feeling light-headed and dizzy after standing for several minutes in one place. She states that she feels better quickly if she sits down. She denies confusion or loss of bowel and bladder continence after these episodes. What is this patient probably experiencing?

    a. Orthostatic hypotension
    b. Cardiac arrhythmia
    c. Hypoglycemia
    d. Vasovagal syncope

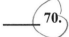

70. A 54-year-old female has macrocytic anemia. Which of the following laboratory tests would be most appropriate for the nurse practitioner to order to identify the cause of this anemia?

    a. Schilling test
    b. Hemoglobin electrophoresis
    c. TIBC
    d. Serum Fe level

71. All of the following are included in the differential diagnosis of hyperthyroidism *except*:

    a. Plummer's disease.
    b. hypersomnia.
    c. thyrotoxicosis.
    d. multinodular goiter.

72. What information would best help the parent who is concerned about a school-age child's eating habits?

    a. A child who is allowed to eat whatever he wants will usually be well-nourished.
    b. The school-age child's nutritional requirements are the same as for adults.
    c. The school-age child requires 50 kilocalories per pound daily.
    d. Establish a consistent schedule for meals and allow the child to participate in meal planning.

73. A 15-year-old has had a 4 day bout of diarrhea with pale greasy stools and abdominal cramping. He is still having symptoms today when he visits the nurse practitioner. What should the nurse practitioner suspect as the cause?

    a. *Giardia*
    b. *Salmonella*
    c. *Shigella*
    d. *Rotavirus*

74. The first step when taking a patient history is the:

    a. review of systems (ROS).
    b. chief complaint (CC).
    c. introductory information.
    d. past medical history.

75. Persons of Mediterranean descent have an increased incidence of which of the following?

    a. Thalassemia
    b. Pernicious anemia
    c. Sickle cell anemia
    d. Leukemia

76. Acute lymphocytic leukemia is usually diagnosed by:

    a. a complete blood count (CBC) with differential.
    b. magnetic resonance imaging (MRI).
    c. a nuclear bone scan.
    d. bone marrow examination.

77. A 75-year-old female with history of CHF presents to a family practice clinic with breathlessness, falling, confusion, and palpitations. What is an appropriate response by the nurse practitioner?

    a. Myocardial infarction (MI) can be ruled out immediately because these are not the symptoms of MI.
    b. These are expected problems in this 75-year-old. Refer the patient to occupational therapy for instructions on use of a walker.
    c. Suspect MI and arrange transportation to the nearest emergency department.
    d. Request a computerized tomography (CT) scan of the head.

78. The nurse practitioner suspects migraine in a 6-year-old male with a 2 month history of recurrent headache. What finding would support a diagnosis of migraine headache?

    a. Family history of migraine headaches
    b. Localized facial pain and ataxia
    c. Problems at home, school, and with peers
    d. Ipsilateral weakness and papilledema

79. Which of the following diagnostic assessments must be considered before developing any plan of care for a 27-year-old female presenting to a family practice clinic?

    a. Pregnancy test
    b. Family social history
    c. Hematocrit and hemoglobin
    d. Blood pressure

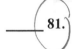

80. Considering mortality statistics for the adolescent age group, education targeted toward this group should first focus on:

    a. sexually transmitted diseases.
    b. sports safety.
    c. automobile safety.
    d. alcohol abuse.

81. A diagnostic finding of Hodgkin's lymphoma is the presence of:

    a. granulocytopenia.
    b. Reed-Sternberg cells.
    c. lymphoblasts.
    d. Howell-Jolly bodies.

82. A 14-year-old develops otitis externa with swelling, erythema, and pain. To facilitate antibiotic delivery to the canal, the nurse practitioner should:

    a. use a cotton tipped swab to apply medication.
    b. insert a wick by gently twisting it into the canal.
    c. prescribe an oral antibiotic.
    d. prescribe an oil-based otic antibiotic to seep into the canal.

83. A 69-year-old patient with chronic obstructive pulmonary disease (COPD) presents for a routine health check. The nurse practitioner encourages him to get an influenza vaccination. How long will it take before the vaccination becomes protective?

    a. 2 to 3 hours
    b. 2 to 3 days
    c. 2 to 3 weeks
    d. 2 to 3 months

84. Upon ophthalmoscopic examination of a 78-year-old patient, the nurse practitioner observes dark spots against a red retina. What diagnosis is this finding most consistent with?

    a. Glaucoma
    b. Retinal detachment
    c. Cataract
    d. Macular degeneration

85. For the general adult population, total dietary fat intake should be no more than what percent of total daily calories?

    a. 10%
    b. 20%
    c. 30%
    d. 40%

86. The correct order of physical examination of the abdomen is:

    a. inspection, palpation, percussion, auscultation.
    b. inspection, auscultation, percussion, palpation.
    c. auscultation, inspection, palpation, percussion.
    d. palpation, percussion, inspection, auscultation.

87. Which of the following may be caused by long term glucocorticoid treatment?

    a. Cushing's syndrome
    b. Skeletal hypertrophy
    c. Hypoglycemia
    d. Hyperkalemia

88. Instillation of silver nitrate ophthalmic solution, or erythromycin, in the eyes of a newborn is recommended to protect against:

    a. gonococcal ophthalmia neonatorum.
    b. chlamydial conjunctivitis.
    c. ophthalmia neonatorum treponema.
    d. vernal conjunctivitis neonatorum.

89. In the differential diagnosis of thyroid dysfunction, the typical patient with hypothyroidism has all of the following characteristic features *except*:

    a. dry course hair and skin.
    b. facial puffiness and periorbital edema.
    c. thinning of the outer 1/3 of the eyebrows.
    d. nervousness and tremor.

90. Which term most accurately describes the prostate gland of a patient with prostate cancer?

    a. Hard
    b. Rubbery
    c. Boggy
    d. Spongy

91. Which of the following is true about cognitive abilities in the elderly?

    a. Most decline occurs in the sixth decade, but persons in later decades show little change.
    b. Skills training and motivational incentives have no effect on memory.
    c. Elderly adults perform poorly in comparison to young adults on tests of verbal skills.
    d. Apprehension about competitive situations has little effect on performance.

92. What is the optimum time to start antiviral therapy in patients with *herpes zoster*?

    a. Within 48 hours of the appearance of rash
    b. As soon as fever is identified
    c. After the prodromal phase
    d. During the first 3 days of rash

B 93. Which of the following oral medications should be avoided in a child under 9 years-of-age?

    a. sulfisoxazole
    b. tetracycline
    c. rifampin
    d. metronidazole (Flagyl®)

D 94. Which determination will affect the interpretation of a physical examination of an infant?

    a. What was the Apgar score at one minute?
    b. Is the child breast or bottle fed?
    c. Are the immunizations current?
    d. What was the gestational age at birth?

A 95. Which of the following medications has been FDA approved for treatment of osteoporosis?

    a. alendronate (Fosamax®)
    b. tamoxifen (Nolvadex®)
    c. parathyroid hormone analogues
    d. bromocriptine (Parlodel®)

D 96. With an ankle sprain, the nurse practitioner would most likely elicit a history of:

    a. a popping sound.
    b. a clicking sound.
    c. ankle eversion.
    d. ankle inversion.

D 97. What factor has the greatest impact on premature mortality rates in the United States?

    a. Gender
    b. Health care accessibility
    c. Genetics
    d. Lifestyle

98. A 52-year-old woman has a firm, fixed, nontender, one centimeter mass in the right lower quadrant of her breast. There are no palpable axillary lymph nodes. A mammogram is negative. The most appropriate nurse practitioner action today is to:

    a. reassure the patient that the mass is benign.
    b. refer the patient to a surgeon for evaluation.
    c. schedule a follow up appointment in 2 months to re-evaluate the mass.
    d. plan a repeat mammogram in 6 months.

99. A 63-year-old male accountant complains of pain and stiffness in his feet and hands of several years duration. He reports that the pain and stiffness become better with activity. On examination, he is noted to have Heberden's nodes but no other bony deformities. Which of the following is the most probable diagnosis?

    a. Gout
    b. Osteoarthritis (OA)
    c. Rheumatoid arthritis (RA)
    d. Osteoporosis

100. An 85-year-old is diagnosed with shingles. The patient states that she became "miserable" yesterday when the symptoms started. What pharmacologic interventions should the nurse practitioner offer this patient?

    a. NSAIDs for pain and fever
    b. Topical capsaicin cream (Zostrix®) to lesions 4 times a day for 21 days plus NSAIDs for pain and fever
    c. Oral acyclovir (Zovirax®) for 7 to 10 days, NSAIDs, and topical capsaicin cream after resolution of the lesions
    d. Acetaminophen, Burrow's solution compresses, and mupirocin (Bactroban®) to the lesions

101. The nurse practitioner strongly suspects hyperthyroidism in a 62-year-old patient. Which of the following would *not* be an appropriate initial intervention?

    a. Order an ECG.
    b. Schedule a thyroid radio-iodine uptake scan.
    c. Refer the patient to an endocrinologist.
    d. Start thyroxine 0.025 mg (25 mcg) daily and re-assess in 2 weeks.

102. A 26-year-old female has a history of diethylstilbestrol (DES) exposure while in utero. What type of cancer is this patient at increased risk for?

    a. Vaginal
    b. Endometrial
    c. Breast
    d. Cervical

103. A 27-year-old male athlete presents with complaints of exquisite pain over his right shin. He runs an average of 6 to 8 miles per day. He wonders if he has a right tibial stress fracture. Which response by the nurse practitioner is *not* correct?

    a. "X-ray may not reveal a stress fracture even if one is present."
    b. "Bone scan is the most definitive diagnostic test."
    c. "There is no radiological test which will identify a stress fracture."
    d. "Without point tenderness, a stress fracture is unlikely."

104. It is recommended that the therapeutic management of children with juvenile rheumatoid arthritis (JRA) should include:

    a. avoidance of exercise.
    b. immunosuppressant agents.
    c. ophthalmological examination at least annually.
    d. avoidance of aspirin therapy.

105. Factors known to be associated with early sexual activity include:

    a. early development of secondary sex characteristics, living in an urban area, and easy access to contraceptives.
    b. lower socioeconomic status, use of tobacco, alcohol, or other drugs, and single parent household.
    c. legalized abortion, frequent viewing of adult television and movies, and lack of church affiliation.
    d. exposure to sex education information at school.

106. Introduction of solid foods to infants should begin:

    a. at 1 to 2 months-of-age, 1 new food at a time, starting with vegetables.
    b. no earlier than 3 months-of age, beginning with cereal, then meats, one food at a time.
    c. at 4 months-of age, with a variety of fruits and vegetables.
    d. no earlier than 4 to 6 months-of age, beginning with cereal, then fruits, 1 new food at a time.

107. A 16-year-old received stitches in his arm after an accident. He tells the nurse practitioner that his last tetanus shot was "on time." Should he receive one today?

    a. Yes, his last one was probably at 10 years-of-age.
    b. Yes, because there is no documentation of the previous immunization.
    c. No, his last one was probably at 11 to 12 years-of-age.
    d. No, his last one was probably at 9 years-of-age.

108. A 15-year-old male has a history of cryptorchidism which was surgically repaired. Because of this history, it is essential for the nurse practitioner to teach him about:

    a. testicular self-examination.
    b. protection of the testes during sports activities.
    c. risk of testicular torsion.
    d. practicing safe sex.

109. Which disease process may be a predisposing factor for balanitis?

    a. Diabetes mellitus (DM)
    b. Atopic dermatitis
    c. Rheumatoid arthritis (RA)
    d. Psoriasis

110. Which of the following factors is(are) associated with increased incidence of cervical cancer?

    a. Smoking and sexual activity at an early age with multiple partners
    b. Routine use of barrier contraceptives, such as diaphragm and/or condoms
    c. Dietary factors, such as vitamin and mineral deficiencies
    d. History of pregnancy before the age of 30 years and history of breastfeeding

111. A 49-year-old man sees the nurse practitioner for evaluation of a 2 mm macular lesion on his back. The lesion is brown with regular borders. The most appropriate action for the nurse practitioner to take is to:

    a. refer the patient to a dermatologist for excision.
    b. reassure the patient that this lesion is not suspicious for pathology.
    c. re-evaluate the lesion in 2 months.
    d. perform cryosurgery on the lesion.

A   112. A 12 month old has conjunctivitis in his right eye with a mucopurulent discharge. The mother asks if the child can forego the antibiotic eye drops because he doesn't like drops put in his eyes. The nurse practitioner replies:

    a. "If untreated, conjunctivitis may permanently damage the cornea."
    b. "Conjunctivitis is usually caused by a virus. Let's wait a few days."
    c. "If no one else at the daycare has it, we can wait a few days."
    d. "An oral antihistamine may be prescribed instead of eye drops."

D   113. A new patient presents to the nurse practitioner clinic stating she wants a second opinion. A week ago, she started propylthiouracil (PTU) 75 mg 3 times a day as therapy for newly diagnosed Graves' disease. She still feels irritable and jittery. How should the nurse practitioner respond?

    a. Obtain a serum TSH and serum T_4 today.
    b. Increase the PTU dose to 100 mg 3 times a day.
    c. Recommend radioactive iodine therapy.
    d. Inform the patient that improvement requires 2 to 3 weeks.

B   114. The diagnosis of Meniere's disease is based on:

    a. magnetic resonance imaging (MRI) findings.
    b. exclusion of other pathologies.
    c. the presence of high frequency hearing loss.
    d. the presence of central vertigo.

C   115. A 16-year-old has had diarrhea and malaise without fever for 10 days following a camping trip. Stool specimen analysis reveals giardiasis. After treatment has been completed, when should follow up stool specimens be checked?

    a. No follow up is needed
    b. 7 to 14 days
    c. 3 to 4 weeks
    d. Anytime after completion of treatment

B   116. Which of the following has been shown by research to be most influential in promoting smoking cessation in the adolescent population?

    a. Cigarette smoking causes lung diseases such as emphysema and cancer.
    b. Cigarette smoking contributes to yellow teeth, bad breath, and decreased capacity to perform sports activities.
    c. Cigarette smoking pollutes the environment.
    d. Cigarette smoking during pregnancy affects infant birth weight.

117. The reason beta-adrenergic blockers should be avoided in patients with diabetes is because they may:

   a. potentiate hyperglycemia.
   b. interfere with the action of insulin and oral hypoglycemics.
   c. mask symptoms of hypoglycemia.
   d. stimulate hepatic glucose secretion.

118. A patient presents with a normal complete blood count (CBC) and a positive stool for occult blood. The nurse practitioner decides to repeat the stool for occult blood after having the patient eliminate certain foods from the diet for 72 hours. Which of the following should be included in the list of foods to omit?

   a. Fish
   b. Bananas
   c. Carrots
   d. Steak

119. A 50-year-old female with varicose veins should be taught to:

   a. massage her legs each night.
   b. elevate the head of her bed.
   c. avoid long periods of standing.
   d. apply support stockings at bedtime.

120. Long-range disease prevention programs are most likely to be successful if:

   a. only long-range goals are included.
   b. the programs are designed to fit the cultural and health profiles of the population.
   c. the practitioner convinces individuals that their beliefs are incorrect.
   d. emphasis is placed on future time.

121. The nurse practitioner notes a decreased digoxin level of 0.5 ng/dL in a 70-year-old who has had stable digoxin levels for the past 3 years. A possible cause is:

   a. blood loss.
   b. hypokalemia.
   c. decreased urine creatinine clearance.
   d. antacid use.

_____122. A 35-year-old female has a history of rheumatic fever with resultant valvular heart disease. She is scheduled for major dental work in 1 month. Which of the following medications is appropriate dental prophylaxis for this patient?

    a. gentamicin (Garamycin®)
    b. tetracycline
    c. cefaclor (Ceclor®)
    d. amoxicillin (Amoxil®)

_____123. According to Erikson, the developmental task of the elderly adult is:

    a. intimacy vs. isolation.
    b. ego integrity vs. despair.
    c. industry vs. self-doubt.
    d. trust vs. mistrust.

_____124. A 24-year-old female taking an oral contraceptive missed her last 2 pills. What should the nurse practitioner advise her to do to minimize her risk of pregnancy?

    a. Take today's dose and do not miss any more during this month.
    b. Double today's dose and use a barrier method for the rest of this month.
    c. Double today's dose and tomorrow's dose and use a barrier method for the rest of this month.
    d. Stop the pills today and restart a new pill pack in 1 week.

_____125. Lead screening of a 12 month old child reveals a capillary lead level of 15 mcg/dL. How should the nurse practitioner proceed?

    a. Consider this a normal capillary lead level.
    b. Confirm the results with a venous blood sample.
    c. Refer the child for chelation therapy.
    d. Have the home inspected for lead contamination.

_____126. The initial step in the management of encopresis is:

    a. patient and family education.
    b. bowel cleansing.
    c. psychosocial evaluation of the patient.
    d. dietary changes.

_____127. A patient presents with a furuncle in his right axilla. The nurse practitioner should prescribe an oral antibiotic and:

    a. frequent warm moist compresses.
    b. benzoyl peroxide.
    c. topical mupirocin ointment (Bactroban®).
    d. topical hydrocortisone cream.

_____128. An 86-year-old Caucasian male requests screening for prostate cancer. What is the best approach to his request?

    a. Give him objective information about the potential benefits and harms of early detection and treatment.
    b. Tell him that screening is only done for men with a life expectancy greater than 10 years.
    c. Perform a digital rectal exam (DRE), obtain a prostatic specific antigen (PSA), and order a transrectal ultrasound (TRUS) at this time.
    d. Perform a DRE and PSA at this visit, reserving the TRUS for patients with abnormal DRE or PSA.

_____129. Patients with human immunodeficiency virus (HIV) are at increased risk for *Pneumocystis carinii* pneumonia (PCP) which is associated with significant morbidity and mortality. For this reason, prophylaxis is recommended. Which of the following is an appropriate drug for PCP prophylaxis?

    a. penicillin
    b. trimethoprim-sulfamethoxazole (Bactrim®)
    c. erythromycin
    d. zidovudine (Retrovir®)

_____130. Which physical finding in an elderly adult warrants further study?

    a. Symmetrically diminished Achilles tendon reflexes
    b. Gynecomastia in a male
    c. Facial hair on the chin of a female
    d. Dimpling in the right breast of a female

_____131. Anticipatory guidance for children 4 to 12 years-of-age should focus primarily on:

    a. infectious disease prevention.
    b. discipline.
    c. injury prevention.
    d. nutrition.

_____132. An 8-year-old female has been brought to the nurse practitioner on 5 occasions in the past 9 weeks with a complaint of abdominal pain. The evaluation each time is negative, but her mother is convinced the child is truly experiencing pain. The most likely diagnosis is:

    a. somatization disorder.
    b. recurrent abdominal pain.
    c. latent appendicitis.
    d. Munchausen by proxy syndrome.

_____133. The nurse practitioner assesses a 10-year-old who has never received any immunizations. Which immunization is *not* recommended from the first series for this patient?

    a. IPV
    b. Measles, mumps, rubella (MMR)
    c. Tetanus, diphtheria (Td)
    d. Influenza type b (Hib)

_____134. The Patient Self-Determination Act of 1991 requires all health care agencies receiving Medicare or Medicaid funds to give patients written information about their rights to make decisions regarding their medical care. A document which declares in advance what type of medical care a person wants to be provided or withheld, should he or she be unable to express his or her wishes, is called:

    a. an advance directive.
    b. a durable power of attorney.
    c. informed consent.
    d. a right to die statement.

_____135. Which of the following statements is true regarding asymptomatic bacteriuria in institutionalized older women?

    a. Treatment has not been shown to decrease mortality.
    b. Treatment has been shown to decrease morbidity.
    c. Screening should be done at least every 3 months.
    d. Treatment will usually eradicate the organisms.

_____136. A father brings his African-American child to the nurse practitioner because he wonders if it is normal for his 3-year-old to still have an umbilical hernia. The hernia is easily reducible and has not increased in size. What response by the nurse practitioner is correct?

    a. "This is a normal finding in your child. It will probably resolve before he is 5 years old."
    b. "This is a normal finding in your child. If it has not resolved in the next 6 months, he will be referred to a surgeon for repair."
    c. "This is an abnormal finding at his age. I will refer him to the surgeon of your choice."
    d. "This is an abnormal finding, but it will probably resolve by using an umbilical belt at night while he sleeps."

_____137. How early should fluoride be added to the diet of an infant whose water supply has inadequate fluoride?

    a. 2 weeks
    b. 2 months
    c. 6 months
    d. 1 year

_____138. Which of the following drugs has a beneficial effect on benign prostatic hyperplasia (BPH)?

    a. doxazosin (Cardura®)
    b. nifedipine (Procardia®)
    c. propranolol (Inderal®)
    d. nadolol (Corgard®)

_____139. A 30-year-old woman comes into a clinic with classic signs and symptoms of appendicitis. The nurse practitioner fails to refer the patient to a surgeon. The appendix ruptures and the woman dies. This is an example of:

    a. failure of diligence.
    b. professional liability.
    c. negligence.
    d. limited scope of practice.

_____140. A 68-year-old female presents with complaints of yellowed and thickened toenails. The nurse practitioner diagnoses onychomycosis and prescribes an oral antifungal agent. The patient asks "how long before this is cured." The nurse practitioner responds:

a. "about 3 to 4 weeks."
b. "about 2 to 3 months."
c. "about 6 months."
d. "probably 9 to 12 months."

_____141. Of the following characteristics, which are most closely associated with risk for becoming an abusive parent?

a. Older, following the example set by the previous generation
b. Young, isolated, with unreasonable expectations of the child
c. Working full time, feeling pressure to perform multiple duties
d. Single, working part time, living with parents, attending school

_____142. Which of the following has been shown to be most effective in the early treatment of Parkinson's disease?

a. carbidopa/levodopa (Sinemet®)
b. selegiline (Eldepryl®)
c. bromocriptine (Parlodel®)
d. amantadine (Symmetrel®)

_____143. A 55-year-old male presents for a routine health examination. After a thorough history, it is determined that the patient does not have any significant risk of developing clinical heart disease. Should an electrocardiogram (ECG) be included in the examination to screen for asymptomatic coronary artery disease (CAD)?

a. Yes, the patient's age places him in the early age category for development of CAD.
b. Yes, routine screening for all male patients should start at 50 years-of-age.
c. No, the Report of the U.S. Preventive Task Force does not recommend screening of asymptomatic men for CAD.
d. No, an ECG is only warranted if symptoms (e.g., chest pain, shortness of breath) develop.

____144. A significant barrier to treatment of depression in the elderly population is:

    a. the belief that depression is an inevitable part of aging.
    b. the serious side effects associated with antidepressant medications.
    c. the high rate of resistance to medications in this age group.
    d. poor patient compliance as a result of cognitive impairment.

____145. Criteria for the diagnosis of Alzheimer's disease include:

    a. metabolic derangements.
    b. slowing of brain wave activity on EEG.
    c. insidious and progressive decline of cognitive functions.
    d. significant disturbances of consciousness.

____146. During a sports physical on a 15-year-old, the nurse practitioner hears an S4 heart sound. The nurse practitioner should:

    a. refer the patient to a cardiologist.
    b. consider this a normal finding.
    c. recheck the patient in 1 to 3 months.
    d. assess the patient for fluid overload.

____147. Which of the following physical findings is consistent with a diagnosis of β-thalassemia major?

    a. Bronze skin color
    b. Expressionless facies
    c. Lymphadenopathy
    d. Extremity pain

____148. The most common cause of obesity is:

    a. lack of adequate exercise.
    b. medication that increases appetite or decreases metabolic rate.
    c. hypothyroid function.
    d. caloric intake which exceeds caloric expenditure.

____149. A common pathological finding in patients with asthma is:

    a. necrosis of small airways.
    b. absence of goblet cells.
    c. absence of ciliary regeneration.
    d. hypertrophy of smooth muscle.

_____150. A 16-year-old athlete complains of pain underneath his heel every time he walks. There is a verrucous surface level with the skin of the heel. What pharmacologic intervention(s) should the nurse practitioner prescribe for this patient?

    a. salicylic acid plasters
    b. NSAIDs and referral to a dermatologist
    c. hydrocortisone cream
    d. mupirocin (Bactroban®) ointment

Practice Exam I
Answers and Rationales

1. *c* *Herpes zoster* infection can be an indication of an immunocompromised host. With a history of IV drug use an HIV test is warranted.

2. *d* Stress incontinence is not associated with lower abdominal pain.

3. *a* The CAGE questions are about alcohol intake. Have you ever felt you should <u>C</u>ut down on drinking? Have people <u>A</u>nnoyed you by criticizing your drinking? Have you ever felt bad or <u>G</u>uilty about your drinking? Have you ever had a drink first thing in the morning to steady your nerves or to get rid of a hangover (<u>E</u>ye-opener)?

4. *d* Signs of congestive heart failure include presence of an S3 heart sound, unexplained weight gain, and crackles.

5. *b* Payment for services provided to Medicare recipients is divided into parts. Part A provides payment to hospitals for inpatient services. Part B pays those providers noted in *a, c,* and *d.*

6. *c* Symptoms usually abate within 3 days. A warm room, especially a humid bathroom, may make breathing more difficult for the child who is wheezing. Cool humidified air is easier to breathe for someone in respiratory distress. Alternation between acetaminophen and ibuprofen is not recommended by the American Academy of Pediatrics because of risk of medication errors.

7. *c* Inderal® is indicated for symptomatic relief of tachycardia secondary to cocaine overdose.

8. *a* Because back pain tends to recur, the most important patient teaching focus is how to prevent back injuries in the future. Muscle strengthening and flexibility exercises, safe lifting techniques, and a weight loss program will be most beneficial in preventing future injury.

9. *b* Gestational diabetes does not increase risk for placenta previa. Cephalopelvic disproportion, macrosomia, and maternal and neonatal hypoglycemia are all common complications of gestational diabetes.

10. *a* Serious consideration should be given to the presence of an underlying but undiagnosed disease (diabetes, HIV). Laboratory testing is directed at identifying an underlying cause. Referral to another provider may be indicated as part of this patient's plan of care.

11. *d* Metformin may be used concurrently with a sulfonylurea to improve glucose control and may be tried before instituting insulin therapy. Glipizide is a sulfonylurea and would not offer any additional benefit. A glitazone might also be considered.

12. *a* A Heberden's node is enlargement of the distal interphalangeal joint (DIP). It is rarely seen in any other condition except osteoarthritis (OA).

13. *d* Since he was asymptomatic for 6 weeks, it is likely that the initial infection cleared and there were no live mites remaining. However, he was probably re-infected from contaminated clothes, bed linens, or other personal items. Decontamination and re-treatment is indicated.

14. *c* Cluster headaches are characterized by sudden onset of severe common unilateral headache. They most commonly occur in males in their thirties. Cluster headaches typically last less than 3 hours. They are aborted with inhaled nasal oxygen or triptans.

15. *d* Periorbital cellulitis signals an emergent condition which may warrant hospitalization and intravenous antibiotics. This patient is diabetic which contributes to his high risk status and possible difficult treatment course.

16. *c* Diarrhea without systemic symptoms and fever should resolve in 3 days. If it does not, laboratory studies and further testing may be necessary to identify the causative organism.

17. *b* There is usually no detectable genital injury in children, who have been sexually abused.

18. *a* Growing pains, typical in 3 to 5-year-old children, present at night and do not involve joints. They are usually bilateral and intermittent. Acetaminophen along with heat and massage at bedtime may be helpful.

19. *d* Patients with unstable angina require urgent care.

20. *b* Some infants may sit unassisted at 6 months, however, others may not sit without support until about 8 or 9 months-of-age. The nurse practitioner should assess other developmental achievements typical of 4 month olds.

21. *a* Presence of hepatitis B surface antigen at this time indicates chronic infection with hepatitis B. Lab studies indicating positive surface antigen on 2 separate occasions at least 6 months apart indicate chronic infection. Vaccination produces positive hepatitis B antibodies. Hepatitis B surface antigen would not be present in a person who has recovered from hepatitis B infection. This case would not be an acute episode because of the history of hepatitis B infection 2 years prior.

22. *c*   Timolol and propranolol are both β-blockers and may potentiate each other. This could precipitate bradycardia or hypotension.

23. *b*   Koilonychia ("spoon nail") occurs because of thinning of the nail plate. This can be caused by iron deficiency anemia or local exposure to irritants.

24. *c*   Transmission of the blood-borne AIDS virus occurs through a) sexual intercourse with an infected person, male or female, b) contact with items contaminated with blood, and/or c) from a mother to her newborn during pregnancy, delivery, or while breastfeeding. The virus has been isolated in semen, vaginal secretions, blood, saliva, and tears. There are no documented cases of transmission other than the ways listed.

25. *a*   Clotrimazole cream is a topical medication which is not absorbed systemically. The other choices are pregnancy category C or D drugs.

26. *a*   In approximately 70% of cases, neither cause(s) nor risk factors can be identified as correlates to cerebral palsy.

27. *c*   Oral acyclovir or other oral antiviral agents are treatments of choice for primary and recurrent *herpes simplex II* infection. Primary infection may be treated with 200 mg 5 times per day for 7 to 10 days or 400 mg TID for 7-10 days. Recurrent infections may be treated with 400 mg TID for 5 days. Topical acyclovir has not been found to be as effective as oral treatment. Burrow's solution and nonsteroidal anti-inflammatory drugs are used for symptom management.

28. *b*   The patient's age, gender, recent loss of spouse, and hopelessness about the future are all risk factors for suicide. When a patient exhibits risk factors, the nurse practitioner must explore whether the patient is actually considering suicide and if he has a plan.

29. *a*   Diabetic retinopathy is rare before puberty, and in patients who have had diabetes mellitus for less than 5 years. However, the American Diabetes Association recommends a dilated exam at the time of diagnosis, annually, and any time there is a vision problem.

30. *a*   Drugs that readily penetrate prostate membranes, have demonstrated high prostatic fluid levels, and have good gram negative coverage are preferred for treatment of chronic prostatitis. Ciprofloxacin and trimethoprim-sulfamethoxazole meet these criteria.

31. *b*   Growth of the testes and scrotum occurs in both Tanner stages 2 and 3, but enlargement of the penis occurs primarily in stage 3.

32. *b* The personal best value is the highest PEFR measurement value that an individual has achieved. It provides the most accurate comparison. If personal best is not available, predicted ranges for height may be used.

33. *d* Topical estrogen cream or oral estrogen therapy may be used for atrophic vaginitis associated with menopause. With this patient's history of breast cancer, topical estrogen is a safer choice.

34. *b* Traditionally, mothers who would be 35 years-of-age or older at the time of delivery were considered candidates for prenatal diagnosis. With advances in technologies, the risk of pregnancy loss has decreased. Thus, prenatal diagnosis is currently offered to mothers who would be 33 years-of-age at the time of delivery.

35. *b* Hydrocele is a very common finding in an infant. It should resolve by 6 months-of-age. If it is still present at 6 months, the infant should be referred for possible surgical repair.

36. *a* Atopic dermatitis is a familial disorder with unknown etiology. It is intensely pruritic. In infants it presents on the cheeks, forehead, scalp, trunk or extremities. It is often associated with asthma and allergy.

37. *c* A rubella titer > 1:10 indicates immunity. That is, mother and fetus are protected from rubella infection even after recent exposure.

38. *c* Amylase is produced by the pancreas and salivary glands. A diagnosis of pancreatitis can be made with a high degree of certainty from an elevated serum amylase level and can be ruled out with a normal level.

39. *b* Barotrauma in infants secondary to mechanical ventilation increases risk of bronchopulmonary dysplasia (BPD). The other items are not causes of BPD.

40. *d* Glycosylation of hemoglobin occurs throughout the life of an RBC (about 90 to 120 days). It is not indicative of recent changes in blood sugar levels. HbA_{1C} reflects average hemoglobin glycosylation for the past 1 to 3 months. HbA_{1C} of 12% means the average glucose exceeds 300 mg/dl.

41. *c* Nurse practitioner certification is conferred by professional bodies such as the American Nurses Credentialing Center (ANCC) and the American Academy of Nurse Practitioners (AANP). Licensure is conferred by individual states.

42. *a* Endometriosis commonly presents with deep pelvic pain, particularly during sexual intercourse.

43. *a* Mean corpuscular volume (MCV) is helpful in the differentiation of macrocytic, microcytic, and normocytic anemias.

44. *b* A glycosylated hemoglobin value reflects the average serum glucose for the past 60 to 90 days. It is an excellent tool to evaluate overall glucose control in diabetic patients. Avoidance of diabetic complications as a result of prolonged hyperglycemia is the best long term measure of the patient's glucose control.

45. *c* By 45 years-of-age, the lens becomes more rigid and the ciliary muscle of the iris becomes weaker. These ocular changes, termed presbyopia, cause diminished near vision.

46. *c* Tympanometry is non-invasive, readily available, and an easily interpreted tool to document the presence of fluid in the middle ear.

47. *d* Information from the sexual history can improve screening strategies, but the most sensitive and specific test is direct culture. DNA probe and enzyme immunoassay are less accurate. A lone finding of leukocyte esterase in urine indicates nonspecific urethritis.

48. *b* Anticholinergics such as ipratropium are very effective in the treatment of emphysema. Epinephrine, cromolyn, and zafirlukast do not have a role in the treatment of emphysema.

49. *d* The 3 leading causes of morbidity and mortality are cardiovascular disease, cancer, and osteoporosis. Routine screenings should be directed toward these diseases.

50. *c* An inhaled β_2-agonist administered 20 to 30 minutes before exercise is the treatment of choice for exercise-induced asthma.

51. *a* Secondary prevention is early diagnosis and treatment of a disease that is already present.

52. *b* The dying patient often gives subtle clues that he wishes to discuss death. It is appropriate to pursue such comments.

53. *c* Avoidance of all methylxanthines (e.g., coffee, tea, chocolate) has been shown to reduce breast pain in women with fibrocystic breast disease. It is usually a benign condition, not a precursor of malignancy. Mammography is recommended once at age 35 years, at least every 1 to 2 years after age 40 years, and then annually beginning at 50 years-of age. Oral contraceptives may help reduce cyclical pain and swelling.

54. *b* Innocent (functional) heart murmur is a common clinical finding in children 3 to 7 years-of-age. Thrill is only present with heart murmurs graded IV-VI/VI. Heart murmurs which occur in diastole and have associated radiation of sound, thrill, and/or cyanosis indicate pathology and require immediate referral.

55. *c* High risk infants include African-Americans, those living in poverty, immigrants from developing countries, preterm and low birth weight babies, and infants who are fed cow's milk exclusively.

56. *a* Primary prevention consists of activities that decrease the probability of occurrence of specific illness. Folic acid 1 mg daily during pregnancy decreases the likelihood of fetal neural tube defects.

57. *c* The National Cholesterol Education Program guidelines for treatment of hypercholesterolemia recommend dietary therapy for persons without coronary heart disease with less than 2 risk factors and whose low density lipoproteins are < 160 mg/dL.

58. *b* Coarctation of the aorta is a pinching or narrowing of the aortic lumen which occurs during fetal development. This condition is characterized by upper extremity hypertension and lower extremity hypotension. It is assessed by palpating the brachial and femoral arteries simultaneously and comparing the intensity of each. If femoral pulses are diminished, delayed or absent, coarctation of the aorta should be suspected.

59. *b* The most common cause of hyperthyroidism is Graves' disease. The body's tissues are exposed to an increased level of circulating thyroid hormone. As a result, there is an excessive metabolic rate in all of the body's tissues characterized by this patient's classic symptoms.

60. *a* The first phase of therapy for gastroesophageal reflux disease (GERD) in the adult is lifestyle and diet modifications plus an antacid or over-the-counter H_2-blocker.

61. *d* This 2-year-old has roseola, a human herpes virus. Since the fever has resolved and the rash will last another day or two, no pharmacologic intervention is needed. Fluids should be encouraged because there may be some residual dehydration from the 3 days of fever.

62. *a* Papilledema represents swelling of the optic disc. It is associated with increased intracranial pressure, not diabetes.

63. *a* It is important to cleanse the skin with water and let it dry completely at each diaper change and prior to applying the medication.

64. *b* Good periorbital hygiene should prevent recurrence of the hordeolum.

65. *a* Research shows that low birth weight infants born to disadvantaged families, who received sensory stimulation in the nursery and throughout the first year of life, perform better on intelligence tests at the end of the first year.

66. *b* Patients with acute anxiety need a medication that is fast-acting. The action of buspirone is delayed. Paroxetine is indicated for GAD (generalized anxiety disorder) and imipramine is a TCA with sedation as a side effect. Neither are indicated for acute anxiety.

67. *b* Most guidelines for outpatient treatment of pneumonia in non-smokers, without comorbidity and 60 years-of-age or younger, recommend erythromycin or another macrolide. Penicillin is indicated for patients with pneumococcal pneumonia and ciprofloxacin is recommended for the *Legionella* species.

68. *b* Anticonvulsants are rarely indicated in febrile seizures. Prevention by fever reduction is usually accomplished with acetaminophen or ibuprofen. Aspirin should not be given to children with febrile illnesses due to the association with Reye's syndrome.

69. *d* Vasovagal syncope, or the common faint, occurs only when the patient is seated or standing. Typical symptoms are those described in the question. Orthostatic hypotension occurs immediately on rising to sitting or standing.

70. *a* The Schilling test is ordered to assist with diagnosis of pernicious anemia, a macrocytic anemia. The other tests would not be helpful to differentiate a macrocytic type of anemia.

71. *b* Plummer's disease is a form of hyperthyroidism due to a single hyper-functioning (hot nodule) thyroid adenoma. Approximately half of the cases of hyperthyroidism in adults over 60 years-of-age are due to multinodular goiter (which may have been previously present, but euthyroid, for years). Thyrotoxicosis, also referred to as "thyroid storm," is a potentially fatal complication of excess thyroid hormone production.

72. *d* Such activities help the child develop a healthy sense of industry and independence and allow the child to talk and participate in a group.

73. *a* *Giardia lamblia* is the leading parasitic cause of diarrhea in the United States. Contaminated water supplies are the usual source. Symptoms of giardiasis include abdominal cramping, diarrhea, and greasy stools.

74. *c* Steps in the patient history are introductory information (including name, age, gender, source and reliability), chief complaint, history of present illness, past medical history, family history, social history, review of systems, and conclusion(s).

75. *a* Thalassemias are a group of inherited disorders which lead to deficient hemoglobin synthesis. They typically present in persons from the Mediterranean region, Southeast Asia, and the Middle East.

76. *d* Bone marrow examination will show infiltration of blast cells in leukemia which is indicative of acute lymphocytic leukemia (ALL).

77. *c* One of the most important principles of geriatric medicine is that there may be an altered presentation of disease. Symptoms exhibited may not be typical of the organ system involved.

78. *a* The most common recurrent headache in children is migraine. There is a positive family history in 75% of cases.

79. *a* Before initiating any procedure or treatment, women of reproductive age should be evaluated for pregnancy. The intervention may be deleterious to a developing fetus.

80. *d* Alcohol is the most commonly used psychoactive substance in the United States today. It is used by about 90% of adolescents by age 16 years. Motor vehicle accidents related to driving under the influence of alcohol are the leading cause of death in the 15 to 24 year age group.

81. *b* A finding of Reed-Sternberg cells is diagnostic for Hodgkin's lymphoma.

82. *b* A wick is used to facilitate passage of the antibiotic into the canal. The child or parent should place the antibiotic drops on the wick positioned in the canal by the practitioner. The wick will fall out spontaneously as swelling resolves.

83. *c* The vaccination takes 2 to 3 weeks to provide immunity and generally protects for 5 to 6 months.

84. *c* A cataract opacity is seen as a dark disruption of the red reflex on ophthalmoscopic exam.

85. *c* Clinical trials suggest that heart disease mortality rates in the United States could be lowered by 5 to 20% if all Americans restricted their fat intake to less than 30% of total daily calories, < 7 % from saturated fat.

86. *b* Percussion or palpation may change intestinal motility; therefore, auscultation should be performed first to yield a more accurate assessment of the patient's "normal" bowel sounds at the moment.

87. *a* Long term glucocorticoid therapy may cause Cushing's syndrome, hyperglycemia, bone loss, and/or hypokalemia.

88. *a* The Centers for Disease Control and Prevention (CDC) recommends, and most states require by law, the prophylactic administration of silver nitrate or an ophthalmic antibiotic ointment such as tetracycline or erythromycin within 1 hour of delivery to protect against gonococcal ophthalmia neonatorum.

89. *d* Anxiety, nervousness, tremor, atrial fibrillation and tachycardia, anorexia, frequent stools or diarrhea, and weight loss are characteristic findings associated with hyperthyroidism. Generally, signs and symptoms associated with hypothyroidism are decreases in functioning.

90. *a* Malignancy of the prostate gland causes the gland to feel hard. In prostatitis, the prostate gland feels boggy. The normal prostate gland feels rubbery.

91. *a* Skills training and apprehension are significant factors affecting outcomes of tests of cognitive abilities. Elderly adults do not lose their verbal abilities. The sixth decade has been found to be the most significant period of cognitive decline.

92. *a* When initiated early, within 48 hours of the appearance of rash, antivirals are effective in relieving symptoms and speeding resolution of rash.

93. *b* Tetracyclines are extensively incorporated into bones and teeth and, if given during the period of enamel formation, may cause tooth discoloration. The risk extends from the 4th month of gestation to 8 years-of-age, at which time the enamel has completely formed in all but the third molars.

94. *d* Developmental assessment of the neonate must begin with the determination of gestational age. All findings must be interpreted in relation to gestational age.

95. *a* Alendronate has been approved for the treatment of osteoporosis.

96. *d* Inversion injuries are far more common than eversion injuries. Eversion accounts for only about 10% of ankle sprains.

97. *d* According to the Centers for Disease Control and Prevention (CDC), 50% of premature mortality in the United States is due to lifestyle, 20% to human biology, and 10% to health care.

98. *b* Any palpable breast lump with these characteristics should be biopsied regardless of mammography findings.

99. *b* Although his vocation involves sedentary activity, this patient is not at great risk for osteoarthritis (OA). However, Heberden's nodes are associated with OA. Rheumatoid arthritis (RA) is characterized by several joint deformities, usually bilaterally symmetrical. RA is characterized by inflammatory processes, while OA is not. RA and OA are chronic conditions. Gout is characterized by acute exacerbations related to a defect in purine metabolism, increased uric acid production, or decreased uric acid excretion.

100. *c* For immunosuppressed patients and the elderly, antiviral therapy is recommended when the patient presents within 72 hours of the onset of symptoms. Acyclovir, famciclovir, or valacyclovir are the oral drugs of choice. NSAIDs are used for their analgesic effect in the acute phase, and capsaicin cream is used for post-herpetic neuralgia.

101. *d* A common finding in hyperthyroidism is atrial fibrillation. A beta-adrenergic blocker will treat the atrial fibrillation and help control the anxiety and nervousness associated with uncontrolled hyperthyroidism. A thyroid scan with radio opaque iodine will reveal any thyroid nodule (seen as a "hot spot"). The patient may require medical ablation or surgical removal of the thyroid gland, so referral to an endocrinologist is indicated.

102. *a* Diethylstilbestrol (DES) exposure of females in utero increases their risk for vaginal cancer. DES exposure of males in utero increases their risk of infertility.

103. *c* There is exquisite point tenderness when a stress fracture is palpated. With early stress fracture, x-ray may be negative. A bone scan is usually definitive, but expensive.

104. *c* Children with systemic and polyarticular JRA should have an annual ophthalmological examination. Those with pauciarticular JRA should be examined 4 times per year.

105. *b* Factors found to be associated with early sexual activity are lower socioeconomic status, use of tobacco, alcohol, or other drugs, and belonging to a single parent household.

106. *d* The introduction of solid foods should be based on readiness of the infant, but not before 4 to 6 months-of-age. Cereals should be offered first (specifically rice cereal), then fruits. One food at a time should be introduced, to observe for allergy or intolerance before introducing another.

107. *b* If there is an uncertain history of tetanus prophylaxis, a Td should be administered now.

108. *a* Cryptorchidism, even with surgical repair, is associated with increased risk for testicular cancer.

109. *a* Balanitis is an inflammation of the glans penis and prepuce. This may be caused by an infectious or a noninfectious agent. A predisposing factor is diabetes mellitus.

110. *a* Smoking is associated with an increased risk of invasive cervical cancer. Women who were sexually active at an early age and with multiple sex partners have increased risk of developing cervical cancer. The use of barrier contraceptives and increased dietary intake of vitamin C are associated with a decreased risk of cervical cancer.

111. *b* Lesions that are less than 5 millimeters, flat, with regular borders and even color, are not suspicious for malignancy. This patient should be reassured.

112. *a* A mucopurulent discharge may suggest a bacterial infection. This patient needs an antibiotic in the form of topical drops. Although complications are rare, corneal damage can occur as the infection spreads beyond the conjunctiva.

113. *d* Because anti-thyroid drugs block the synthesis of thyroid hormone but do not interrupt the release of stored hormone, clinical improvement is delayed for 2 to 3 weeks. A euthyroid state can be expected in 4 to 6 weeks.

114. *b* Most cases of Meniere's disease are idiopathic and diagnosis is based on exclusion of other pathologies. Central vertigo is present with many vestibular problems. Low frequency hearing loss is more commonly associated with Meniere's disease. MRI is helpful to rule out acoustic neuroma, but not to diagnose Meniere's disease.

115. *c* Follow up with repeat stools for ova, cysts, and parasites should be planned for 3 to 4 weeks after symptoms have abated.

116. *b* Pender's Health Promotion Model emphasizes importance of the individual's perception about the benefits of health promoting behavior.

117. *c* Beta-blockers may mask the peripheral signs of hypoglycemia like jitteriness and tachycardia. However, beta-blockers will not mask diaphoresis. Therefore, diabetics on beta-blockers should be taught to look for this specific symptom as a possible indication of hypoglycemia.

118. *d* A diet free of red meat is recommended for 72 hours prior to testing stool for occult blood to decrease the incidence of false positive. Vitamin C rich foods should be avoided also.

119. *c* Patients with varicose veins should be taught to avoid long periods of standing to reduce venous pooling. Massaging the legs is of no benefit. Elevating the head of the bed promotes venous pooling, not venous return. Support stockings should be applied in the morning before lowering the legs from the bed.

120. *b* A prevention program must be shaped to fit the cultural and health profile of the population. Long-range prevention goals should be combined with measures to meet immediate needs.

121. *d* Antacid use decreases digoxin absorption which results in decreased serum level and reduced clinical effect.

122. *d* Amoxicillin is one of the drugs recommended as prophylaxis prior to surgery or procedures when there is a history of rheumatic fever or valvular disease.

123. *b* Ego integrity is the coming together of all previous phases of the life cycle. Without a sense of ego integrity the person may feel a sense of self-disgust.

124. *c* If 2 pills are missed on consecutive days, the next 2 days' dosage should be doubled and a barrier method recommended for the remainder of the cycle.

125. *b* Screening for elevated lead level at least once at 12 months-of-age is recommended for children at increased risk for lead exposure. If capillary blood is used, elevated lead levels should be confirmed with a venous sample. Correlates of high lead levels include minority race, central city residence, low income, low education level, and residence in the northeast region of the United States.

126. *a* The initial step in management of encopresis is patient and family education. Successful outcome is dependent on family understanding of the condition. It is essential that the family not blame or chastise the child.

127. *a* Warm moist compresses may provide some relief from pain and promote drainage. If the furuncle is not draining, topical antibiotic ointments are of no benefit.

128. *a* The American Cancer Society recommends an annual digital rectal examination (DRE) for prostate cancer beginning at age 40 years. Annual examination of men age 50 years and older should include a serum prostate specific antigen (PSA). The best approach is to screen with DRE and PSA. ACS recommends screening only for men with a life expectancy greater than 10 years.

129. *b* Trimethoprim-sulfamethoxazole, aerosolized pentamidine, or dapsone are indicated for *Pneumocystis carinii* pneumonia (PCP) prophylaxis in HIV-positive patients.

130. *d* All of these could be normal findings in elderly adults except choice *d*. Any dimpling, mass, or discharge from the breast should be explored regardless of the patient's age. The incidence of breast cancer increases with age and mortality increases with delayed detection and treatment.

131. *c* The leading cause of death and disability in children is motor vehicle accident. Fire and burns, firearms, drowning, bicycle injury, and poisoning also contribute significantly to accidental injury and death.

132. *b* Recurrent abdominal pain is defined as at least 3 episodes of abdominal pain over a 3 month period. The physical examination is normal. Explanation of the condition and reassurance is given to the parent.

133. *d* When a child is > 7 years old at the time of first visit for immunizations, the recommended vaccinations are the HBV series, Td, IPV, MMR.

134. *a* Some examples of treatment directives are living will, durable power of attorney for health care directives, and declaration of desire for natural death.

135. *a* Treatment of asymptomatic bacteriuria in institutionalized older adults has not been shown to decrease morbidity or mortality, or to lead to periods without bacteriuria. There are no recommendations for screening elderly institutionalized women.

136. *a* Umbilical hernias are a common finding in children under 2 years-of-age. In African-American children, the hernia may be present up to 7 years-of-age.

137. *c* Infants younger than 6 months-of-age should not receive fluoride supplementation. This includes breastfed babies. These are American Dental Association recommendations.

138. *a* Doxazosin, an α-1-adrenergic blocker, is indicated for relief of obstruction caused by prostatic hyperplasia. It does not decrease blood pressure in a normotensive patient.

139. *c* Negligence is the failure of an individual to do something that a reasonable person would do that results in injury to another.

140. *d* Length of treatment depends on rate of growth of the nail. Treatment is usually 1 to 3 months for fingernails, 3 to 6 months for toenails. The time for new nail growth is longer than the treatment period.

141. *b* Typically, the abuser manifests the following characteristics: young, emotionally unstable, inadequately mothered, isolated, ignorant of child development, having been a victim of abuse, low self-esteem, expects the child to be perfect, and/or perceives the child as different.

142. *c* The dopamine agonists (such as Parlodel®) are recommended as first-line drugs for treatment of Parkinson's disease because they are thought to be neuroprotective.

143. *c* *The Guide to Clinical Preventive Services, a Report of the U.S. Preventive Services Task Force*, does not recommend screening with electrocardiogram (ECG) for asymptomatic men or women. Routine screening should be based on patient history, patient risk factors, and likelihood of development of coronary artery disease based on patient risk factors.

144. *a* Only 10% of elderly adults who suffer from depression receive treatment. This is largely because many health care providers and elderly patients mistakenly believe depression is an inevitable and normal result of aging.

145. *c* There are 6 clinical assessment criteria for the probable diagnosis of Alzheimer's disease. These are dementia, deficits in 2 or more areas of cognition, progressive worsening of memory and other cognitive functions, no disturbance of consciousness, onset between the ages of 40 and 90 years, and absence of a systemic disorder which may account for the deficits.

146. *b* An S4 in children and adolescents is a common normal finding. In patients older than age 30 years, this finding might indicate a "stiff" ventricle, an abnormal finding.

147. *a* Persons with β-thalassemia major have a peculiar skin color, usually described as "bronze," caused by icterus, pallor, and increased melanin deposits. Enlargement of the malar bones often give a characteristic appearance, but elongation is not present. Lymphadenopathy and extremity pain have no known association with β-thalassemia major.

148. *d* Dietary practice is clearly the usual cause of obesity. Other less common causes are hypothalamic injury, hypothyroidism, Cushing's syndrome, gonadal failure, medication, and genetic syndromes.

149. *d* Histological findings in patients with long-standing asthma demonstrate hypertrophy of bronchial smooth muscle, hyperplastic vessels, and thickening of the basement membrane. These changes are brought about because of chronic inflammation in the bronchial branches.

150. *a* This patient has a plantar wart, an epidermal tumor caused by a virus. Daily or every other day application of a salicylic acid plaster will help to remove a large part of the wart. Rubbing with a pumice stone will help remove a large part and also give this patient some pain relief. Total length of treatment is usually 6 to 8 weeks.

Practice Exam II

_____ 1. An obese patient presents with intertrigo under her breasts. The nurse practitioner prescribes an antifungal cream and encourages her to:

   a. return if there is no improvement in 1 month.
   b. change her brassiere at least twice per day.
   c. expose the intertriginous areas to light and air 3 times a day.
   d. wear her bra to bed.

_____ 2. A 25-year-old complains of fever and throat pain. The tonsils have exudate bilaterally. The patient describes having an anaphylactic reaction to penicillin in the past. What antibiotic should the nurse practitioner prescribe if she believes the causative agent is bacterial?

   a. amoxicillin (Amoxil®)
   b. erythromycin
   c. cefadroxil monohydrate (Duricef®)
   d. ceftriaxone (Rocephin®)

_____ 3. A 17-year-old female presents with painful vesicular lesions on her vulva. Which of the following would be the most definitive diagnostic test?

   a. KOH prep
   b. Tzanck prep
   c. Gram stain
   d. Pap smear

_____ 4. Educating parents to avoid putting their children to bed with a baby bottle:

   a. helps to prevent tooth decay.
   b. decreases the incidence of "crib death."
   c. prevents babies from becoming overweight.
   d. prevents infantile colic.

_____ 5. Patients with benign prostatic hyperplasia (BPH) should be taught to avoid which one of the following drug classes?

   a. α-1-adrenergic antagonists
   b. Anti-androgen agents
   c. Tricyclic antidepressants (TCAs)
   d. Sulfonamides

_____ 6. A 6-year-old patient presents to the nurse practitioner's health clinic with a 1 x 1 inch honey-colored crust on his right shin. The nurse practitioner diagnoses impetigo. Following debridement with soap and water, the most appropriate pharmacological treatment is:

    a. cephalexin 250 mg orally 4 times a day for 7-10 days.
    b. mupirocin (Bactroban®) ointment applied to the lesion 2-3 times a day for 10 days.
    c. ciprofloxacin (Cipro®) 500 mg orally 2 times a day for 10 days.
    d. miconazole nitrate (Monistat®) ointment applied to the lesion 4 times a day for 10 days.

_____ 7. A 60-year-old patient is screened for hypercholesterolemia. His total cholesterol is 250 mg/dL. What should the nurse practitioner do next?

    a. Recommend a fasting lipid profile.
    b. Refer the patient to a cardiologist for further evaluation.
    c. Prescribe a lipid-lowering agent.
    d. Recommend a diet with fat content < 10% of total calories.

_____ 8. Risk factors for elder abuse do *not* include:

    a. dependency.
    b. mental impairment.
    c. age 65 to 70 years.
    d. lower socioeconomic group.

_____ 9. An 8-year-old is sent home from school with a mucopurulent discharge from his eye. He is brought to the nurse practitioner for treatment. What is the most appropriate intervention?

    a. Cromolyn sodium ophthalmic solution (Opticrom®) for 4 days
    b. Doxycycline (Vibramycin®) orally for 10 days
    c. Bacitracin/polymyxin (Polysporin®) ophthalmic solution for 7 to 10 days
    d. No pharmacologic intervention is needed because the condition will resolve quickly without treatment

_____ 10. Patients who have been diagnosed with malignant melanoma should be taught:

    a. that only raised lesions need to be evaluated.
    b. to have a skin examination every 2 years.
    c. to conduct weekly skin self-examination.
    d. that a topical anti-neoplastic agent is the treatment of choice.

_____ 11. For which patient group does the U.S. Preventive Services Task Force recommend routine screening for asymptomatic bacteriuria?

    a. Pregnant women
    b. Children
    c. Patients with diabetes
    d. Patients over 70 years-of-age

_____ 12. When prescribing an iron supplement for a child, it is *most* important to tell the mother:

    a. the best time to give the iron is in between meals.
    b. to keep this and all other medications out of the reach of children.
    c. to watch for constipation.
    d. that iron may stain the teeth.

_____ 13. The nurse practitioner examines a 2 month old with unequal gluteal and thigh skin folds. What should the nurse practitioner do next?

    a. Send the infant for x-rays of the hips.
    b. Send the infant for ultrasound of the hips.
    c. Perform Ortolani and Barlow tests.
    d. Examine the infant for unequal arm length.

_____ 14. Which of the following would the nurse practitioner *not* recommend to the parents of a child with asthma?

    a. Eliminate air conditioning in the child's room.
    b. Encase the child's mattress in a sealed vinyl cover.
    c. Remove carpeting from the child's bedroom.
    d. Do not allow smoking in the home.

_____ 15. A mother complains that her 3 month old infant becomes constipated easily. She states she has been using the 4-year-old sibling's suppositories, but they make the baby "fussy" and have diarrhea stools. The nurse practitioner should recommend:

    a. obtaining a stool specimen to check for an infectious process.
    b. adding 1 to 2 teaspoons of corn syrup to the infant's bottle twice a day.
    c. obtaining stool for ova, cysts, and parasites.
    d. cutting the suppository in half.

_____ 16. A 45-year-old female in good health complains of "pink-tinged" urine. There is no costovertebral angle tenderness and vaginal exam is unremarkable. Urinalysis demonstrates alkaline urine and positive nitrite and leukocyte esterase. The most likely diagnosis is:

    a. kidney stone.
    b. a sexually transmitted disease (STD).
    c. bladder neoplasm.
    d. urinary tract infection (UTI).

_____ 17. A 54-year-old female's blood pressure is 145/95 mmHg during a routine annual evaluation. She has no previous history of hypertension. Appropriate management of this patient would be to:

    a. recheck the blood pressure within 8 weeks.
    b. start the patient on diuretic therapy.
    c. start the patient on lifestyle modifications.
    d. order an electrocardiogram (ECG).

_____ 18. In the United States, occupational licensure is a responsibility of:

    a. the states.
    b. state and local governments, cooperatively.
    c. the federal government.
    d. national professional organizations.

_____ 19. An asymptomatic 4-year-old has developmental delays. The child lives with his parents in a home that is 35 years old. The child's parents make ceramics in their home workshop for extra income. What tests should the nurse practitioner order?

    a. Complete blood count (CBC) and lead level
    b. Evaluation of Intelligence Quotient
    c. Erythrocyte sedimentation rate (ESR) and urinalysis (UA)
    d. CBC, blood urea nitrogen (BUN), and serum creatinine

_____ 20. A 20-year-old male complains of a "skin rash" on his knees and elbows. The lesions have silvery scales and are pruritic. A positive Auspitz sign is present. What is the most likely diagnosis?

    a. Eczema
    b. Lichen planus
    c. Tinea corporis
    d. Psoriasis

21. A 10-year-old female's mean corpuscular volume (MCV) is 73 fl. What type anemia would the nurse practitioner suspect?

    a. Folate deficiency
    b. Vitamin B-12 deficiency
    c. Iron deficiency
    d. Reticulocytosis

22. What is the most common cardiac defect presenting in childhood?

    a. Patent ductus arteriosus (PDA)
    b. Tetralogy of Fallot
    c. Ventricular septal defect (VSD)
    d. Tricuspid atresia

23. A 50-year-old male patient complains of a 2 month history of hearing loss in his left ear. The nurse practitioner notes absence of canal obstruction and hearing loss in both ears. Physical exam is normal. Which of the following actions by the nurse practitioner is most appropriate?

    a. Consult an otolaryngologist.
    b. Refer the patient to an audiologist.
    c. Reassure him that this is a normal part of aging.
    d. Re-evaluate the patient in 4 weeks.

24. The nurse practitioner assesses an asymptomatic 43-year-old male and determines that he is at minimal risk for a myocardial infarction (MI). The patient asks whether he would benefit from taking aspirin 325 mg every day to prevent an MI. What should the nurse practitioner recommend?

    a. "Take a daily aspirin because it will decrease your overall risk of death and prevent any complications from heart attack."
    b. "Take a daily aspirin because there are numerous studies which support that people who do not have heart symptoms benefit from one aspirin per day."
    c. "It is not necessary to take a daily aspirin as there is insufficient evidence at this time for primary prevention of heart attack in people without heart symptoms."
    d. "Do not take a daily aspirin until you reach 55 years-of-age."

_____ 25. Practitioners working with physically active girls need to be aware of the "female athlete triad" in order to develop an effective plan for prevention, recognition, and treatment. The components of the female athlete triad are:

    a. distorted body image, low self-esteem, and generalized anxiety.
    b. stress fractures, osteoarthritis, and plantar fasciitis.
    c. eating disorder, amenorrhea, and osteoporosis.
    d. iron deficiency anemia, steroid abuse, and bradycardia.

_____ 26. A 78-year-old female is suspected of having renal failure. Which of the following is the best diagnostic test to assess the patient's renal function?

    a. Blood urea nitrogen (BUN)
    b. Serum creatinine
    c. A 24 hour creatinine clearance
    d. Serum uric acid

_____ 27. Screening for increased intraocular pressure or early glaucoma is:

    a. recommended annually beginning at 40 years-of-age.
    b. indicated only if symptoms such as eye pain or blurred vision are noted.
    c. best performed by an eye specialist.
    d. part of the routine physical examination of an adult.

_____ 28. The nurse practitioner must increase a patient's dosage of theophylline to achieve a therapeutic level. After the dosage has been increased, serum theophylline level should be checked:

    a. in about 7 to 10 days.
    b. before breakfast in 14 days.
    c. just prior to the fifth dose.
    d. anytime before the next office visit.

_____ 29. Which of the following therapies is appropriate for initial treatment of an 8 week old infant diagnosed with gastroesophageal reflux (GER)?

    a. Smaller and more frequent feedings thickened with rice cereal
    b. Cimetidine (Tagamet®) orally every 8 hours
    c. Change to a soy formula
    d. Left lateral position after feedings

____ 30. A patient requests information about foods to include in his diet while vacationing in Mexico to avoid "Montezuma's revenge." The nurse practitioner should advise him to ingest only:

   a. milk, cooked vegetables, and pasta salad.
   b. fresh fruits, fish, and local cuisine in restaurants.
   c. eggs, increased fluids, and tortillas.
   d. cooked vegetables in soup, bottled water, and wine.

____ 31. A 15-year-old female reports she is a strict vegetarian. Which of the following is the most appropriate response by the nurse practitioner?

   a. "Include a wide variety of legumes, enriched grains, nuts, and seeds in your diet."
   b. "It is impossible for anyone to get adequate nutrients from a strict vegetarian diet."
   c. "You should eat fish at least 3 to 4 times a week."
   d. "Consume as many dairy products as possible."

____ 32. On examination, a 67-year-old patient is noted to have high-tone hearing loss. This finding is consistent with what diagnosis?

   a. Otosclerosis
   b. Cerumen impaction
   c. Presbycusis
   d. Conductive hearing loss

____ 33. In which choice below is alkaline phosphatase (ALP) most likely normal (and not elevated)?

   a. adolescents and children.
   b. pregnant women in the third trimester.
   c. Paget's disease.
   d. nephrotic syndrome.

____ 34. When discussing treatment options with a patient, the nurse practitioner would be correct to say that surgery can be curative for:

   a. ulcerative colitis.
   b. irritable bowel syndrome (IBS).
   c. Crohn's disease.
   d. inflammatory bowel disease.

_____ 35. The most effective prevention of skin cancer is to educate the public about:

    a. using tanning parlors as opposed to natural sun tanning.
    b. the ABCD of melanoma recognition.
    c. periodic skin self-examination.
    d. limiting exposure to natural solar radiation.

_____ 36. An anxious parent brings her 3-day-old female infant to see the nurse practitioner because of a serosanguineous vaginal discharge. The nurse practitioner tells the mother:

    a. this is a normal finding in female newborns.
    b. a vaginal exam is necessary.
    c. the discharge should be cultured for bacteria.
    d. the discharge should be checked for occult blood.

_____ 37. A 64-year-old female has sudden onset of right eye pain, blurred vision, and dilated pupil. The most likely diagnosis is acute:

    a. open-angle glaucoma.
    b. angle-closure glaucoma.
    c. retinal detachment.
    d. uveitis.

_____ 38. The mother of an 18 month old child is in the office. She has not yet immunized her child because the child's grandmother "doesn't believe in that." The nurse practitioner should:

    a. respect her opinion and discuss the subject no further.
    b. provide education and recommend beginning the series of vaccines.
    c. ask her to talk to her friends about immunizations.
    d. plan to address the subject at a future visit.

_____ 39. Which of the following is the most common presenting sign of substance abuse in adolescents?

    a. Dental erosion
    b. Hypersomnia
    c. Increased blood pressure
    d. Changes in behavior

_____ 40. A 62-year-old female has been diagnosed with osteoporosis. She refuses hormone replacement therapy as well as new medication shown to increase bone density. Important education for this patient should include:

   a. information about joint replacement surgery.
   b. the need for annual bone density assessment.
   c. the benefits of increasing calcium intake and daily weight-bearing exercise.
   d. avoidance of calcium robbing foods.

_____ 41. Which of the following physical examination findings is abnormal?

   a. 20 teeth in a 2-year-old
   b. 4+ tonsillar hypertrophy in a 4-year-old
   c. Nonpalpable thyroid gland in a 6-year-old
   d. Visual acuity 20/40 in a 3-year-old

_____ 42. A 38-year-old patient has folliculitis on a bearded part of his face. The nurse practitioner prescribes delayed-release erythromycin and tells the patient:

   a. erythromycin may upset his stomach, so it should be taken with food.
   b. taking erythromycin should clear the affected area in 3 days.
   c. the problem will recur unless he remains beardless.
   d. to avoid shaving the affected area until the infection has cleared.

_____ 43. At 20 weeks gestation, fundal height is expected to be:

   a. 12 cm (at the symphysis pubis).
   b. 20 cm (in the hypogastric region).
   c. 24 cm (at the umbilicus).
   d. 28 cm (above the umbilicus).

_____ 44. Which of the following is *not* a component of the CAGE questionnaire?

   a. Have you ever felt the need to cut down on drinking?
   b. Have you gotten into fights when drinking?
   c. Have you ever taken a morning eye-opener?
   d. Have you ever felt annoyed by criticism of drinking?

_____ 45. A common finding associated with temporal arteritis is:

    a. severe headache.
    b. facial nerve paresis or paralysis.
    c. paresthesia.
    d. macular degeneration.

_____ 46. One exception to the recommendation to limit dietary fat intake is:

    a. adolescents during a growth spurt.
    b. anyone undergoing chemotherapy for cancer.
    c. school-age children who are under-weight for age.
    d. children under 2 years-of-age.

_____ 47. A 23-year-old male complains of severe headache localized to the left frontal and parietal area with blurred vision. The nurse practitioner identifies vesicular lesions on his forehead. The most appropriate interventions are:

    a. acyclovir, and referral to an ophthalmologist.
    b. topical cortisone cream, and referral to a neurologist.
    c. topical mupirocin (Bactroban®), and referral to a dermatologist.
    d. ibuprofen and cool compresses.

_____ 48. A nurse practitioner who orders fluoride supplements for a child is practicing:

    a. health self-determination.
    b. preventive dentistry.
    c. primary prevention.
    d. secondary prevention.

_____ 49. An important factor to consider when interviewing the geriatric patient is that:

    a. elders are less skilled than young adults at decision-making.
    b. the capacity to learn, re-learn, synthesize, and problem-solve diminishes in old age.
    c. there is considerable variation in general health, mental status, and functional ability among elders.
    d. abstract reasoning and conceptual skills decrease with advanced age.

_____ 50. The nurse practitioner examines a 6-year-old who has had sore throat and fever for less than 24 hours. Based on the most common cause of pharyngitis in this age group, the most appropriate action is to:

a. prescribe amoxicillin in a weight-appropriate dose.
b. ask if any other family members have the same symptoms.
c. encourage supportive and symptomatic care.
d. prescribe an antihistamine and decongestant.

_____ 51. The screening test most commonly used for diabetes mellitus is:

a. a fasting blood sugar (FBS).
b. hemoglobin A_{1C}.
c. oral glucose tolerance test (GTT).
d. random blood glucose.

_____ 52. What is the confirmatory test for human immunodeficiency virus in a patient over 18 months-of-age?

a. Enzyme linked immunosorbent assay (ELISA)
b. CD4 cell count
c. Western blot
d. Rapid plasma reagin (RPR)

_____ 53. The nurse practitioner assesses a patient who has a laterally displaced apical impulse. What finding should be suspected?

a. Cardiomegaly
b. Atrial fibrillation (AF)
c. Congestive heart failure (CHF)
d. Hepatomegaly

_____ 54. What are the current recommendations for the use of live attenuated varicella vaccine?

a. Serologic testing is recommended before vaccination of children 18 months-of-age and < 12 years-of-age.
b. Children vaccinated at 12 to 18 months-of-age will need a booster at 12 years-of-age.
c. Varicella vaccine has been approved for routine use in all healthy children > 12 months-of-age.
d. Children with a positive history of varicella infection are still considered susceptible and should be vaccinated.

_____ 55. Which antihypertensive drug would be *least* appropriate to prescribe during pregnancy?

   a. metoprolol (Lopressor®)
   b. propranolol (Inderal®)
   c. methyldopa (Aldomet®)
   d. verapamil (Calan®)

_____ 56. The type of assessment found to be most effective when screening for domestic violence is:

   a. routine questioning about abuse.
   b. a written self-report.
   c. reflection as part of the interview.
   d. careful physical examination.

_____ 57. Which of the following accurately describes the appropriate use of influenza vaccine?

   a. Influenza vaccine is recommended on a one time only basis for all persons aged 65 years or older and to persons 6 months or older who are residents of chronic care facilities or who suffer from chronic cardiopulmonary disorders, metabolic diseases, hemoglobinopathies, or immunosuppression.
   b. Influenza vaccine should be administered annually to all persons aged 65 years and older, and to persons 6 months or older who are residents of chronic care facilities, or who suffer from chronic cardiopulmonary disorders, metabolic disorders, hemoglobinopathies, or immunosuppression.
   c. Influenza vaccine should be administered to all persons born after 1956 who lack evidence of immunity to influenza.
   d. Influenza vaccine should be administered intranasally to all young adults not previously immunized and also to susceptible adults in high risk groups including homosexual men, intravenous drug users, and persons in health-related jobs with frequent exposure to influenza.

_____ 58. Which of the following is true concerning sensitivity and specificity?

a. Assessment techniques must be highly sensitive and highly specific to be useful.
b. Sensitivity relates to the reliability of a technique to give a positive result when the finding is present. Specificity relates to the reliability of a technique to successfully rule out a finding.
c. Sensitivity relates to the reliability of a technique to successfully rule out a finding. Specificity relates to the reliability of a technique to give a positive result when the finding is present.
d. A test of high sensitivity will fail to determine a finding in many patients. A test of high specificity tends to produce false positive results.

_____ 59. An adolescent goes to Colorado for a ski trip. He is unaccustomed to the high altitude and very dry air. He develops epistaxis (nose bleeds) and visits the nurse practitioner. What intervention is *least* effective?

a. Use phenylephrine (Neo-Synephrine®) nose spray and pressure against the bleeding site for 5 to 10 minutes.
b. Avoid aspirin use for aches, pains, or headaches until the problem has resolved.
c. Apply a lubricant liberally in the nares.
d. Drink adequate water to promote hydration of the nares.

_____ 60. The major health risk(s) associated with oral contraceptive therapy is(are):

a. hypertension.
b. vascular events.
c. infertility.
d. weight gain.

_____ 61. The Dubowitz Clinical Assessment is a:

a. standardized scoring system for assessing gestational age of newborns.
b. scale developed for rating the newborn's appearance, heart rate, reflexes, activity, and respirations.
c. system for identifying children who have been sexually or physically abused.
d. screening system to identify congenital anomalies.

_____ 62. The nurse practitioner is initiating levothyroxine for primary hypothyroidism in a 71-year-old female. The usual starting dose of levothyroxine is 50 to 100 mcg (0.05 to 0.100 mg) per day. What would be the most appropriate initial therapy for this patient?

    a. 25 mcg (0.025 mg) per day
    b. 50 mcg (0.05 mg) per day
    c. 75 mcg (0.075 mg) per day
    d. 100 mcg (0.100 mg) per day

_____ 63. A 35-year-old woman with prior history of "extreme nervousness" has been treated with daily diazepam (Valium®) for one week. She reports improvement. Today her pulse is 130 bpm and blood pressure is 140/98 mmHg. She is 5'4" and weighs 98 pounds. What is the most likely diagnosis?

    a. Anxiety
    b. Somatization
    c. Cushing's syndrome
    d. Hyperthyroidism

_____ 64. Which of the following findings is consistent with otitis externa?

    a. Fever
    b. Rhinorrhea
    c. Dizziness
    d. Pain

_____ 65. A PPD is considered positive at 5 millimeters or more for which population?

    a. Intravenous drug users who are known to be HIV-negative, occupants of long term care facilities, age < 4 years, groups with high prevalence for tuberculosis (TB) infection, the medically underserved
    b. Persons with no known risk factors
    c. Immigrants, low income populations, persons who received prior BCG vaccination
    d. Confirmed or suspected HIV infection, intravenous drug users, close contacts of a TB case, persons with chest x-ray suggestive of TB

_____ 66. Which of the following therapies is *not* appropriate management for a person with degenerative joint disease (DJD)?

    a. Aspirin
    b. Corrective surgery
    c. Physical therapy
    d. Oral steroid therapy

_____ 67. A nurse practitioner palpates a nodule during a prostate exam. What other clues may indicate prostate cancer?

    a. Elevated PSA and hematuria
    b. Freely movable cystic mass and non-viable sperm
    c. Urethral discharge and elevated PSA
    d. Urinary retention and scrotal pain

_____ 68. Which of the following laboratory tests, if positive, is part of the diagnostic criteria for systemic lupus erythematosus in an adult?

    a. Anti-nuclear antibody (ANA)
    b. Rheumatoid factor (RF)
    c. Erythrocyte sedimentation rate (ESR)
    d. HLA-B27

_____ 69. Bouchard's nodes are most commonly associated with what disease process?

    a. Rheumatoid arthritis (RA)
    b. Juvenile rheumatoid arthritis (JRA)
    c. Osteoarthritis (OA)
    d. Psoriatic arthritis

_____ 70. Which of the following indicates need for further evaluation?

    a. A 7-year-old girl with vaginal bleeding
    b. A 7-year-old girl with no true pubic hair
    c. A 12-year-old boy with sparse, slightly pigmented pubic hair
    d. A 12-year-old girl with breast buds

_____ 71. A 15-year-old male presents to the school-based health clinic with complaints of diarrhea and fever. Which factor supports a viral cause of the diarrhea?

    a. Household contact with diarrhea
    b. Abrupt onset
    c. Fever 103° F (39.4°C)
    d. Presence of neurological deficits

_____ 72. A 4-year-old child received immune globulin (IG) at a relatively low dose for tetanus today. What is the minimum amount of time she should wait before receiving the MMR vaccine?

    a. 3 months
    b. 5 to 6 months
    c. 8 to 10 months
    d. 1 year

_____ 73. An asymptomatic 76-year-old man reports a history of 3 acute episodes of gout in the past 3 months. He was treated with nonsteroidal anti-inflammatory agents (NSAIDs) during each episode. He states, "I'm really worried about the next attack." Which of the following is the drug treatment of choice for this patient today?

    a. allopurinol (Zyloprim®)
    b. colchicine
    c. prednisone (Deltacortisone®)
    d. methotrexate (Amethopterin®)

_____ 74. A 16-year-old sexually active student presents with complaint of a malodorous greenish-gray frothy vaginal discharge and vaginal itching. The nurse practitioner should suspect:

    a. bacterial vaginosis (BV).
    b. trichomoniasis.
    c. syphilis.
    d. gonorrhea.

_____ 75. Which of the following signs and symptoms is typical of hyperthyroidism?

    a. Heat intolerance
    b. Constipation
    c. Hyporeflexia
    d. Weight gain

_____ 76. Which of the following is the most prevalent skeletal problem in the United States?

   a. Osteoarthritis
   b. Fracture
   c. Osteoporosis
   d. Rheumatoid arthritis

_____ 77. Breastfed infants may need which one of the following vitamin or mineral supplements?

   a. Iron, as breast milk contains less iron than does infant formula.
   b. Calcium, because it is less easily absorbed from breast milk than in formula.
   c. Vitamin D, if the infant is not exposed to sunlight.
   d. Vitamin C, to promote better absorption of iron.

_____ 78. A 2-year-old has iron deficiency anemia and has not had an increase in hemoglobin for the past 2 months despite iron supplementation. The nurse practitioner should:

   a. repeat the hemoglobin and hematocrit.
   b. obtain a diet history from the caregiver.
   c. listen to the chest for a systolic flow murmur.
   d. consult a physician for further assessment.

_____ 79. A 2-year-old is being evaluated by the nurse practitioner. Child abuse has been suspected in the past. Which of the following findings would warrant further evaluation for possible abuse?

   a. Small teeth marks on the child's forearm
   b. Multiple bruises on the child's knees and elbows
   c. Absence of crying or protesting when an immunization is administered
   d. Daytime and nocturnal enuresis

_____ 80. What is an appropriate drug for prophylactic treatment of migraine headache in a 17-year-old female?

   a. sumatriptan (Imitrex®)
   b. propranolol (Inderal®)
   c. ibuprofen (Motrin®)
   d. dihydroergotamine (DHE®)

_____ 81. The main component of oral hygiene that reduces the incidence of tooth decay is:

    a. fluoride in the toothpaste, water, and/or supplement.
    b. the mechanical action of tooth brushing.
    c. rinsing with an antimicrobial mouthwash.
    d. flossing between the teeth.

_____ 82. A 14-year-old high school freshman sprained his ankle 1 week ago. He had immediate pain, was unable to bear weight, but had no joint instability. X-rays were negative. He has used crutches since sustaining the injury. He returns to see the nurse practitioner and reports that the ankle has improved "very little." The nurse practitioner should:

    a. order a second set of x-rays of the ankle.
    b. insist that he use crutches for 1 more week.
    c. refer him to an orthopedist.
    d. consult physical therapy.

_____ 83. Which of the following lifestyle changes has demonstrated effectiveness in the prevention of coronary disease, hypertension, obesity, diabetes, osteoporosis, and some mental disorders?

    a. Limiting dietary fat to 30% of total daily calories
    b. Daily social interaction
    c. Smoking cessation
    d. Regular physical activity

_____ 84. A significant finding in the history of a patient with a suspected cerebral vascular accident (stroke) is:

    a. family history of cerebral aneurysm.
    b. urinary incontinence.
    c. history of atrial fibrillation.
    d. chest pain with inspiration.

_____ 85. A 30-year-old salesman complains of heartburn after meals. He takes over-the-counter medicines which provide temporary relief, but the heartburn symptoms always return. The nurse practitioner discusses lifestyle changes and prescribes a proton pump inhibitor daily. When should the nurse practitioner follow up with this patient?

    a. 1 to 2 days
    b. 1 to 2 weeks
    c. 1 to 2 months
    d. No follow up is needed

_____ 86. A patient newly diagnosed with type 2 diabetes mellitus is referred to a diabetes nurse educator and completes the initial educational program. A need for further education is indicated when the patient says which of the following?

a. "My body has developed resistance to my own insulin."
b. "I may notice some weight loss as my diabetes gets under better control."
c. "One of my medicines could make my blood sugar drop too low, so I will keep some candy in my purse."
d. "One of my medicines helps my body use my blood sugar for energy better."

_____ 87. The finding which is most consistent with a diagnosis of benign prostatic hyperplasia is digital palpation of a prostate gland that is:

a. enlarged, symmetrical, semi-firm, and nontender.
b. enlarged, symmetrical, boggy, and exquisitely tender.
c. asymmetrical and nodular.
d. exquisitely tender with absence of median sulcus.

_____ 88. A 2-year-old has several discrete, shiny, flesh-colored papules with dome-shaped tops and firm, waxy center. The area surrounding them is erythematous and the child scratches them frequently. The mother asks, "What should be done for my child?" The nurse practitioner responds:

a. "They may regress spontaneously in 6 to 9 months, but cryosurgery will eliminate them."
b. "Salicylic acid patches will clear them in several days."
c. "Hydrocortisone cream will prevent itching and clear the lesions in several weeks."
d. "These are benign epidermal tumors which are usually inherited. They will resolve on their own without treatment."

_____ 89. Primary prevention of human papilloma virus (HPV) infection requires educational efforts directed toward:

a. receiving annual screening examinations.
b. self-examination to detect signs of infection.
c. receiving a vaccination on an annual basis.
d. delaying the onset of sexual activity and using barrier methods of contraception.

_____ 90. An early sign of multiple sclerosis (MS) is:

    a. acute monocular vision loss.
    b. memory loss.
    c. personality changes.
    d. brief losses of consciousness.

_____ 91. The mother of a 6 month old infant asks about the use of an infant walker. The most appropriate response is to:

    a. discourage the use of walkers and encourage parental holding and floor play.
    b. encourage the use of walkers as a safe precursor to walking alone.
    c. suggest that walker use be limited to 20 minute periods.
    d. suggest waiting to use the walker until the infant is bearing full weight.

_____ 92. A mother calls the office reporting that her child has burned his finger by touching a hot pot about 1 hour ago. She describes the burn as red, painful, and without blistering. The child cried at the time of the accident and is complaining of pain now. The nurse practitioner should instruct the mother to:

    a. apply cool water compresses and administer ibuprofen.
    b. bring the child to the clinic for evaluation.
    c. apply cooking oil.
    d. apply moisturizing lotion.

_____ 93. A 17-year-old male visits the clinic with his mother who says, if there are no medical consequences or risks known, she will allow her son to get a tattoo. How should the nurse practitioner respond?

    a. "Tattoos distort one's body image resulting in a high incidence of depression."
    b. "Tattoos and body piercing are possible sources of hepatitis C infection if there is common use of contaminated needles."
    c. "The tattoo should be applied to an area that will not be exposed to sun to avoid increased risk of skin cancer."
    d. "The only medical consequence of tattooing is the scarring associated with removal."

94. An active 82 year male in good health complains "I don't see as well as I used to and my eyes are very sensitive to glare." His near and distant visual acuity is diminished and he has a bilateral white pupillary reflex. The most likely diagnosis is:

    a. ocular tumor.
    b. open-angle glaucoma.
    c. cataract.
    d. retinal detachment.

95. A characteristic of delirium that is typically absent in dementia is:

    a. acute onset of confusion in a previously alert and oriented patient.
    b. gradual loss of short-term memory.
    c. loss of language skills.
    d. long term memory gaps filled in with confabulation.

96. An older patient is taking warfarin (Coumadin®) for chronic atrial fibrillation. When teaching the patient to notify the nurse practitioner of changes in his health or plan of care, what is *least* important for him to report?

    a. Chest pain
    b. A missed dose of warfarin
    c. Shortness of breath
    d. Ankle swelling

97. The nurse practitioner treats a family of 4 with mebendazole (Vermox®) for pinworms. General measures to prevent reinfection have been explained and the mother understands them. The nurse practitioner tells the mother that:

    a. reinfection is not very likely.
    b. the itching may continue for another 2 weeks.
    c. family members may experience diarrhea.
    d. family members often need several treatments.

98. Which of the following findings would raise the nurse practitioner's suspicion of bulimia in a 17-year-old female?

    a. Hyperkalemia
    b. Emaciation
    c. Scars on her knuckles
    d. Dental caries

_____ 99. Which of the following is a "red flag" indicating possible developmental delay?

    a. A 5 month old does not roll from supine to prone.
    b. A 16 month old is unable to walk backwards.
    c. A 36 month old has a 50-word vocabulary and 50% of speech is intelligible.
    d. Absence of voluntary bladder and bowel control in a 2½ year old.

_____ 100. A nurse practitioner is providing guidance to a newly diagnosed diabetic patient who is being treated with insulin. The nurse practitioner would be correct to tell the patient to self-treat signs and symptoms of hypoglycemia with:

    a. "100 grams of sugar, or 1 chocolate candy bar."
    b. "50 grams of sugar, or 1 tablespoon of granulated sugar."
    c. "15 grams of sugar, or 5 lifesavers."
    d. "5 grams of sugar, or 1 lifesaver."

_____ 101. A 50-year-old female complains of urinary incontinence. Which patient response supports a diagnosis of stress incontinence?

    a. "It burns when I urinate."
    b. "I'm only incontinent at night."
    c. "I'm incontinent when I laugh, cough, or sneeze."
    d. "It's hard to predict when I will be incontinent."

_____ 102. The gold standard for cervical cancer screening is:

    a. vaginal examination.
    b. the Papanicolaou smear.
    c. colposcopy.
    d. serum carcinoembryonic antigen (CEA).

_____ 103. One of the most important aspects of caring for patients with sickle cell anemia is prevention of infection. What is the recommended prophylaxis drug of choice for infants with sickle cell anemia?

    a. penicillin
    b. erythromycin
    c. trimethoprim-sulfamethoxazole (Bactrim®)
    d. cephalexin (Keflex®)

_____104. The nurse practitioner should refer the pregnant patient for ultrasound and amniocentesis when the patient:

    a. has a history of high risk sexual behavior.
    b. received a blood transfusion after 1989.
    c. has a history of a neural tube defect in a previous pregnancy.
    d. has unsensitized Rh-negative blood.

_____105. The parents of a 2-year-old report that she is not saying any words, but makes sounds, babbles, and understands simple commands from her parents. The parents are not concerned. The nurse practitioner responds:

    a. "Your child should be saying a few words by this time. She should be referred for further assessment."
    b. "Your child should be saying a few words by this time. We will wait another 3 to 6 months and observe her progress."
    c. "Your child's language skills are not as developmentally advanced as we would expect. She will need speech therapy."
    d. "Your child should be referred to an ear, nose, and throat specialist to assess her hearing."

_____106. A 26-year-old patient, 18 weeks pregnant with twins, has been healthy and has followed the recommendations of her nurse midwife. She is in the office to discuss results of her maternal serum α-fetoprotein (MSAFP) test which show an elevation. In this particular pregnancy:

    a. elevated MSAFP is an indicator of Down syndrome.
    b. low MSAFP is expected at 18 weeks gestation.
    c. neural tube defect is highly probable.
    d. elevated MSAFP is an expected finding.

_____107. An 8 month old male presents with hemarthrosis of both knees and hematuria. The parents give no history of trauma, but report "he has always bruised easily." The most likely diagnosis is:

    a. physical child abuse.
    b. idiopathic thrombocytopenia (ITP).
    c. a type of hemophilia.
    d. a form of leukemia.

_____108. The nurse practitioner has treated an infant for the last 3 weeks for thrush with nystatin (Mycostatin®) oral suspension. The mother returns today and states that the problem continues despite using the medicine. What diagnostic test could the nurse practitioner perform which might quickly confirm a diagnosis of oral candidiasis?

    a. A potassium hydroxide (KOH) slide preparation
    b. Venous blood cultures
    c. Normal saline microscopic examination
    d. A Giemsa stain of oral scrapings

_____109. A 32-year-old mother and her 10-year-old child each have a round, reddened patch on the trunk. There is central clearing in the lesion. Different lesions run parallel to each other in a Christmas tree pattern. The mother has been treating the "ringworm" with an antifungal cream for 7 days without success. The nurse practitioner's best response is:

    a. "The antifungal cream you have been using is not strong enough. Prescription strength should clear this up."
    b. "No medication will help this to clear. It must clear on its own and may take 4 to 8 weeks."
    c. "Since you and your daughter both have this, it is most probably a contagious viral rash. We will treat the symptoms."
    d. "This is highly unusual to occur in both of you. Perhaps a dermatologist should biopsy the lesions."

_____110. Which of the following tests is(are) diagnostic for cystic fibrosis?

    a. Serum amylase
    b. Fecal fat excretion
    c. Pulmonary function studies
    d. Sweat test

_____111. Given appropriate patient education by the primary care provider, poor compliance with medical recommendations is most often due to:

    a. willful disobedience.
    b. vision and/or hearing deficits.
    c. anxiety.
    d. limited cognitive ability.

_____112. A 50-year-old farmer who wears a hat every day is diagnosed with tinea capitis. Griseofulvin 250 mg daily for 4 weeks is prescribed. After 2 weeks of therapy, the patient has not improved. What course of action should the nurse practitioner take?

    a. Add 2.5% selenium sulfide shampoo twice weekly to the patient's treatment regimen.
    b. Have the farmer shave his head and warn him that hair re-growth will be slow.
    c. Initiate a short course of oral steroids to reduce inflammation and prevent scarring.
    d. Consider increasing the griseofulvin to 500 mg per day, screen for diabetes mellitus, and re-evaluate in 1 to 2 weeks.

_____113. A patient presents with classic signs and symptoms of Graves' hyperthyroidism. Which laboratory test(s) is (are) needed to confirm the diagnosis?

    a. Radioactive iodine uptake.
    b. Serum TSH, serum free T_4, and T_3.
    c. Total serum T_4 and a radioactive thyroid scan.
    d. Serum TSH and serum free T_4 index.

_____114. Strabismus is observed in a 13 month old child. The most appropriate action for the nurse practitioner is to:

    a. refer the patient to an ophthalmologist.
    b. patch the child's affected eye.
    c. follow the child closely for 2 more months.
    d. teach the patient and parent eye muscle exercises.

_____115. What is the law concerning informed consent and childhood vaccines?

    a. Because childhood vaccines are required for school, a consent form is considered redundant.
    b. All health care providers are required to use standard consent forms.
    c. Public health department nurses are required to use consent forms but this is optional for practitioners in the private sector.
    d. A standard general immunization consent is required for the first vaccine only.

_____116. A 78-year-old man has a diagnosis of emphysema. It is imperative that the nurse practitioner teach him to:

    a. use oxygen at home during the night.
    b. call the office at the first sign of infection.
    c. limit intake of high protein foods.
    d. be immunized annually with the polyvalent pneumococcal vaccine.

_____117. A 44-year-old patient has a dark multi-colored mole on his back which is about eight millimeters in diameter and has an irregular border. The nurse practitioner should:

    a. have the patient return in 3 months to check the mole for changes.
    b. have the patient use sunscreen when in the sun.
    c. refer the patient to a surgeon or dermatologist for biopsy.
    d. take skin scrapings from the mole for laboratory analysis.

_____118. Ideally, antepartum care should begin:

    a. as soon as the pregnancy is identified.
    b. at 6 weeks gestation.
    c. with preconception counseling.
    d. in the first trimester.

_____119. Patients diagnosed with polycystic ovarian disease should be taught that they are at increased risk for developing which of the following?

    a. Diabetes mellitus
    b. Cervical cancer
    c. Endometriosis
    d. Cushing's syndrome

_____120. A 25-year-old female complains that she never had a bladder infection before she became sexually active, but now she has had 3 in 1 year. What intervention is especially important for the nurse practitioner to teach this patient to help prevent recurrence of bladder infections?

    a. Drink a glass of water before sexual intercourse and urinate within 15 minutes after.
    b. Do not douche or use feminine hygiene sprays or deodorants.
    c. Wear nylon underwear and wipe well after bowel movements.
    d. Urinate frequently to avoid a full bladder.

_____121. The most successful patient interview is likely to:

    a. be the "find it, tell what to do" model.
    b. be a collaborative process.
    c. yield a complete and accurately detailed history.
    d. be completely objective.

_____122. A 74-year-old female complains of pain bilaterally in her lower legs while walking. The pain disappears at rest. There is absence of edema and erythema. What is the most likely diagnosis?

    a. Deep vein thrombosis (DVT)
    b. Arterial embolism
    c. Peripheral arterial insufficiency
    d. Osteoarthritis (OA)

_____123. Regarding the effectiveness of spermicides and female barrier methods against gonorrhea and chlamydia, spermicides and diaphragms or cervical caps:

    a. have no effect on reducing the risk of gonorrhea and chlamydia.
    b. can reduce risk but are not as effective as properly used male condoms.
    c. when properly used, are just as effective in reducing the risk of gonorrhea and chlamydia as the male condom.
    d. are as effective as male condoms in reducing the risk of gonorrhea and chlamydia as well as HIV and other sexually transmitted diseases.

_____124. A first-time mother asks the nurse practitioner how much her baby will grow in the first 3 months of life. The nurse practitioner explains that the normal baby will grow:

    a. ½ to 1 ounce per day.
    b. 1 to 2 ounces per week.
    c. 1 inch per week.
    d. more than 6 inches.

_____125. A patient with a history of cerumen impaction in the past presents with a feeling of fullness, itching, and decreased hearing bilaterally. The nurse practitioner describes the irrigation and tells the patient which of the following?

    a. "I'm going to use cool water to irrigate your ear."
    b. "This will probably hurt, but it will only last a few seconds."
    c. "Let me know if you feel nauseated or dizzy."
    d. "I recommend using a cerumen solvent weekly for this problem."

_____126. A 2 week old African-American male infant has ecchymotic-like marks over his lower back and upper buttocks. The most appropriate intervention is to:

    a. report the finding to child protection services.
    b. order bleeding studies and a complete blood count.
    c. reassure the infant's mother that this is a normal finding.
    d. recommend a genetics consultation.

_____127. A 15-year-old swim team member presents with mild "swimmer's ear." Vital signs are normal. What is the most appropriate therapy for this patient?

    a. Oral amoxicillin-clavulanic acid (Augmentin®)
    b. Oral cefaclor (Ceclor®)
    c. Keep the ear canals dry at all times until the condition resolves on its own
    d. Hydrocortisone/bacitracin/polymyxin B (Cortisporin®) otic suspension

_____128. A 73-year-old with a history of congestive heart failure (CHF) controlled with ACE inhibitors presents to the clinic with symptoms of shortness of breath on exertion. After assessing the patient, the nurse practitioner determines that he is in mild exacerbation of chronic CHF because of recent dietary indiscretions. What action should the nurse practitioner consider to relieve the patient's symptoms?

    a. Increase the patient's dose of ACE inhibitor for the next 3 days.
    b. Prescribe a daily diuretic for the next 3 days.
    c. Prescribe a daily diuretic to be taken for the next week.
    d. Add daily digoxin to the patient's regular medication regimen.

_____129. Which patient would *not* be considered at high risk for development of tuberculosis infection?

    a. A patient with cancer
    b. A prison inmate
    c. An HIV-infected patient
    d. A homeless person

_____130. Among adolescents in the U.S., the greatest known risk factors for contracting hepatitis B (HBV) is(are):

    a. homosexual activity.
    b. intravenous drug use.
    c. heterosexual activity.
    d. alcohol and designer drug use.

_____131. According to the Standards of Advanced Practice Nursing developed by the American Nurses Association (ANA), an advanced practice registered nurse (APRN) who informs the patient of the risks, benefits, and outcomes of a health care regimen is following which standard of practice?

    a. Leadership
    b. Research
    c. Interdisciplinary process
    d. Ethics

_____132. An elderly patient has just been placed on a calcium channel blocker for treatment of hypertension and angina. The nurse practitioner informs the patient to expect any of the following *except*:

    a. constipation.
    b. peripheral edema.
    c. decreased heart rate.
    d. nocturnal cough.

_____133. The most common breast cancer risk factor is:

    a. a family history of breast cancer.
    b. a family history of breast and ovarian cancer.
    c. nulliparity.
    d. advancing age.

_____134. Which of the following medication classifications has been found to be most helpful in managing the problems associated with congestive heart failure (CHF)?

    a. ACE inhibitors
    b. β-blockers
    c. Central α-agonists
    d. Calcium channel blockers

_____135. Which choice below is *not* a contraindication to receiving the diphtheria, acellular pertussis, and tetanus (DTaP) vaccine?

    a. Current antibiotic use
    b. Acute febrile illness
    c. An evolving neurological condition
    d. A severe reaction to DTaP in the past

_____136. The Centers for Disease Control and Prevention (CDC) recommends which of the following strategies for preventing neonatal group B streptococcal (GBS) infection?

    a. Provide antibiotic prophylaxis to all women who have risk factors for GBS.
    b. Culture all pregnant women at 35 to 37 weeks gestation for GBS and administer antibiotics intrapartum to those who test positive.
    c. Order antibiotic prophylaxis for those with risk factors or culture all pregnant women and treat those who test positive.
    d. Prescribe prophylactic antibiotics for all women at 35 to 37 weeks gestation.

_____137. Adolescents are at increased risk for contracting the human immunodeficiency virus (HIV) due to:

    a. immaturity of their immune systems.
    b. increased sexual experimentation.
    c. pubertal changes in body composition.
    d. inadequate primary health care for adolescents.

_____138. A 65-year-old patient comes to the health clinic during December and requests the "flu and pneumonia shots." He reports to the nurse practitioner that he got both shots last year, was healthy, and now he wants them every year. The nurse practitioner responds:

    a. "It's a good idea to get them both again."
    b. "It's too late to get the flu shot, but the pneumonia shot can be given today."
    c. "I will give you the flu shot, but you only need the pneumonia shot once in a lifetime."
    d. "They cannot be given at the same time, but I will give you the flu shot today."

_____139. Which of the following diagnostic tests provides the most precise assessment of left ventricular function?

    a. Electrocardiogram
    b. Echocardiogram
    c. Exercise stress test
    d. Plethysmography

_____140. An appropriate initial treatment for benign positional vertigo is:

    a.   a sodium-restricted diet.
    b.   a systematic exercise program.
    c.   prednisone (Deltasone®).
    d.   meclizine (Antivert®).

_____141. A 17-year-old presents with a wound received while building a fence. He completed a primary vaccination series and he had a Td booster 3 years ago. Does he need a Td booster today?

    a.   No, expert opinion supports vaccination after a contaminated wound when more than 5 years has elapsed since the last Td vaccine.
    b.   Yes, and he should also receive tetanus immune globulin (TIG) prophylaxis.
    c.   Maybe, the answer is dependent on whether the wound is considered contaminated.
    d.   Yes, a booster is recommended at the time of injury if greater than 3 years has elapsed since the last Td.

_____142. A 16-year-old sexually active female presents to the clinic. She has never had vaccinations for hepatitis A or B, she has had 1 MMR immunization, and her last tetanus vaccination was 4 years ago. Which vaccination would be contraindicated without further testing?

    a.   Hepatitis B
    b.   Hepatitis A
    c.   MMR
    d.   tetanus

_____143. A 29-year-old homeless male's blood pressure is 160/108 mmHg in his right arm and 158/104 mmHg in his left arm. He gives a history of being hypertensive in the past, but has never taken blood pressure medication. On physical examination, the nurse practitioner auscultates a vascular bruit in the left upper quadrant of his abdomen. This patient's blood pressure elevation is most likely:

    a.   essential hypertension.
    b.   due to coarctation of the aorta.
    c.   a function of left ventricular failure.
    d.   caused by renal artery stenosis.

_____144. A 47-year-old female's total cholesterol is 250 mg/dL. The nurse practitioner should:

    a. begin pharmacologic therapy with nicotinic acid (niacin).
    b. order a complete lipoprotein analysis.
    c. start the patient on the AHA Step 2 low fat diet.
    d. order an electrocardiogram (ECG).

_____145. Babies should begin oral iron supplementation:

    a. when they are able to eat iron-enriched cereal.
    b. at 2 months-of-age.
    c. at 4 to 6 months-of-age.
    d. anytime after their teeth have erupted.

_____146. Which of the following is the only drug class proven to decrease cardiovascular mortality in hypertensive patients?

    a. Alpha blockers
    b. Calcium channel blockers
    c. Loop diuretics
    d. Beta-adrenergic blockers

_____147. The mechanism by which nurses are held accountable for practice, based on the quality of nursing care in a given situation in accordance with established standards of practice, is:

    a. outcome criteria.
    b. process criteria.
    c. peer review.
    d. quality improvement.

_____148. Patients with congestive heart failure should be taught to:

    a. restrict fluids to 1000 ml per day.
    b. notify the nurse practitioner of any sudden weight increase.
    c. strictly limit physical activity between exacerbations.
    d. adhere to a 1000 mg sodium restricted diet.

_____149. Which of the following diuretics does *not* cause loss of potassium?

    a. furosemide (Lasix®)
    b. spironolactone (Aldactone®)
    c. hydrochlorothiazide (Hydrodiuril®)
    d. bumetanide (Bumex®)

150. According to the American Nurses Association (ANA), the role of the nurse practitioner who provides primary health care is the:

    a. nurse educator.
    b. direct nursing care role.
    c. indirect nursing care role.
    d. administrator.

Practice Exam II
Answers and Rationales

1. *c*   Exposure of these areas to light and sun will help the area to heal. Encouraging weight reduction would also be of benefit to her. Sleeping with a brassiere increases moisture retention and should be avoided.

2. *b*   This patient had a severe reaction to penicillin in the past. Choices *c* and *d* are both cephalosporins which have a 2% to 10% cross-reactivity with the penicillins. The safest choice in this situation is to avoid penicillin and cephalosporins.

3. *b*   Tzanck prep is the only test in this list which is diagnostic for *herpes simplex*. KOH prep is used to diagnose candidal and bacterial vaginosis. Gram stain is used to distinguish Gram positive and Gram negative organisms. The Papanicolaou (Pap) smear is used to screen for cervical dysplasia and cancer.

4. *a*   Regular brushing and flossing, brushing with a fluoride-containing toothpaste, or using an appropriate dietary supplement of fluoride all help to prevent tooth decay.

5. *c*   Tricyclic antidepressants should not be used by men with benign prostatic hyperplasia because of the increased risk of urinary retention secondary to the anticholinergic effects of TCAs.

6. *b*   Cephalexin could be used to treat impetigo. A topical, however, would be a better choice because the infected area is small and oral antibiotics could present unnecessary systemic effects.

7. *a*   Coronary heart disease risk associated with elevated total cholesterol is primarily due to elevated LDL cholesterol and is inversely related to HDL cholesterol. The primary evidence to support cholesterol screening is the ability of cholesterol-lowering interventions to reduce coronary heart disease (CHD) risk.

8. *c*   Elder abuse is more common in the very old (mean age 84 years). Other risk factors are financial or physical dependence and mental or physical impairment. There is also a higher rate of elder abuse in the lower socioeconomic population.

9. *c*   This patient probably has bacterial conjunctivitis. Polysporin® is an effective agent for bacterial ophthalmic infections. Although bacterial conjunctivitis will eventually resolve spontaneously without treatment, ophthalmic antibacterial treatment will speed resolution and the child will be able to return to school sooner.

10. *c* All suspicious lesions need to be evaluated for possible malignancy. The skin should be carefully and thoroughly examined by a health care provider every 3 to 6 months after diagnosis of malignant melanoma. Thorough skin self-examination should be performed weekly. Early surgical excision is the treatment of choice for malignant melanoma.

11. *a* An increased incidence of bacteriuria is found in all the populations listed. However, bacteriuria in pregnant women increases the mother's risk of delivering a low birth weight infant. The risk of pre-term delivery is also increased, which then increases perinatal and fetal morbidity and mortality. The recommended time for screening is at 12 to 16 weeks gestation.

12. *b* Unintentional poisoning is the third leading cause of unintentional injury and death. Periodic counseling of parents with young children, regarding measures to reduce risk of unintentional household injury, is recommended by the U.S. Preventive Services.

13. *c* Gluteal and thigh skin fold asymmetry may indicate congenital hip dysplasia. X-ray studies are not useful before 3 months-of-age because the femoral head has not completely ossified.

14. *a* Air conditioning is beneficial for patients with asthma as it decreases the amount of outdoor irritants and allergens in the indoor air. Air conditioning also decreases humidity which reduces mold and mite growth.

15. *b* Corn syrup acts as an osmotic agent to increase water concentration in fecal material, stimulate peristalsis and, thus, a bowel movement.

16. *d* Hematuria is a diagnosis of exclusion, but the urinalysis findings strongly support a diagnosis of UTI. Patients who are treated for uncomplicated UTI should be followed up in 2 to 3 weeks for resolution of the hematuria and other urinalysis findings because hematuria could be indicative of an underlying malignancy.

17. *a* Patients with blood pressure 140-159 mmHg systolic and/or 90-99 mmHg diastolic should have this confirmed within 2 months. Treatment is not started until elevated blood pressure has been confirmed with additional measurements.

18. *a* Occupational licensure is regulated by each individual state. Although this policy could potentially result in wide variation in scope of practice, in reality, it does not. A statute that works well in a given state may be copied by other states, resulting in similar regulations.

19. *a*   There are 3 clues to possible lead poisoning in this patient. The 4-year-old has developmental delays, lives in a house older than 30 years with possible lead paint and iron soldered pipes, and has parents who may have significant lead exposure due to possible lead glazes used on ceramics. A lead level should be checked and should be less than 10 mcg/dL. A complete blood count (CBC) is ordered to assess for microcytic anemia which can result from inhibition of hemoglobin synthesis.

20. *d*   Psoriasis is characterized by silvery scales most commonly in a knee, elbow, and scalp distribution. It is pruritic. Positive Auspitz sign (bleeding when the lesions are scraped) is a hallmark of psoriasis.

21. *c*   A mean corpuscular volume (MCV) 73 fl indicates microcytic anemia. Iron deficiency is the only microcytic anemia listed. The other anemias are macrocytic.

22. *c*   Ventricular septal defect (VSD) is the most common cardiac defect seen in childhood. Manifestations are frequent respiratory infections, poor weight gain, fatigue, and a harsh, high-pitched, holosystolic murmur at the left lower sternal border. Surgical closure is recommended in the first year of life for large defects.

23. *b*   More detailed information is needed about this patient's hearing loss. Referral to an audiologist for testing and then to an otolaryngologist, if indicated, would be appropriate. There is no benefit to waiting 4 more weeks, particularly because the hearing loss has been present for about 8 weeks already. Hearing loss is not necessarily a normal part of aging and should be evaluated for a pathological disease process.

24. *c*   According to the *Guide to Clinical Preventive Services*, there is insufficient evidence at this time to support the use of aspirin for MI prophylaxis in asymptomatic men. Aspirin use for secondary prevention is associated with positive outcomes with stroke and cardiac events.

25. *c*   The position of the American College of Sports Medicine is that pressure placed on young, female sports participants to maintain unrealistic low body weight is the basis for the development of this triad. Health care professionals should educate young women about these risks.

26. *c*   A 24-hour urine for renal creatinine clearance is the best test for assessing renal function. Creatinine clearance approximates glomerular filtration rate. Serum creatinine level is less accurate. BUN is primarily a measure of overall hydration.

27. *c*   There is currently no reliable method for primary care practitioners to screen efficiently for glaucoma. Accurate screening is best performed by an eye specialist with access to specialized equipment.

28. *c*   The half-life of theophylline is 8 to 9 hours. A steady state is reached after 4 to 5 doses. The lowest steady state, or trough, is measured before the 5th dose.

29. *a*   Small frequent feedings, frequent burping, and thickening the formula with rice cereal, are initial therapies for infants with GER. Infants should be positioned on the right side with head of bed elevated after feeding. Changing to soy formula has not been shown to reduce the incidence of GER in infants.

30. *d*   Cooked food and bottled water or wine are less likely to contain harmful bacteria than milk and raw fruits and vegetables.

31. *a*   A wide variety of legumes, grains, nuts, seeds, and vegetables can supply adequate amounts of required nutrients, especially iron.

32. *c*   Presbycusis is the form of hearing loss usually associated with normal aging. Perception of high-frequency tones is impaired.

33. *d*   Alkaline phosphatase (ALP) is elevated in conditions where rapid bone growth occurs and during pregnancy (because the placenta produces ALP).

34. *a*   Ulcerative colitis is amenable to surgical resection, usually a total colectomy. Surgery for Crohn's disease is not curative, but may be indicated in certain situations. Surgery is not indicated for irritable bowel syndrome (IBS).

35. *d*   Primary prevention of skin cancer includes limiting sun exposure, avoiding tanning facilities, and applying sunscreen. Examining the skin and recognizing melanoma are both secondary prevention measures.

36. *a*   This is a normal finding during the first few days of life and occurs because of estrogen influence from the mother. The discharge should abate in a few days.

37. *b*   Acute angle-closure glaucoma causes ocular pain, blurred vision, and a fixed mid-dilated pupil.

38. *b*   According to the U.S. Preventive Services Task Force, all children without established contraindications should receive the DTP, IPV, MMR, Hib, hepatitis B, and varicella vaccines in accordance with recommended schedules.

39. *d* There are usually no physical findings associated with substance abuse in adolescents. The clinical manifestations are usually behavior changes.

40. *c* Observational data suggest that postmenopausal women already diagnosed with osteoporosis may benefit to an extent from calcium supplementation and weightbearing exercise.

41. *b* Children commonly have enlarged tonsils as a normal variant. However, 4+ tonsil size (often called "kissing tonsils") indicates the tonsils meet at mid-line in the posterior oropharynx. This may be significant for obstructive apnea (e.g., sleep apnea).

42. *a* Erythromycin may cause stomach upset, which can be decreased when taken with food. The absorption of delayed release erythromycin is not affected by food intake.

43. *b* This is an application of McDonald's rule. Between 16 and 34 weeks, the height of the fundus approximately equals the number of weeks gestation. Measurements are taken from the top of the symphysis pubis to the top of the fundus in a straight vertical line. The patient's bladder should be empty for accurate measurement.

44. *b* The question "Have you gotten into fights when drinking" is not part of the CAGE questionnaire. It is part of the Michigan Alcoholism Screening Test. The CAGE questionnaire is composed of 4 questions, and the fourth question is "Have you ever had guilty feelings about drinking?"

45. *a* Temporal arteritis is almost exclusively a disease of the elderly. Symptoms include severe headache, scalp tenderness, and visual disturbances.

46. *d* In order for myelinization of the nervous system to occur, children under 2 years-of-age require > 30% daily dietary fat.

47. *a* The patient has a *herpes zoster* infection affecting the optic nerve. Oral and topical antivirals are indicated as well as evaluation and further treatment by an ophthalmologist. If severe optic neuritis develops, the patient can lose vision in the effected eye.

48. *c* Primary prevention consists of activities that decrease the probability of occurrence of specific illness. Fluoride supplementation decreases the probability of occurrence of dental caries.

49. *c* Studies indicate that elderly adults are equivalent to young adults in memory and decision-making skills. The capacity to learn, re-learn, synthesize and problem-solve continues into old age. The normal aging brain may function as effectively as the normal young adult brain except for speed and recent memory. Individuals age 65 years and older are members of a group that experience considerable variation in general health, mental status, and functional abilities.

50. *c* The most common cause of pharyngitis in this age group is viral (80-90%). Based on this knowledge, the nurse practitioner should recommend supportive and symptomatic care with acetaminophen or ibuprofen and hydration. A throat swab for a rapid strep screen and/or culture may be indicated to detect *Streptococcus* sp.

51. *a* Fasting blood glucose is usually used for diabetes mellitus screening because of simplicity and accuracy. It has been found to be more sensitive and more specific than HgA_{1C} for screening. Random blood glucose is only 25% sensitive for screening. An oral glucose tolerance test (GTT) confirms the diagnosis.

52. *c* ELISA is the initial screening test for HIV. The Western blot is then ordered for confirmation of a positive ELISA. Rapid plasma reagin (RPR) is the screening test for syphilis. CD4 cell count is used to monitor the immune status of HIV-positive patients.

53. *a* A left laterally displaced apical impulse suggests cardiomegaly. The apical impulse, or point of maximal impulse (PMI), is the location of maximum outward movement of the apex of the heart with each beat. It is normally at the 4th or 5th left intercostal space at the midclavicular line.

54. *c* Varicella virus vaccine has been approved for use in healthy children > 12 months-of-age. Children 12 months to 12 years-of-age should receive a 0.5 ml dose of the vaccine subcutaneously. Serologic testing is not warranted. Vaccination is not necessary for children who have a reliable history of varicella. Persons 13 years-of-age and older should be given two 0.5 ml doses of the vaccine, 4 to 8 weeks apart.

55. *d* β-blockers and methyldopa may be safely used in pregnancy. Verapamil (Calan®) is a calcium channel blocker and, therefore, contraindicated in pregnancy.

56. *a* The large majority of abuse victims favor routine questions about abuse, with half indicating they would volunteer information about domestic abuse only if specifically asked. Directly asking individuals about abuse has been shown to elicit more positive reports (29%) than the use of written self-reports (7%). The Abuse Assessment Screen, containing 5 open-ended questions, has been validated in pregnant women against more comprehensive instruments. The effectiveness of screening for abuse with physical examination is not known.

57. *b* Influenza vaccine should be administered annually to all persons age 65 years and older, and to persons 6 months-of-age or older who are residents of chronic care facilities, or who suffer from chronic cardiopulmonary disorders, metabolic diseases, hemoglobinopathies, or immunosuppression. Influenza vaccine is also recommended for those who suffer from renal dysfunction, and for health care providers caring for high risk patients. Vaccination for members not described above should be on a case-by-case basis, depending on local disease activity, vaccine coverage, feasibility, and supply.

58. *b* Sensitivity relates to the reliability of a technique to give a positive result when the finding is present. Specificity relates to the reliability of a technique to successfully rule out a finding. A technique is rarely both very sensitive and very specific; therefore, several techniques must be used for an appropriate assessment. A test of high sensitivity is useful for screening, but tends to produce false positive results. A test of high specificity will produce many false negative results.

59. *d* Drinking an adequate amount of water may help hydrate the patient, but it is the least effective way to hydrate the nasal passages.

60. *b* The risk of thromboembolism, stroke, and myocardial infarction (MI) is greater in oral contraceptive users than in non-users.

61. *a* The Dubowitz Clinical Assessment is a standardized scoring system for assessing the gestational age of neonates based on 10 neurological signs and 11 external signs.

62. *a* A principle of pharmacotherapeutics in the elderly is "start low and go slow." In older patients, starting at 50% of the lowest usual adult dose is an appropriate starting dose. Larger doses may precipitate tachycardia and chest pain.

63. *d* All of the signs and symptoms are indicative of hyperthyroidism. This patient should be evaluated for this condition.

64. *d* Fever, rhinorrhea, and dizziness are common clinical findings associated with otitis media. Tragal pain is a common finding in otitis externa.

65. *d* A PPD is considered positive at 5 millimeters or greater induration for confirmed or suspected human immunodeficiency virus (HIV) infection, intravenous drug users with indeterminate HIV status, close contacts of TB cases, and chest x-ray suggestive of previous TB. A PPD greater than or equal to 10 mm induration is considered positive for intravenous drug users known to be HIV-negative, occupants of long term care facilities, age less than 4 years, groups with a high prevalence for TB, the medically underserved, and health care workers. A PPD is considered positive at 15 mm or more in those with no known risk factors.

66. *d* Systemic steroids are not recommended for use in the treatment of degenerative joint disease (DJD). Aspirin, physical therapy, and corrective surgery are all appropriate therapies.

67. *a* A typical malignant prostate gland feels hard on digital examination and is nontender. Hematuria, elevated PSA, and urinary retention are common. Scrotal pain is common with infectious processes and testicular torsion. Spermatocele should be considered with a freely movable cystic mass and non-viable sperm.

68. *a* A positive anti-nuclear antibody (ANA) is 1 of 11 criteria for the diagnosis of systemic lupus erythematosus (SLE). Rheumatoid factor (RF) is used in the diagnosis of rheumatoid arthritis (RA). Erythrocyte sedimentation rate (ESR) is not part of the criteria, but may be elevated. HLA-B27 is not useful for diagnosing SLE.

69. *c* Bouchard's nodes are enlarged proximal interphalangeal (PIP) joints. These are rarely observed in conditions other than osteoarthritis (RA).

70. *a* In 66% of cases, vaginal bleeding in girls under 9 years-of-age is due to infection or presence of a foreign object. Trauma accounts for 16%.

71. *c* A household contact may be suggestive of viral infection but should prompt questions regarding commonly eaten foods among those with symptoms. Typically, bacterial agents are more common during warm months and fever ranges from 101° to 102° F (38.3°C to 38.8°C). Neurological deficits may indicate a neurotoxic agent and immediate, emergency intervention is required.

72. *a* Children who receive a relatively low dose of IG for tetanus or hepatitis prophylaxis may receive the MMR vaccine 3 months later. Children should wait 5 to 6 months after a large dose of IG for measles or varicella prophylaxis. Children receiving replacement therapy on a monthly basis should wait 8 to 10 months.

73. *a* A person having 3 episodes of gout in 3 months needs prophylactic treatment. Corticosteroids have not been shown to be effective in the treatment of gout. Colchicine is often used during an acute attack but may be used for prophylaxis. Allopurinol is more commonly used for prophylaxis because it is better tolerated.

74. *b* The cardinal symptoms of infection with *Trichomonas vaginalis* (a flagellated protozoan) is a frothy, greenish-gray discharge with a fishy odor. The vagina may be very edematous and red. The cervix may be friable with petechiae ("strawberry cervix").

75. *a* Frequent stools, heat intolerance, weight loss, and anxiety or nervousness are indicative of hyperthyroid function. Constipation, cold intolerance, weight gain, lethargy, and impaired concentration are indicative of hypothyroid function.

76. *c* As life expectancy for women has increased, osteoporosis has reached epidemic proportions especially among elderly Caucasian women.

77. *c* Breastfeeding meets the nutritional requirements of healthy infants in most instances. Vitamin D supplements are needed if the infant is not exposed to sufficient sunlight, or if the mother's nutrition is poor. Although both calcium and iron are lower in breast milk, absorption from breast milk is better. Breast milk is high in vitamin C.

78. *d* During iron supplementation, hemoglobin should increase about 1.0 g/dL or more in 1 month. If hemoglobin concentration has not increased, referral should be made to a physician.

79. *c* Overly compliant, withdrawn, or apathetic behavior should be investigated for possible abuse. Small teeth marks on forearms are often from other children. Multiple bruises on the child's knees and elbows are typically associated with unintentional injuries commonly occurring during usual childhood activities and play. Nocturnal enuresis is a normal finding in a 2-year-old.

80. *b* Propranolol is the only medication choice listed for prophylactic treatment of migraine headache. Sumatriptan and DHE are abortive therapies. Ibuprofen is indicated for palliative treatment.

81. *a* Tooth brushing and flossing are very important to prevent tooth decay and periodontal disease. However, fluoride has the greatest influence on reduction of dental caries. Antimicrobial mouth rinses have been shown to reduce gingivitis and plaque.

82. *c*   The lack of improvement after 1 week on crutches and his inability to bear weight are signs indicating a more severe sprain than previously thought. Although there may still be some discomfort, there should be noticeable improvement after 1 week.

83. *d*   Regular physical activity has been proven to reduce the risk of these 6 chronic conditions. Beginning moderately vigorous physical activity during adulthood may reduce the risk of coronary heart disease to the level of those who have been active for many years.

84. *c*   Patients with atrial fibrillation are at increased risk for cerebral vascular accident (CVA) and are candidates for anticoagulation therapy.

85. *b*   It will be important for the nurse practitioner to follow up after 1 to 2 weeks because, if symptoms are controlled, treatment can be continued for 6 to 8 weeks. If symptoms are not controlled, then a different drug therapy regimen should be instituted or the patient should be referred.

86. *b*   As glucose uptake and utilization by the cells of the body improves, weight is gained, not lost. Patients taking metformin (Glucophage®-XR) may experience weight loss, but with the use of most anti-hyperglycemic agents for treatment of type 2 diabetes mellitus, weight gain may occur.

87. *a*   BPH is characterized by an enlarged, symmetrical, semi-firm, and nontender prostate gland. Pain and bogginess is associated with infection. Asymmetry, hardness, and/or nodularity are associated with prostate cancer.

88. *a*   These lesions are typical of molluscum contagiosum. Destruction of lesions will prevent them from spreading, but they usually regress on their own.

89. *d*   There is a strong causal link between human papilloma virus (HPV) and sexual activity. Screening exams and self-examination are secondary prevention measures. At present, there is no prophylactic immunization for HPV. Condom use is the most effective method of prevention.

90. *a*   Acute monocular vision loss may be seen in 15% to 20% of patients with multiple sclerosis (MS). Memory loss and personality changes appear later in the course of the disease. Loss of consciousness is not usually associated with multiple sclerosis.

91. *a*   Baby walkers are a significant cause of injury in young children. Their use should be discouraged and parental holding and floor play should be encouraged instead.

92. *a* Cooking oil may help prevent pain because it prevents air from reaching sensitive skin; however, it has no therapeutic value and may hinder later treatment if the burn is severe. Cool water decreases the temperature of the burned area, prevents further thermal injury, and provides some analgesia.

93. *b* Tattoos and body piercing are potential sources of hepatitis C virus infection if there is common use of contaminated needles. The person receiving the tattoo should make sure the tattooing needles are sterile.

94. *c* The patient's age and symptoms, and the finding of a white pupillary reflex instead of a red reflex, are hallmark physical findings in a patient with cataract. Lens opacity is consistent with cataract. Patients may not be aware of changing vision because age-related cataracts usually develop slowly.

95. *a* Delirium is usually acute with sudden onset, whereas the development of dementia is insidious.

96. *b* Chest pain, shortness of breath, and swollen ankles are all possible indicators of worsening in the patient's cardiac status. While it is important not to omit doses of warfarin, this is the least important of all the choices.

97. *c* After administration of mebendazole, diarrhea and abdominal pain may occur in extreme cases.

98. *c* Scars on the knuckles from induced vomiting are often found on persons with bulimia nervosa. Hypokalemia may be present. Persons with anorexia nervosa are commonly emaciated, but those with bulimia nervosa typically have normal weight. Frequent vomiting causes erosion of dental enamel.

99. *c* The ability to roll from supine to prone (typically achieved by 4.8 [SD 1.4] months) and walk backwards (typically achieved by 14.3 [SD 2.4] months) are examples of gross motor milestones measured by the Denver II Developmental Screening Test (DDST-R). The Early Language Milestone Scale (ELM) measures language development (expressive, receptive, visual language, intelligibility) from birth to 36 months-of-age. Typically, a 50-word vocabulary is achieved by about 24 months-of-age and by 30 months-of-age, most children have a vocabulary of over 400 words with 75% intelligible speech.

100. *c* Hypoglycemia may be appropriately self-treated with 5 lifesavers, which are 3 g of sugar each.

101. *c* Stress incontinence is triggered by straining (e.g., coughing, sneezing, laughing), seldom occurs at night, and is not accompanied by dysuria.

102. *b* The Papanicolaou (Pap) smear is the gold standard for cervical cancer screening. Screening should begin at 21 years-of-age or when the patient becomes sexually active.

103. *a* It is extremely important for patients with sickle cell anemia to avoid infection. Penicillin is the recommended prophylaxis drug for patients with sickle cell anemia. Dosage is based on age, is usually started at 4 months of age and continued until about 5 years-of-age.

104. *c* Women with a history of bearing an infant with a neural tube defect are at increased risk for recurrence in subsequent pregnancies. Ultrasound and amniocentesis can identify whether the fetus has a neural tube defect.

105. *a* By 2 years-of-age, the child should have a vocabulary of at least 20 or more words and should refer to herself by name. She should be referred for a speech and hearing evaluation, but it is not necessary to refer her to an ear, nose, and throat (ENT) specialist yet.

106. *d* Elevated MSAFP levels may indicate underestimation of gestational age, multiple gestation (this particular case), threatened abortion, Rh incompatibility, or a congenital abnormality including neural tube defect.

107. *c* Hemophilia is usually diagnosed within the first year of life. It commonly presents with hemarthrosis, bleeding into soft tissue, hematuria, and prolonged bleeding times.

108. *a* Potassium hydroxide (KOH) breaks down cell walls and allows yeast to be more easily identified with microscopic exam. Inability to visualize hyphae does not rule out fungal infection.

109. *b* The illness described is pityriasis rosea. The origin of this disease is unknown, but is commonly thought to be viral. The "herald patch" typically appears on the trunk and precedes the Christmas tree distribution of lesions by 1 to 30 days. Lesions last 4 to 8 weeks, may be mildly pruritic, and resolve spontaneously without treatment.

110. *d* The quantitative pilocarpine iontophoresis sweat test is the diagnostic test specific for cystic fibrosis. While the other tests may contribute useful information to the overall evaluation, none provide a definitive diagnosis.

111. *d* In the National Adult Literacy Survey, 75% of Americans with chronic physical or mental health problems scored in the lowest 2 out of 5 skill levels. This translates to marginal functional literacy. Among the elderly, minorities, and low income groups, 2 out of 5 cannot read the simplest brochure. Most patients are not likely to volunteer this information.

112. *d* Tinea capitis is unusual in this age group. It usually occurs in children between 2 and 10 years-of-age. There may be an underlying immune or other medical disorder.

113. *d* Laboratory tests needed to confirm the diagnosis of Graves' disease are serum TSH and serum free T_4 index. The T_3 should be measured if both the T_4 and TSH are low and there are clinical manifestations of hyperthyroidism.

114. *a* Any ocular deviation beyond 6 months-of-age is considered abnormal and the patient should be referred to an ophthalmologist for evaluation.

115. *b* The National Childhood Vaccine Injury Act became effective in 1988. It calls for standard consent forms to be used by all health care providers to fulfill their duty to inform the public.

116. *b* Infection is common and can be life-threatening to persons with chronic obstructive pulmonary disease (COPD). It is imperative to treat the infection aggressively. Oxygen is not always indicated. A well-balanced high protein diet is suggested. Polyvalent pneumococcal vaccine is administered once in a lifetime unless the patient is immunocompromised.

117. *c* Malignant melanoma tends to have an irregular border, color variation, and size greater than 6 millimeters in diameter. This patient should be referred for biopsy. Applying sunscreen is a good habit, but does not address the current problem.

118. *c* Traditionally, antepartum care began as soon as the pregnancy was identified. The new recommendation is for every woman who desires pregnancy to undergo preconception counseling for the purpose of evaluating nutritional and psychosocial needs, and assessing medical problems prior to pregnancy.

119. *a* Polycystic ovarian disease is associated with increased insulin resistance and development of diabetes mellitus. The risk of endometrial and breast carcinoma is also increased, but not cervical cancer.

120. *a* Bacteria from the skin around the genitals and anal area enter the urinary tract and may cause a urinary tract infection (UTI). Nylon underwear without a cotton crotch, and nylon panty hose, prevent perspiration and moisture from evaporating. This moist environment is an excellent medium for bacterial growth.

121. *b* Interviewing patients is most successful when the process is collaborative. Patients need to express all their concerns and associated feelings. When these needs are not met, patients are less likely to comply with clinical recommendations.

122. *c* Peripheral arterial insufficiency causes leg pain with walking. Blood flow is generally adequate for basic metabolic demands at rest, but is insufficient to meet the demands of exercise. Edema is usually absent, although dependent rubar is a common feature.

123. *b* Spermicides and female barrier methods can reduce the risk of gonorrhea and chlamydia but are not likely to be as effective reducing transmission of gonorrhea, chlamydia, human immunodeficiency virus (HIV) and other sexually transmitted diseases as male condoms.

124. *a* The average growth rate for a term infant is ½ to 1 ounce per day and one inch per month during the first 3 months of life. After this period, the rate of growth slows.

125. *c* Cool or warm water lavage may cause nausea and/or dizziness. Lukewarm water is recommended. The instillation of cerumen solvent without water irrigation to follow may compound the problem.

126. *c* Mongolian spots are normal variants seen in non-Caucasian infants (particularly African-American, native-American, and Asian infants). They appear as "bruised" areas on the lower back and buttocks and usually fade spontaneously.

127. *d* "Swimmer's ear" is otitis externa. There are no indications that this infection is severe enough to necessitate systemic antibiotics. The infectious organism is usually bacterial or fungal, and choice *d* represents the best treatment option.

128. *b* It is unlikely that this patient's CHF exacerbation is due to a deterioration in his condition. Rather, his dietary indiscretions have caused him to become fluid over-loaded. He needs an intervention that will decrease the amount of fluid his heart must pump. A short-term thiazide or loop diuretic will reduce circulating fluid volume, thereby decreasing cardiac workload.

129. *a* About 30% of the cases of tuberculosis (TB) in the United States occur in HIV-infected patients, African-Americans, Hispanics, foreign-born immigrants, and the homeless. Prison populations are at increased risk for tuberculosis infections due to extended living in close proximity. HIV-infected patients are at highest risk for developing TB.

130. *c* In 1990, heterosexual activity accounted for 27%, homosexual activity accounted for 11%, and intravenous drug use accounted for 14% of cases of infection with hepatitis B. No associated risk factor can be identified for over 30% of patients with HBV infection.

131. *d* Standard 5 on Ethics of the Standards for Advanced Practice Nurses, states that the advanced practice registered nurse (APRN) integrates ethical principles and norms in all areas of practice. One of the outcome measures of this standard is that the advanced practice registered nurse informs the patient of the risks, benefits, and outcomes of health care regimens.

132. *d* Cough is sometimes associated with the use of ACE inhibitors, not calcium channel blockers.

133. *d* The risk of developing breast cancer increases from 0.49% during the period from 20 to 40 years to 5.48% during the period from 65 to 85 years-of-age.

134. *a* ACE inhibitors have been shown to reduce mortality and improve functional status in patients with heart failure.

135. *a* Choices *b*, *c*, and *d* are all contraindications for receiving DTaP. Antibiotic use is not a contraindication.

136. *c* The Centers for Disease Control and Prevention (CDC) offers a choice of 2 strategies for prevention of Group B streptococcal infection: 1) provide antibiotic prophylaxis to pregnant women who have risk factors for GBS or 2) perform a culture for GBS on all pregnant women at 35 to 37 weeks gestation and administer antibiotics to those who test positive. Those at risk are women who go into preterm labor, have ruptured membranes for > 18 hours, women who have had a previous child with GBS, and those who have a urine culture positive for the organism during pregnancy.

137. *b* Adolescence is a time when risk-related sexual practice usually begins.

138. *c* The pneumococcal pneumonia vaccine should only be given once in a lifetime unless the patient has a marked decline in immune function.

139. *b* Echocardiogram with doppler allows the most precise assessment of left ventricular function. A reduction in ejection fraction is seen in congestive heart failure on doppler ultrasound.

140. *d* The initial treatment of benign positional vertigo is bed rest and a vestibular suppressant drug such as an anticholinergic or antihistamine. A systematic exercise program may be of benefit for persons whose vertigo persists beyond 7 to 10 days. A sodium-restricted diet is indicated with Meniere's disease, but not with benign positional vertigo. Prednisone is not indicated for benign positional vertigo.

141. *a* Re-vaccination is indicated when more than 5 years has lapsed since the last Td and the wound is considered contaminated or "major."

142. *c* MMR vaccination is absolutely contraindicated during pregnancy. Before this patient receives the MMR vaccine, it should be made certain that she is not pregnant and does not plan to get pregnant in the subsequent month.

143. *d* A secondary cause of hypertension is suspected because of the patient's age and past history of hypertension. Renal artery stenosis produces a bruit in the right or left upper quadrant as the blood flows through the narrowed vessel.

144. *b* Persons with a cholesterol of 240 mg/dL or greater should have a lipoprotein analysis before the initiation of any treatment.

145. *c* Generally, full term infants who are breastfed have sufficient stores of iron to last through the first 4 to 6 months of life. Earlier supplementation may be necessary for premature infants, infants who are breastfed exclusively beyond the first 6 months-of-age, and infants who begin drinking cow's milk prior to 1 year-of-age.

146. *d* Thiazides, *β*-blockers, and ACE inhibitors are the only agents demonstrated to reduce cardiovascular morbidity and mortality.

147. *c* Peer review is the process by which registered nurses, who are actively engaged in the practice of nursing, appraise the quality of nursing care in a given situation in accordance with established standards of practice.

148. *b* A sudden and unexplained weight gain of 2 to 3 pounds can signify early exacerbation of congestive heart failure. Fluids do not need to be restricted unless the heart failure is complicated by hyponatremia. Patients with congestive heart failure should be encouraged to exercise within their limits except when exacerbations occur. The usual dietary sodium restriction is 2000 mg/day.

149. *b* Spironolactone is a potassium-sparing diuretic. The other diuretics listed are not potassium-sparing and, therefore, predispose the patient to hypokalemia.

150. *b* The nurse practitioner with a traditional direct nursing care role is a primary health care provider. Increasing numbers of nurse practitioners are assuming indirect roles such as educator, administrator, researcher, and consultant.

Practice Exam III

_____ 1. Acute rheumatic fever is diagnosed using the modified Jones criteria. Which is *not* a major criterion in the Jones System?

    a. Jaundice
    b. Polyarthritis
    c. Subcutaneous nodules
    d. Carditis

_____ 2. A patient with past history of documented coronary arterial blockage less than 70% complains of chest pain several times per day (while at rest) which is relieved with nitroglycerin. What is the most appropriate action for the nurse practitioner?

    a. Refer the patient to a cardiologist as soon as possible.
    b. Prescribe long-acting nitroglycerin.
    c. Order a treadmill stress test.
    d. Prescribe an ACE inhibitor and re-evaluate in 24 to 48 hours.

_____ 3. Which of the following may predispose the patient to hyperglycemia?

    a. Glucocorticosteroids
    b. Beta-adrenergic blockers
    c. Alcohol
    d. High-dose salicylates

_____ 4. An urgent call is received from a patient's wife who states that her husband is having chest pain unrelieved by 5 sublingual nitroglycerin tablets. The nearest hospital is 40 minutes away. What intervention can the nurse practitioner suggest which might facilitate a positive outcome?

    a. Have the patient chew an aspirin on the way to the hospital.
    b. Have the patient continue to take sublingual nitroglycerin every 5 minutes until reaching the hospital.
    c. Guide his wife through a cursory assessment (color, respirations, pulse) over the telephone.
    d. Ask the wife what her husband ate that day to rule out gastroesophageal reflux (GER).

_____ 5. Diagnosis of systemic lupus erythematosus (SLE) is made:

    a. on the basis of demonstrable anti-nuclear antibodies (ANA).
    b. considering symptom complex with confirmation by laboratory tests.
    c. using renal function studies and rheumatoid factor (RF) for confirmation.
    d. on the basis of renal or cutaneous biopsy.

_____ 6. **What type of question is most useful when initiating an interview?**

    a. "Yes-No"
    b. Clarifying
    c. Direct
    d. Open-ended

_____ 7. **An example of primary prevention is:**

    a. providing an adolescent with information about sexually transmitted diseases.
    b. performing a testicular exam on an adolescent during a sports physical.
    c. instructing a 16-year-old female how to perform self breast exam.
    d. performing a urine pregnancy test on a 14-year-old sexually active female.

_____ 8. **A 12-year-old presents with ear pain of 36 hours duration. The nurse practitioner diagnoses acute otitis media because the:**

    a tympanic membrane is bulging and glossy with tiny bubbles visible posteriorly.
    b. tympanic membrane is retracted against the bony landmarks.
    c. bony landmarks are obscured and the tympanic membrane is mildly erythematous, dull, and immobile.
    d. canal is narrowed, erythematous, and exquisitely tender on speculum contact.

_____ 9. **The nurse practitioner correctly teaches the patient with diabetes mellitus that if blood glucose is less than 100 mg/dL prior to exercise, the patient should first consume 15 grams of carbohydrates, such as:**

    a. 15 saltine crackers.
    b. 5 small pretzels.
    c. a peanut butter and jelly sandwich.
    d. 1 slice of bread.

_____ 10. The most appropriate first-line drug treatment for elderly African-American patients diagnosed with hypertension is:

a. a calcium channel blocker (CCB), demonstrated by research to be the most effective antihypertensive drug class for this population.
b. an angiotensin converting enzyme inhibitor (ACE-I), because African-Americans are typically high renin-producers.
c. an angiotensin converting enzyme inhibitor (ACE-I), because African-Americans are typically low renin-producers.
d. a thiazide diuretic, demonstrated by research to be the most effective first-line treatment for all ethnic populations.

_____ 11. Which of the following signs and symptoms are typical of hypothyroidism?

a. Constipation
b. Heat intolerance
c. Weight loss
d. Nervousness

_____ 12. Alpha-adrenergic blockers increase urine outflow in males by:

a. improving detrusor muscle stability.
b. shrinking the prostate gland.
c. relaxing prostate smooth muscle.
d. dilating the urethral vasculature.

_____ 13. A healthy 4-week-old infant presents with continuous ipsilateral eye tearing for the past 3 days. There is absence of purulence, erythema, and swelling. The nurse practitioner diagnoses dacryostenosis and most appropriately recommends:

a. regular nasolacrimal duct massage.
b. an ophthalmic antibacterial agent.
c. no treatment, as the condition will resolve spontaneously.
d. an ophthalmic antibiotic/steroid combination.

_____ 14. A patient is diagnosed with primary hypertension. Blood pressure readings for the previous 3 months were 154/100, 148/102, and 158/104. How is this patient's hypertension categorized?

a. Stage 1
b. Stage 2
c. Stage 3
d. Stage 4

_____ 15. The developmental task for the family of an adolescent is to:

    a. provide the adolescent with limits and restrictions.
    b. encourage the adolescent's mastery of physical skills.
    c. enable the adolescent to form a lasting relationship with another person.
    d. allow the adolescent increasing freedom and responsibility.

_____ 16. The initiation of an antidepressant medication in a patient with bipolar disorder may:

    a. trigger anxiety or mania.
    b. improve the depression.
    c. relieve symptoms of both.
    d. precipitate a suicide attempt.

_____ 17. A professional liability insurance policy that provides coverage only if an injury occurs, and the claim is reported to the insurance company, during the active policy period or during an uninterrupted extension (policy tail) of the policy, is termed a(an):

    a. individual policy.
    b. occurrence-based policy.
    c. supplemental policy.
    d. claims-made policy.

_____ 18. The nurse practitioner correctly teaches an elderly patient with pernicious anemia that food sources of vitamin B-12 include:

    a. red meat, poultry, fish, eggs, dairy products.
    b. canned and frozen fruit.
    c. whole grain breads, cereals, and pastas.
    d. fresh vegetables.

_____ 19. Which of the following activities is *not* included in the assessment of Independent Activities of Daily Living (IADLs)?

    a. Preparation of meals
    b. Bathing and dressing
    c. Adherence to medication regimen
    d. Money management

_____ 20. The most important factor in development of peptic ulcer disease (PUD) is:

a. dietary intake of spicy foods.
b. obesity.
c. *Helicobacter pylori.*
d. NSAID use.

_____ 21. A patient complains of "stomach pains on and off" for the past month. In distinguishing between a gastric and duodenal ulcer, what question is *least* important to ask?

a. "Have you been out of the country in the past several months?"
b. "Have you had dark, tarry, or bloody stools?"
c. "Is your stomach pain made worse by eating?"
d. "Does your stomach pain wake you up in the early morning?"

_____ 22. The mother of a 3-year-old male asks about her son's nocturnal enuresis. Which of the following responses is appropriate?

a. Suggest waking the child up mid sleep cycle to urinate.
b. Recommend that the mother require the child to change his own bedding.
c. Prescribe desmopressin acetate (DDAVP®) nasal spray at bedtime.
d. Explain that nocturnal enuresis is generally not considered to be a problem before 6 years-of-age.

_____ 23. The tricyclic antidepressants (TCAs) and selective serotonin reuptake inhibitors (SSRIs) have demonstrated efficacy in the treatment of each of the following conditions *except*:

a. diabetic peripheral neuropathy.
b. migraine prophylaxis.
c. fibromyalgia.
d. gastroesophageal reflux (GER).

_____ 24. An obese 43-year-old has a history of recurrent superficial fungal skin infection over the past 2 years. Today, she presents with intertriginous candida. Her skin is macerated from frequent rubbing and scratching. The plan of care for this patient should include:

a. screening for diabetes mellitus and HIV infection.
b. application of cornstarch or body powder to finger webs, toe webs, and skin folds to absorb moisture.
c. liberal application of a moisturizing cream to affected areas.
d. a topical antibiotic for 7 to 10 days.

_____ 25. According to the JNC-VII guidelines for evaluation of blood pressure, pre hypertension is defined as systolic blood pressure between:

a. 140-159 mmHg.
b. 130-149 mmHg.
c. 120-139 mmHg.
d. 100-119mmHg.

_____ 26. Right-sided heart failure is characterized by all of the following clinical findings *except*:

a. a 4th heart sound.
b. increased JVD or hepatojugular reflux.
c. hepatosplenomegaly.
d. peripheral edema.

_____ 27. Which drug(s) used in the treatment of congestive heart failure (CHF) is(are) *not* associated with decreased mortality?

a. ACE inhibitors
b. Diuretics
c. Beta-adrenergic blockers
d. Digoxin

_____ 28. Your 45-year-old patient with diabetes asks about the medications you have prescribed. You respond:

a. "A daily aspirin will help reduce the risk of cardiovascular complications from diabetes."
b. "ACE inhibitors are no longer renoprotective after albuminuria is present."
c. "Every diabetic should take a lipid-lowering drug to protect the blood vessels from damage."
d. "As long as your blood pressure is normal, you'll never need an ACE inhibitor."

_____ 29. A patient presents to the rural health clinic with severe chest pain. The nurse practitioner places the patient on a cardiac monitor and observes a normal sinus rhythm with elevated ST segments. Blood pressure is 130/75 mmHg. What is the most likely cause of this patient's chest pain?

a. Anxiety
b. Dyspepsia
c. Cardiac ischemia
d. Myocardial infarction

_____ 30. Six weeks gestation is confirmed in a 23-year-old, moderately overweight, patient. She asks the nurse practitioner, "Should I diet so I won't gain too much weight?" The nurse practitioner appropriately responds:

a. "It is probably a good idea to lose a few pounds in the first trimester since it will be harder to control weight gain later."
b. "A weight gain of approximately 25 pounds is ideal for mother and baby."
c. "It doesn't matter how much weight you gain or lose as long as you eat a well-balanced diet."
d. "Just try to limit your weight gain as much as you comfortably are able."

_____ 31. Clinical features associated with a diagnosis of syndrome X include all of the following *except*:

a. tachyarrhythmias and angina.
b. hypertriglyceridemia, reduced HDL, and increased LDL.
c. high levels of serum fatty acids stored as fat.
d. hypertension, atherosclerotic plaque formation, and CAD.

_____ 32. Which drug class is knows to exacerbate hyperglycemia?

a. NSAIDs
b. DMARDS
c. Corticosteroids
d. COX-2 inhibitors

_____ 33. A patient who is taking an oral glucocorticosteroid should be advised to take it:

a. with milk.
b. with a high fat meal.
c. on an empty stomach.
d. with orange juice.

_____ 34. Appropriate treatment for seborrheic dermatitis includes all of the following *except*:

a. a keratolytic agent.
b. a coal tar preparation.
c. oral and/or topical acyclovir.
d. a topical corticosteroid.

_____ 35. An elder's caretaker is planning the elder's menus. The elder is on a bland diet. The nurse practitioner reviews the meal plans and notes that which of the following is *not* appropriate?

    a. Oatmeal, cold cereal, white toast, french toast with syrup
    b. Cream soup, jello, noodles
    c. Scrambled or boiled eggs, cottage cheese, ice cream
    d. Coffee, tea, carbonated beverages, orange juice

_____ 36. Which of the following is appropriate to teach a patient who is using a daily nitrate agent for treatment of chronic angina?

    a. Continuous 24-hour coverage is necessary for maximum protection.
    b. A daily 12-hour nitrate-free period is important to prevent tolerance.
    c. A daily 6-hour nitrate-free period is important to prevent tolerance.
    d. Nitrate-free periods present a potential for developing nitrate tolerance.

_____ 37. A very active 35-year-old male has painful hemorrhoids. His diet has been indiscriminate as his job requires frequent travel. The most appropriate recommendation is for him to select foods that are:

    a. low in fiber such as milk and other dairy products.
    b. high in simple carbohydrates such as white bread and mashed potatoes.
    c. high in fiber such as bran, complex carbohydrates, and fresh fruit.
    d. high in protein such as meat, poultry and fish.

_____ 38. Asthma is:

    a. an obstructive airway disease.
    b. chronic, progressive, irreversible airway disease.
    c. characterized by wheezing without sputum production.
    d. a disease only of childhood and adolescence.

_____ 39. The nurse practitioner notes several patchy, scaly, raised, irregular lesions on sun-exposed areas of an elderly patient's skin. The lesions appear similar except that they are various sizes and shades of black, brown, tan, or yellow. The nurse practitioner refers the patient to a dermatologist for evaluation and treatment because the lesions are most likely:

    a. seborrheic keratoses which are benign, but unsightly.
    b. caused by contact with an allergen and are intensely pruritic.
    c. malignant melanoma, a highly lethal and metastatic skin cancer.
    d. actinic keratoses, and approximately 20% develop into squamous cell carcinoma.

_____ 40. A patient with hepatic cirrhosis presents with pedal edema. He reports that his wife prepares the same lunch for him every day: a ham and cheese sandwich on white bread with mustard, a bowl of fresh vegetable soup, a fresh orange, banana, or grapes, and sweetened iced tea. He denies adding salt to his food. The food that is most likely causing his edema is the:

a. sweetened tea.
b. ham and cheese.
c. fresh vegetable soup.
d. fresh fruit.

_____ 41. A drug used for acute episodes of gout is colchicine. What is the most common early sign of colchicine toxicity?

a. Palpitations
b. Heartburn
c. Diarrhea
d. Headache

_____ 42. A 43-year-old male presents with a large and painful furuncle, the 3rd in the past 6 months. The nurse practitioner should recommend all of the following *except*:

a. incision and drainage (I&D) of the furuncle.
b. a prophylactic antibiotic.
c. screening the patient for diabetes mellitus.
d. advising the patient to apply moist heat compresses to facilitate rupture and drainage of the furuncle.

_____ 43. The nurse practitioner receives a call from a skilled nursing care facility about a 66-year-old male with chronic liver failure. Which of the following symptoms is of greatest concern?

a. Nausea
b. Fatigue
c. Shortness of breath
d. Anorexia

_____ 44. Which of the following is a microcytic hypochromic anemia?

a. Folic acid deficiency anemia
b. Iron deficiency anemia
c. Pernicious anemia
d. Anemia of chronic disease

_____ 45. Which of the following clinical findings is *not* consistent with a diagnosis of pyloric stenosis in a 3-month-old infant?

    a. Projectile vomiting
    b. Severe dehydration as demonstrated by sunken eyeballs and depressed anterior fontanelle
    c. A bloated and tense, tympanic, abdomen
    d. A palpable mass, the size and shape of an olive, in the right upper quadrant of the abdomen

_____ 46. The nurse practitioner correctly teaches an insulin-dependent patient the signs and symptoms of early hypoglycemia, which include:

    a. facial flushing and dilated pupils.
    b. frequent urination and abdominal pain.
    c. diplopia and irregular pulse.
    d. blurred vision, pallor, and perspiration.

_____ 47. The nurse practitioner correctly diagnoses a 2nd degree burn injury, which is described as:

    a. full thickness, waxy or leathery, without vesicles.
    b. partial thickness, with erythema and edema but no vesicles.
    c. partial thickness, involving the dermis and epidermis, with edema and vesicles.
    d. full thickness, with involvement of muscle and bone.

_____ 48. The plan of care for a 75-year-old female with arteriosclerosis obliterans would appropriately include:

    a. maintaining a consistently warm temperature in the home.
    b. wearing support stockings during the daytime.
    c. avoidance of walking as much as possible.
    d. frequent rest periods with legs and feet elevated.

_____ 49. Expected findings associated with a diagnosis of folic acid deficiency include all of the following *except*:

    a. glossitis.
    b. pallor and/or jaundice.
    c. depression and listlessness.
    d. MCV < 80 fl.

_____ 50. Infants with cystic fibrosis are at risk for multiple complications. The most urgent complication of this disease is:

a. iron deficiency anemia.
b. intussusception or volvulus.
c. frequent anorexia, nausea, and vomiting.
d. frequent pulmonary infection.

_____ 51. The nurse practitioner correctly diagnoses iron deficiency anemia in a male patient whose lab report reveals:

a. hemoglobin (Hgb) 15.0 g/dL.
b. a decreased total iron-binding capacity (TIBC).
c. mean corpuscular volume (MCV) < 80 fl.
d. increased mean corpuscular hemoglobin concentration (MCHC).

_____ 52. The nurse practitioner would be correct to include all of the following points in the education of patients with folic acid deficiency anemia *except*:

a. all alcoholic beverages should be eliminated.
b. foods high in folic acid include broccoli, red beans, and oatmeal.
c. oral folate replacement therapy is 0.4 mg per day.
d. folic acid deficiency during pregnancy places the fetus at risk for neurological anomalies including neural tube defects.

_____ 53. Prescriptive authority for APRNs is:

a   legislated and regulated at the state level.
b. uniform for all states.
c. governed by the state medical board.
d. regulated by federal and state laws.

_____ 54. The long term prognosis for a patient with a diagnosis of dementia is:

a. unpredictable, because the condition is characterized by remissions and exacerbations.
b. poor, because the progression of dementia is fairly rapid.
c. good, because it is reversible with appropriate intervention.
d. poor, because gradual deterioration of cognitive function, memory, judgment, and emotional stability is progressive and irreversible.

_____ 55. A mother who has diabetes mellitus wants to breastfeed her infant. The nurse practitioner should:

    a. explain that breastfeeding is contraindicated, because diabetic medications are secreted in breast milk, placing the infant at risk for hypoglycemia.

    b. explain that breastfeeding is unwise, because it places excess physiological stress on the mother.

    c. support the mother's decision and recommend more frequent monitoring of blood sugars.

    d. encourage bottle feeding, as breastfeeding would cause the mother's serum glucose to be too erratic.

_____ 56. What is the anatomical site currently believed to be the best location for subcutaneous insulin administration?

    a. Buttocks

    b. Thigh

    c. Abdomen

    d. Arm

_____ 57. Health Maintenance Organizations (HMOs) and Preferred Provider Organizations (PPOs) are:

    a. managed care systems.

    b. regulated by state law.

    c. cooperatives of fee-for-service providers.

    d. networks of hospitals and clinics.

_____ 58. A 46-year-old female has hypertension which is well controlled with propanolol. Which of the following is a beneficial secondary effect of this drug?

    a. Improved glycemic control

    b. Improved lipid profile

    c. Weight loss

    d. Migraine prophylaxis

_____ 59. Which of the following clinical findings is consistent with a diagnosis of parathyroid tumor?

    a. Headaches and diplopia

    b. Positive Chvostek's sign

    c. Nausea and vomiting

    d. Hypotonic deep tendon reflexes

_____ 60. Of the following factors in a 57-year-old postmenopausal patient's history, which is an additional risk factor for osteoporosis?

   a. Walking slowly on a treadmill for 20 minutes every other day
   b. Prednisone 5 mg every other day
   c. A daily calcium channel blocker for management of hypertension
   d. An 1800 calorie ADA weight-loss diet

_____ 61. The nurse practitioner teaches the parents of a 2-month-old infant with gastroesophageal reflux (GER) that treatment typically includes all of the following interventions *except*:

   a. maintaining the usual feeding regimen and burping the infant well when the feeding is completed.
   b. positioning the infant with head and trunk elevated 30 to 45 degrees both during and after feedings.
   c. thickening the formula with rice cereal.
   d. providing smaller, more frequent, feedings and burping the infant at regular intervals during the feeding.

_____ 62. The nurse practitioner recommends a 24-hour urine for creatinine clearance. Appropriate instructions to the patient are to:

   a. begin the 24-hour time period and collect the next voided urine.
   b. empty the bladder and begin the 24-hour time period, then collect the next voided specimen.
   c. empty the bladder, begin the 24-hour time period at the time of the next voiding and collect that specimen.
   d. begin the 24-hour time period, discard the next voided urine, then collect the next voided specimen.

_____ 63. The primary reason that infants and very young children are at greater risk for acute otitis media than adolescents and adults is because:

   a. infants and very young children do not know how to effectively blow their noses.
   b. adolescents and adults understand the principles of contamination and transmission of microorganisms.
   c. adolescents and adults have more mature immune systems.
   d. the eustachian tubes are narrower and more vertical in infants and young children.

_____ 64. To differentiate testicular torsion from epididymitis, the nurse practitioner should order:

   a. a urinalysis.
   b. scrotal ultrasound.
   c. a urine Gram stain.
   d. a CT scan.

_____ 65. The nurse practitioner correctly diagnoses pernicious anemia when:

   a. the patient's tongue is smooth, glossy, and beefy red.
   b. the patient has hypoesthesia of the distal extremities.
   c. the patient's Schilling test reveals excessive renal excretion of radiolabeled B-12.
   d. the patient's MCV is < 80 fl.

_____ 66. Which drug class should be avoided in patients with a diagnosis of osteopenia or osteoporosis?

   a. Glucocorticoids
   b. DMARDS
   c. COX-2 inhibitors
   d. NSAIDs

_____ 67. Which age group is at highest risk for testicular cancer?

   a. < 20 years-of-age
   b. 20 to 40 years-of-age
   c. 40 to 60 years-of-age
   d. > 60 years-of-age

_____ 68. Which of the following is true regarding Medicaid?

   a. The primary recipients are adults over 65 years-of-age.
   b. Beneficiaries 21 years-of-age and older are allowed a specified number of outpatient visits per year.
   c. The provider may bill the patient for services and medications that are not reimbursed by Medicaid.
   d. Coverage and reimbursement is established at the federal level and is the same for all states.

_____ 69. Of the following risk factors associated with cervical cancer, which two factors represent the highest risk?

1. Smoking
2. History of multiple sexual partners
3. Early age at first intercourse
4. Multiparity
5. African-American descent
6. Low socio-economic income status

a. 1, 2   c. 5, 6
b. 3, 4   d. 1, 6

_____ 70. A patient presents with a chief complaint of heat intolerance and weight loss. These symptoms may be associated with:

a. Hashimoto's disease
b. iodine deficiency
c. autoimmune thyroiditis
d. Grave's disease

_____ 71. What is the most common chronic condition in the elder population in the United States?

a. Hypertension
b. Arthritis
c. Cataract
d. Diabetes mellitus

_____ 72. Of the following 4 malpractice issues for which an APRN may incur liability, which is the most prevalent cause of action?

a. Failure to refer when the APRN's skills are exceeded
b. Failure of the APRN to adequately diagnose
c. Conduct exceeding the APRN's scope of expertise that causes harm
d. Conduct within the APRN's scope of practice which results in death of a patient

_____ 73. Trophic changes associated with chronic arterial insufficiency include all of the following lower extremity characteristics *except*:

a. dry ulcerations with round smooth edges.
b. edema and weeping ulcerations.
c. sparse or absent hair.
d. pronounced malleoli and MTP joints.

_____ 74. On clinical examination of the skin of an elderly patient, the nurse practitioner knows that all of the following are normal benign variants associated with the aging process, and require no pharmacotherapeutic treatment, *except*:

    a. xerosis.
    b. cherry angiomas and senile purpura.
    c. senile keratoses and senile lentigines.
    d. dermatophytoses.

_____ 75. A 73-year-old patient, without teeth or dentures, presents with a very sore, glossy, smooth, beefy-red tongue, chronic dry mouth, decreased sense of taste, cracked corners of the mouth, and persistent lip smacking. This clinical presentation most likely reflects:

    a. pernicious anemia, due to insufficient intrinsic factor.
    b. secondary hypothyroidism.
    c. cheilosis, a condition of the lips.
    d. a neurological disorder such as Parkinson's disease.

_____ 76. The nurse practitioner wants to assess intactness of a patient's cerebellar function. Which of the following clinical tests will provide information relative to cerebellar function?

    a. Kinesthesia
    b. Stereognosis
    c. Romberg
    d. Graphesthesia

_____ 77. On examination of the skin of a 65-year-old male, the nurse practitioner notes erythematous eruptions with scaly and flaky, but oily, yellowish plaques over the nasolabial folds, scalp, and area of the eyebrows. The patient reports the condition is always present and is exacerbated by stress. What is the most likely diagnosis?

    a. *Herpes zoster* (shingles)
    b. Tinea corporis
    c. Seborrheic dermatitis
    d. Psoriasis

_____ 78. A father brings in his 4-year-old child who sustained a dog bite to his forearm 1 hour earlier. Two wounds are each 0.5 cm and appear as deep puncture wounds. After exploration, debridement, and cleansing, the most appropriate intervention is to:

a. suture the wounds.
b. apply a topical antibiotic and occlusive dressing without suturing.
c. apply a topical antibiotic and leave the wounds uncovered.
d. suture the wounds, instruct the father to keep the sites clean and uncovered, and prescribe an oral antibiotic.

_____ 79. An adult patient has an S4 heart sound and the PMI is located at the 5th left ICS, left of the MCL. What are these findings associated with?

a. Congestive heart failure
b. Mitral insufficiency
c. Hypertension
d. Aortic insufficiency

_____ 80. The retinopathy most specifically associated with chronic hypertension is(are):

a. microaneurysms.
b. cotton wool spots.
c. AV nicking.
d. dot and blot hemorrhages.

_____ 81. The nurse practitioner is inspecting the skin on a 63-year-old patient and notes a single pearly-gray papule with a raised border, central clearing, and telangiectasis. The lesion is located on the patient's posterior neck. What is the most likely diagnosis?

a. Basal cell carcinoma
b. Malignant melanoma
c. Common nevus
d. Squamous cell carcinoma

_____ 82. All of the following agents are generally contraindicated in pregnancy *except*:

a. angiotensin converting enzyme inhibitors (ACE-I), angiotensin II receptor blockers (ARB), warfarin.
b. oral anti-seizure medications, oral anti-diabetes agents, oral estrogen.
c. fluoroquinolones, tetracyclines, ibuprofen.
d. cephalosporins, parenteral insulin, parenteral heparin.

_____ 83. A 15-year-old high school student presents with mild sore throat and low grade fever that has persisted for about 2 weeks. She reports general malaise, fatigue, and loss of appetite. The nurse practitioner suspects mononucleosis. Which of the following is the *least* appropriate intervention?

    a. Palpate the lymph nodes and spleen.
    b. Examine the posterior oropharynx for petechiae.
    c. Obtain a CBC, throat culture, and heterophil antibody test.
    d. Obtain a urinalysis and serum for LFTs and amylase.

_____ 84. Physical examination findings consistent with emphysema include all of the following *except*:

    a. increased anterior-posterior chest diameter.
    b. hyper-resonant percussion sounds.
    c. decreased diaphragmatic excursion and flattening of the diaphragm.
    d. pallor and cyanosis of the mucosa and nail beds.

_____ 85. A 3½-year-old presents in the emergency department complaining of arm pain. History is negative for blunt trauma or fall. She holds the arm in flexed position against her body with the opposite forearm and hand. After much persuading, she allows the nurse practitioner to examine the arm. She is not able to supinate the hand. There is absence of crepitus and absence of palpable bony deformity. The most likely diagnosis is:

    a. fracture of the distal humerus.
    b. subluxation of the proximal radial head.
    c. contusion or fracture of the olecranon process.
    d. fracture of the distal radius or ulna.

_____ 86. An 18-year-old patient is diagnosed with classic migraine headache. Her headaches are frequent and debilitating. She is offered an abortive therapy, but says she would rather take a medication for prophylaxis. The nurse practitioner would recommend:

    a. a "triptan."
    b. B vitamins.
    c. calcium channel blocker.
    d. an angiotensin receptor blocker.

_____ 87. Two siblings, 4 years old and 8 years old, present with impetigo. The older sibling has multiple lesions over the arms and legs and some are confluent. The younger sibling has 3 minor lesions on 1 leg. The most appropriate intervention is to advise the mother to wash the lesions thoroughly and:

    a. administer the prescribed oral antibiotic to both children.
    b. apply a topical antibacterial ointment to the lesions on both children.
    c. apply a topical antibacterial ointment to the lesions on both children and administer an oral antibiotic to the older child.
    d. apply a topical antibacterial ointment to the lesions on the older child and simply keep the lesions on the younger child clean and dry.

_____ 88. History and clinical findings consistent with a diagnosis of Marfan's syndrome include:

    a. tall stature with disproportionately long arm and fingerlength.
    b. restricted joint range of motion.
    c. increased anterior/posterior to transverse (AP/T) chest diameter.
    d. hypotension and cardiac arrhythmias.

_____ 89. The adult child of a 79-year-old disabled Medicare beneficiary notifies the nurse practitioner that her father's home health agency has terminated his services without prior notification. The nurse practitioner contacts the agency and is told that services were terminated because the patient's care had become economically burdensome with recent changes in Medicare reimbursement. The home health agency's action is:

    a. malpractice.
    b. negligence.
    c. abandonment.
    d. legal.

_____ 90. Which of the following is *not* true regarding the diagnosis of scoliosis in children?

    a. Scoliosis is most apparent during the pre-adolescent growth spurt.
    b. Scoliosis may be evidenced by unequal shoulder, scapula, or iliac crest height with the child standing.
    c. Kyphosis in the adolescent indicates scoliosis.
    d. Routine screening for scoliosis should begin at 10 to 12 years-of-age, with forward bending touching the toes, and unclothed examination of the spine.

_____ 91. A patient with active tuberculosis (TB) has a negative PPD skin test. This phenomenon may be explained by any of the following *except*:

    a. oral steroid treatment.
    b. chronic antihistamine use.
    c. HIV infection.
    d. malnourishment due to anorexia nervosa.

_____ 92. All of the following are characteristic of macular degeneration *except*:

    a. it is a leading cause of legal blindness among the elderly.
    b. normal peripheral vision.
    c. it is a usual consequence of diabetic retinopathy.
    d. distorted size and shape of objects.

_____ 93. The nurse practitioner suspects a TMJ disorder. As the patient slowly opens and closes the lower jaw, the nurse practitioner palpates the temporomandibular joint (TMJ) bilaterally:

    a. anterior to the mastoid process.
    b. anterior to the tragus.
    c. at the lower border of the lobule.
    d. at the angle of the jaw.

_____ 94. A patient presents with distorted areas and blind spots in the visual field. The painless condition was first noticed on awakening this morning. The nurse practitioner would most appropriately include all of the following in the plan of care *except*:

    a. refer the patient to an ophthalmologist if the condition has not resolved in 24 hours.
    b. refer the patient for a fluorescein angiogram and exam by soon as possible.
    c. examine the retinal field for edema, infarcts, exudates, and retinal detachment.
    d. screen the patient for diabetes mellitus.

_____ 95. Which of the following is *not* true of presbycusis?

    a. It involves a low frequency hearing loss.
    b. It is more prevalent with advancing age.
    c. It is a normal part of aging.
    d. The onset is sudden and caused by drug toxicity.

_____ 96. Tinnitus is an audible sound which is not present in the environment. All of the following are true about tinnitus *except* it:

    a. may be described as roaring, ringing, or humming.
    b. may be attributed to excessive ingestion of aspirin.
    c. may be a presenting sign for Meniere's disease, otosclerosis, or presbycusis.
    d. is only audible to the patient.

_____ 97. Correct instructions to give new parents who are transporting their newborn infant are:

    a. a rear facing infant car seat secured in the backseat is required until the infant weighs 20 lbs.
    b. the infant car seat may be secured in the back or front seat, but must be rear facing.
    c. the infant car seat may be front facing when the infant is 1-year-old.
    d. a rear or front facing infant car seat must be secured in the back seat until the infant weighs 20 lbs.

_____ 98. A 16-year-old presents to the clinic for a scheduled immunization. The patient is unaccompanied by an adult. The nurse practitioner's action is based on the knowledge that:

    a. a minor must have the informed consent of a parent or guardian to receive an immunization.
    b. the minimum age of consent is 21 years.
    c. consent is considered "informed" when the patient's mental age is at least 12 years.
    d. consent is considered "informed" when the patient is at least 16 years old.

_____ 99. Untreated infection with human papilloma virus (HPV-16) increases the female's risk for:

    a. infertility.
    b. ovarian cancer.
    c. pelvic inflammatory disease (PID).
    d. cervical cancer.

_____100. Differential diagnosis of heart failure due to a high cardiac output state includes:

a. thyroid storm (thyrotoxicosis).
b. digitalis toxicity.
c. excessive beta receptor blockade.
d. hypervolemia and hypertension.

_____101. A nurse practitioner is examining a 2-month-old infant. What question is most important to ask about the baby?

a. "Does the infant have siblings?"
b. "Has the umbilical cord stump fallen off yet?"
c. "Was the infant full-term at birth?"
d. "Has the baby had a PKU test?"

_____102. Which statement below about breastfeeding is *not* accurate?

a. An infant with hyperbilirubinemia should not be breastfed.
b. A mother with flat or inverted nipples may be able to breastfeed.
c. Improper positioning of the infant can result in the mother having sore nipples.
d. A mother with a plugged milk duct should not stop breastfeeding.

_____103. A mother reports that her infant is making audible clicking sounds throughout breastfeeding. How should the nurse practitioner respond?

a. "This is normal. Continue to breastfeed."
b. "Avoid using pacifiers and bottles because they cause nipple confusion."
c. "The breast milk is probably too thin."
d. "Reposition the nipple in the infant's mouth."

_____104. A patient with diabetes brings his glucose diary from the past 7 days for the nurse practitioner to review and evaluate. What change should be made?

DAY	1	2	3	4	5	6	7
AM	67	52	61	48	39	58	44
PM	138	161	148	168	121	142	176

a. Increase the PM dose of NPH insulin.
b. Increase the PM dose of regular insulin.
c. Decrease the PM dose of NPH insulin.
d. Decrease the PM dose of regular insulin.

_____105. Visible carotid artery pulsations on physical examination of the neck most likely indicate:

    a. right heart failure exacerbation.
    b. pulmonary hypertension.
    c. arteriosclerotic carotid artery disease.
    d. aortic regurgitation.

_____106. Which cranial nerves are responsible for eye movement?

    a. II, III, IV
    b. III, IV, VI
    c. II, IV, VI
    d. III, IV, VII

_____107. A female patient believes that she was exposed to HIV through sexual intercourse several months ago. She requests "the test for AIDS." Which statement is *not* correct?

    a. The ELISA is used for screening, but may yield a false negative this soon after exposure.
    b. The Western blot is an immunofluorescence assay and is used to confirm a positive ELISA.
    c. Either blood or saliva can be used for screening.
    d. She should refrain from all sexual intercourse until results of the test are known.

_____108. A patient takes theophylline twice daily for bronchospastic disease. Today he presents with thick, discolored, tenacious sputum, mild shortness of breath, and fever. What drug should he avoid?

    a. prednisone
    b. clarithromycin (Biaxin® XL)
    c. levofloxacin (Levaquin®)
    d. doxycycline

_____109. When examining a pregnant patient, where should the fundal height be at 22 weeks?

    a. Slightly above the symphysis pubis
    b. At the level of the umbilicus
    c. Midway between the symphysis pubis and umbilicus
    d. Just below the xiphoid process

_____110. Which activity during the first trimester could be deleterious to the fetus?

    a. Sexual intercourse
    b. Jogging
    c. Dieting
    d. Airplane flight

_____111. A patient presents with pruritic lesions on both knees. There are visible silver scales. This condition is most appropriately managed with a(an):

    a. topical antifungal cream or ointment.
    b. oral antibiotic.
    c. topical corticosteroid cream.
    d. topical antifungal/steroid cream.

_____112. What assessment finding is *not* typical of the patient with psoriasis?

    a. Pruritis
    b. Positive Auspitz sign
    c. Pitted nails
    d. Satellite lesions

_____113. Which class of drugs increases a patient's risk for developing rhabdomyolysis?

    a. Antihypertensives
    b. Thiazide diuretics
    c. The "statins"
    d. Anticoagulants

_____114. At what age should an infant be expected to triple his birth weight?

    a. 6 months
    b. 8 months
    c. 9 months
    d. 1 year

_____115. Which drug class is associated with elevated serum lipid levels?

    a. Thiazide diuretics
    b. Potassium-sparing diuretics
    c. Loop diuretics
    d. ACE inhibitors

_____116. Atenolol (Tenormin®) should be avoided in which patient?

    a. A 65-year-old male with renal failure
    b. A 43-year-old female with asthma
    c. A 70-year-old male with alcoholism
    d. A 68-year-old female, post-myocardial infarction

_____117. A 12-year-old patient's fasting serum cholesterol is 190 mg/dL. Her mother asks "is that okay?" The nurse practitioner responds:

    a. "This is acceptable for her age and gender, although less than 200 mg/dL is desirable."
    b. "This is acceptable, but she should increase her fruit and vegetable intake."
    c. "This is unacceptable. The desired level is < 170 mg/dL."
    d. "This is unacceptable, but inappropriate to treat because of her age."

_____118. Which murmur is associated with radiation to the neck?

    a. Pulmonic stenosis
    b. Aortic stenosis
    c. Hypertrophic obstructive cardiomyopathy
    d. Mitral valve insufficiency

_____119. A patient with 20/80 visual acuity can see:

    a. at 20 feet what a person with normal vision can see at 80 feet.
    b. at 80 feet what a person with normal vision can see at 80 feet.
    c. at 80 feet what other people can see at 20 feet.
    d. better than a patient with 20/40 vision.

_____120. A 72-year-old male presents with fluid collected in his scrotum. He states that the size of his scrotum does not fluctuate during the course of a day. He is also likely to describe:

    a. a recent traumatic injury.
    b. a history of testicular torsion.
    c. pain associated with the swelling.
    d. frequent nocturia.

_____121. Which of the following lymph node characteristics are of greatest concern?

    a. Enlarged and mobile
    b. Tender and 0.5 cm in diameter
    c. Firm and nontender
    d. Warm and 1.0 cm in diameter

_____122. A 35-year-old male patient with a past history of glaucoma and frequent sinusitis presents today with hypertension. On his last 2 visits to the clinic, his blood pressures were 150 to 160 systolic and 90 to 98 diastolic. The nurse practitioner decides to treat the hypertension with long-acting propanolol. Before prescribing it, the nurse practitioner should ask:

    a. if other family members are hypertensive.
    b. whether he smokes or consumes alcohol on a daily basis.
    c. what other medications have been prescribed for him.
    d. if he takes a daily antihistamine.

_____123. A male infant had a clinic visit at 2 and 4 months of age. Today, he returns for his 6-month exam. The nurse practitioner notes absence of the red reflex in the patient's right eye. What diagnoses should be included in the differential?

    1. Cataract
    2. Retinoblastoma
    3. Retinal detachment
    4. Iritis

    a. 1 only
    b. 2, 4
    c. 1, 2, 3
    d. all of the above

_____124. A nurse practitioner is examining the gluteal folds of a 2-month-old African-American infant and notices a 7 to 8 cm bluish discoloration in the sacral area. The nurse practitioner should:

    a. discuss discipline with the caregiver.
    b. suspect child abuse and report this to the authorities.
    c. inquire about recent trauma or falls.
    d. consider this a normal finding.

_____125. A 2-year-old has been diagnosed with herpangina. His symptoms began 48 hours ago. He is very irritable and his temperature is 102.8° F. When he is examined by the nurse practitioner, he begins to cry but there are no visible tears. The nurse practitioner knows that this:

    a. is abnormal and indicates anorexia.
    b. child is dehydrated.
    c. is manipulative behavior by the child to stop the examination.
    d. may indicate meningeal irritation.

_____126. Which symptom is *not* typical in a female during the peri-menopausal period?

    a. Vasomotor instability
    b. Paresthesias
    c. Increased vaginal lubrication
    d. Disturbed sleep patterns

_____127. During routine examination of a 65-year-old male, the prostate gland feels hard and asymmetrical. The nurse practitioner suspects prostate cancer. What other finding is likely?

    a. Tenderness on DRE
    b. Hematuria
    c. Nitrites in the urine
    d. PSA 4.0 – 10.0 ng/ml

_____128. A usually very healthy 3-year-old was diagnosed yesterday with acute otitis media. The nurse practitioner prescribed amoxicillin. The child's caregiver calls today to report that the pain has not subsided and his temperature has not decreased. How should the nurse practitioner respond?

    a. Stop the amoxicillin and prescribe a broader spectrum antibiotic.
    b. Have the mother administer ibuprofen or acetaminophen for pain relief for 24 to 48 more hours.
    c. Ask the mother to recheck his temperature and call you back if it is still elevated.
    d. Re-examine the child for a tympanic membrane rupture.

_____129. An elderly patient presents with a gray-white ring around the periphery of the iris. This is probably:

    a. an emerging cataract.
    b. a normal variant associated with the aging process.
    c. indicative of underlying atherosclerotic disease.
    d. iritis or uveitis.

_____130. Which of the following demonstrates that a 30-year-old male has successfully achieved the developmental task of young adulthood?

    a. Is married with 2 children
    b. Lives alone and spends most of his time at home surfing the internet
    c. Has changed careers 3 times in the past 10 years
    d. Lives with his parents and has a girlfriend

_____131. A patient states that he has received the hepatitis B immunization series. What should the nurse practitioner check to determine if he has protection from the immunization?

    a. Hepatitis B surface antigen
    b. Hepatitis B surface antibody
    c. Hepatitis B surface antibody and hepatitis B core antibody
    d. Hepatitis B surface antigen and antibody

_____132. Factors associated with increased risk for osteopenia and osteoporosis include all of the following *except*:

    a. anticonvulsant medication taken for peripheral neuropathy pain.
    b. a hyperthyroid or hyperparathyroid condition.
    c. Caucasian race and early menopause.
    d. oral contraceptive use or postmenopausal hormone replacement therapy (HRT).

_____133. A 55-year-old male patient presents with dysuria, urgency, perineal pain, and temperature 101°F (38.3°). What is the most likely diagnosis?

    a. Cystitis
    b. Epididymitis
    c. Urethritis
    d. Prostatitis

_____134. A 25-year-old male complains of heaviness in his scrotum accompanied by a dull ache. On exam, the nurse practitioner palpates a mass at the inguinal canal. Which of the following would *not* be included in the differential diagnosis for this patient?

    a. Inguinal hernia
    b. Testicular mass
    c. Undescended testicle
    d. Varicocele

_____135. Immediately after receiving 2 immunizations by injection, a 5-year-old became pale and fainted. He was placed on an exam table and in about 15 seconds he regained consciousness. He did not stop breathing. His mother asks what happened. The nurse practitioner correctly explains:

    a. an allergic reaction to the vaccine is the likely cause.
    b. the child became afraid and had a vasovagal episode.
    c. this happens frequently when immunizations are given.
    d. this will likely recur next time the child receives an injection.

_____136. A patient is diagnosed with Bell's palsy. He is placed on high dose steroid therapy. After 4 days of prednisone, the patient states that his eye still will not close completely. How should the nurse practitioner manage the problem?

    a. This patient should be referred to a neurologist.
    b. This is not unusual. He should continue with the treatment plan.
    c. The nurse practitioner should increase the dosage of prednisone.
    d. The patient should have a CT scan to rule out other etiologies.

_____137. Which of the following occurs first in female sexual development?

    a. Pubic hair in a reverse triangle distribution
    b. Presence of breast buds
    c. Secondary mound formed by the areola and papilla
    d. Onset of menses

_____138. Which item below is *not* implicated in erectile dysfunction (ED)?

    a. Diabetes mellitus (DM)
    b. Urinary tract infection (UTI)
    c. paroxetine (Paxil®)
    d. enalapril (Vasotec®)

_____139. A patient's TSH is increased and free T_4 and T_3 are decreased. The nurse practitioner most likely expects the patient to report:

    a.   heat intolerance.
    b.   soft and thin hair and nails.
    c.   warm and moist skin.
    d.   hair loss.

_____140. A patient taking oral contraceptive pills reports that she has forgotten to take her pill for the past 3 days. How should the nurse practitioner advise her today?

    1.   Take 2 tablets today and 2 tablets tomorrow. Then resume the regular schedule."
    2.   Discard the pill pack and begin a new pill pack.
    3.   Use an additional method of contraception for the rest of the pill pack.
    4.   Discard the 3 missed pills and continue as scheduled.

    a.   1
    b.   1, 2
    c.   3
    d.   3, 4

_____141. A patient taking oral contraceptives pills for 3 cycles complains of breast fullness, tenderness, and nausea. The patient is concerned. How should the nurse practitioner manage this complaint?

    a.   Continue the pills for 2 more cycles and then re-evaluate.
    b.   Change the pill to a brand containing less estrogen.
    c.   Change the pill to a brand containing less progesterone.
    d.   Ask her to take the pill at bedtime.

_____142. A patient with moderate persistent asthma will probably be most effectively managed with a daily:

    a.   oral leukotriene blocker.
    b.   short- and long-acting bronchodilator.
    c.   inhaled steroid and long-acting bronchodilator.
    d.   long-acting bronchodilator only.

_____143. Peak flow is determined by:

    a.   age.
    b.   weight.
    c.   height.
    d.   gender.

_____144. A patient is 26 weeks pregnant. She presents today with very tender vesicles on an erythematous base in the genital area. She complains of malaise and fever and states that she's never felt anything like this before. The nurse practitioner would be correct to say the lesions and symptoms should resolve:

    a.   at delivery.
    b.   in about 3 days.
    c.   in about 14 to 21 days.
    d.   in about 7 days.

_____145. The best location to assess a bruit produced by renal artery stenosis is:

    a.   anteriorly, below the umbilicus, at the midclavicular line.
    b.   anteriorly, along a horizontal band crossing the umbilicus.
    c.   posteriorly, immediately below the costovertebral angle.
    d.   posteriorly, at the waistline.

_____146. A 74-year-old widowed male, who lives alone, tells the nurse practitioner "I get enough to eat. I don't need much." He does not prepare food for himself at home, preferring to eat a noon meal at a neighborhood restaurant. Which of the following is the most sensitive indicator of this patient's nutritional status?

    a.   Absence of 3 well-rounded daily meals
    b.   Fatigue and weight loss
    c.   Serum pre-albumin level
    d.   Elevated serum BUN and RBCs

_____147. Which of the following are characteristic of benign breast lesions?

    a.   Solitary with irregular borders
    b.   Movable and "rope-like"
    c.   Hard and attached to adjacent tissue
    d.   Ipsilateral and nontender

_____148. Which of the following liver enzyme values is indicative of alcohol-related hepatitis?

    a.   ALT : AST ratio > 2.0
    b.   AST : ALT ratio > 2.0
    c.   ALT and AST equally elevated
    d.   ALT and AST equally decreased

_____149. Which of the following is considered a noninflammatory disease process?

    a. Osteoarthritis (OA)

    b. Rheumatoid arthritis (RA)

    c. Systemic lupus erythematosus (SLE)

    d. Psoriatic arthritis

_____150. Which of the following is a medication or medication class that does *not* have dizziness and vertigo as potential adverse side effects?

    a. Aminoglycoside antibiotics

    b. High-dose salicylates

    c. Central-acting antihypertensives

    d. meclizine (Antivert®)

Practice Exam III
Answers and Rationales

1. *a* One of the major criteria for diagnosis of acute rheumatic fever using the Jones System is polyarthritis, the most common finding. This usually responds to aspirin therapy within 48 hours. Another common finding is carditis. Other major criteria which are far less common include erythema marginatum and subcutaneous nodules.

2. *a* This patient probably has increased blockage in one or more of his coronary arteries. He should to be referred promptly for further diagnosis and treatment. It would be inappropriate to order any of the other suggested interventions before referral.

3. *a* Nonselective beta-blockers, alcohol, and high dose salicylates may potentiate insulin-induced hypoglycemia.

4. *a* Based on the patient's symptoms and his unrelieved chest pain after 3 sublingual NTG tablets, he is probably having a myocardial infarction. He needs immediate medical intervention, without unnecessary delay, to prevent serious medical complications or death. Since the hospital is 40 minutes away, chewing an aspirin will help with anti-coagulation and possibly prevent damage from myocardial ischemia secondary to clot formation.

5. *b* The American College of Rheumatology has specified 11 criteria to categorize abnormalities associated with systemic lupus erythematosus (SLE). At least 4 of these criteria are required to make the diagnosis. Laboratory tests alone cannot be used for diagnosis of SLE, but anti-nuclear antibodies are part of the criteria.

6. *d* Open-ended questions are most effective when attempting to elicit general information in the beginning of the patient interview.

7. *a* Primary prevention consists of activities that decrease the probability of occurrence of specific illness such as disease prevention education.

8. *c* Serous otitis media, not acute otitis media, typically presents with a flat or bulging tympanic membrane with a fluid line and/or tiny bubbles visible posteriorly. The tympanic membrane may be immobile and retracted against the bony landmarks when the eustachian tube is swollen or congested as with the common cold or allergies. Narrowing of the external canal, with erythema and extreme tenderness of the canal wall, is indicative of otitis externa.

9. *d* Consuming 5 grams of carbohydrate prior to exercise will protect the diabetic patient with a blood glucose less than 100 mg/dL from a hypoglycemic episode. The following foods represent approximately 5 g of carbohydrate: 4 to 6 saltine crackers, 10 to 25 small pretzels, 1 slice of bread.

10. *d* Research has demonstrated that the most effective first-line drug treatment for hypertension in elderly patients of African-American descent is a thiazide diuretic. Calcium channel blockers are also good choices. African-Americans are typically low renin-producers, therefore, angiotensin converting enzyme inhibitors are usually not effective. Beta-blockers and diuretics are recommended as first-line agents for all ethnic populations when there is absence of a comorbid condition that is a contraindication.

11. *a* Frequent stools, heat intolerance, weight loss, and anxiety or nervousness are indicative of hyperthyroid function. Constipation, cold intolerance, weight gain, and lethargy are indicative of hypothyroid function.

12. *c* Alpha-1 blockers are commonly used in the pharmacologic treatment of benign prostatic hyperplasia (BPH). These agents improve urine outflow in males by relaxing prostate smooth muscle. Terazosin (Hytrin®) and doxazosin (Cardura®) are appropriate choices when the patient has comorbid hypertension. The α-1 blockers do not cause hypotension in normotensive patients. Tamsulosin (Flomax®) is an α-1 blocker that is prostate-specific.

13. *a* The condition is not likely an allergic condition, as both eyes would typically be affected. Dacryostenosis is narrowing of the nasolacrimal duct, preventing normal drainage from the eye. The treatment is regular massage to open the duct and maintain patency. Ophthalmic antibacterial agents are appropriate for ophthalmic infections only. Ophthalmic infections typically present with swelling, erythema, pain, and purulence. When an ophthalmic infection presents with extreme swelling and erythema, an ophthalmic antibacterial/steroid combination may be a more appropriate choice.

14. *b* According to the National Heart, Lung, and Blood Institute (NHLBI) and JNC VII, blood pressure is classified:

< 120 systolic and < 80 diastolic:	normal
120-139 systolic or 80-89 diastolic:	pre-hypertensive
140-159 systolic or 90-99 diastolic:	stage 1
>160 systolic or >100 diastolic:	stage 2

15. *d* By increasing freedom and responsibility, the family allows the adolescent to prepare for young adulthood through mastering of the developmental task of identity vs. identity diffusion.

16. *a* Screening for a family or personal history of bipolar disorder should be done for patients who report symptoms of anxiety and depression. The initiation of an antidepressant in these patients may trigger a manic episode.

17. *d* A "claims-made" professional liability insurance policy provides coverage only if an injury occurs, and the claim is reported to the insurance company during the active policy period or during an uninterrupted extension of the policy ("policy tail"). An occurrence-based policy provides coverage for injuries arising out of incidents occurring during the period the policy was in effect, even if the policy subsequently expires or is not renewed by the policyholder.

18. *a* The principal sources of vitamin B-12 (cobalamins) are liver and other organ meats, beef, pork, eggs, milk and milk products. Deficiencies produce a macrocytic anemia.

19. *b* Bathing, grooming, and dressing are activities in the assessment of Activities of Daily Living (ADLs), a lower (less complex) level of functioning.

20. *c* *H. pylori* infection is found in 90 to 95% of patients with duodenal ulcer and in 60 to 70% of patients with gastric ulcers. Obesity plays no role in the development of PUD. NSAID use is an important risk factor for PUD development.

21. *a* The questions in choices *b*, *c*, and *d* are critical questions to ask patients with suspected peptic ulcer disease. A positive response to the question in choice *b* implies GI hemorrhage. A positive response to the question in choice *a* could imply an infectious etiology of the stomach pain and has little bearing on distinguishing between gastric and duodenal ulcer disease.

22. *d* There is a wide range in the age at which urinary continence is established. The incidence of enuresis is estimated to be 40% in 3-year-olds, 10% in 5-year-olds, and 3% in 10-year-olds. For 3 to 5-year-old children, the best approach is a matter-of-fact, non-judgmental, attitude toward "accidents."

23. *d* Randomized controlled trials have demonstrated efficacy of the TCAs and SSRIs in the management of idiopathic symptoms and functional symptom syndromes such as chronic fatigue, tinnitus, peripheral neuropathy, fibromyalgia and other chronic pain conditions, and migraine prophylaxis. Most of these uses are "off -label."

24. *a* Skin infection with *candida albicans*, a fungus, is characterized by shiny, red plaques with papules, and satellite lesions. Frequent fungal infection is an indication for screening for diseases associated with decreased immunity such as diabetes mellitus and HIV infection. Cornstarch powder absorbs and retains moisture and, therefore, should not be used. Application of a moisturizing cream preparation would be contraindicated. A topical antibiotic is only indicated if a superimposed bacterial infection presents.

25. *c* Most learned bodies and specialty organizations recognize 140/90 as hypertension necessitating intervention. For patients with other comorbid conditions such as diabetes, renal failure, CHF, much lower readings are necessary to prevent damage to organs and vasculature. Pre-hypertension is a new classification which describes blood pressure 120-139 or 80-89.

26. *a* Right-sided heart failure is characterized by presence of a 3rd heart sound. The most common cause of right-sided heart failure is left-sided heart failure.

27. *d* ACE-Inhibitors, beta-blockers, and diuretics are associated with decreased morbidity and mortality in heart failure. Digoxin has been shown to reduce morbidity in patients with congestive heart failure, but not to reduce mortality. It was previously thought that beta-blockers were contraindicated in the treatment of CHF and are still to be avoided in acute exacerbations of CHF. Carvedilol (Coreg®) and metoprolol (Toprol® XL) are beta-adrenergic blockers that have FDA indications for chronic CHF treatment. Diuretics reduce pre-load, reducing such symptoms as shortness of breath, orthopnea, and paroxysmal nocturnal dyspnea.

28. *a* The cardiovascular risk in diabetic patients after 30 years-of-age is 2 to 4 times that of non-diabetics. The ADA recommends a daily aspirin provided there are no contraindications. ACE inhibitors are especially beneficial after albuminuria is present. Even if blood pressure is normal, an ACE inhibitor may be used for renoprotection. A "statin" is the drug of choice for hyperlipidemia in diabetes; however, there are many contraindications and a "statin" should not be used when lipids are at target levels.

29. *c* Although he is in a normal sinus rhythm and has a normal blood pressure, this patient's chest pain is due to cardiac ischemia based on his reported symptoms and elevated ST segments. He is at high risk for a myocardial infarction if the ischemia is not reversed.

30. *b* Dieting to induce weight loss is contraindicated at any time during pregnancy. To decrease the risk of prematurity, low birth weight, and stillbirth, a weight gain of approximately 25 lbs is recommended.

31. *a* Syndrome X is also termed "insulin resistance syndrome" and "cardiovascular dysmetabolic syndrome." Although there are cardiovascular and peripheral vascular complications, neither tachyarrhythmias nor angina are associated with this syndrome.

32. *c* Corticosteroids are well known to increase glycemia in susceptible persons and, therefore, should be avoided or used with caution by patients with diabetes. Serum glucose level is not affected by NSAIDs, DMARDS, or COX-2 inhibitors.

33. *a* Glucocorticosteroids are associated with gastric ulcer formation. Taking an oral glucocorticosteroid with milk facilitates maximum absorption while protecting the gastric mucosa.

34. *c* Acyclovir is appropriate treatment for a viral skin infection such as *herpes zoster*, *herpes genitalis*, or severe, recurrent, *herpes labialis*. Keratolytic agents and coal tar preparations are appropriate treatments for seborrheic dermatitis. Topical corticosteroids are also appropriate treatment for allergic dermatitis conditions, such as contact dermatitis and atopic dermatitis.

35. *d* Caffeinated and carbonated beverages, and acidic juices, are contraindicated for the patient on a bland diet. Foods selected should not be raw, spicy, acidic, or gas forming.

36. *b* Continuous 24-hour coverage increases tolerance to the effects of nitrates. A daily 12-hour nitrate-free period is important to prevent this potential problem.

37. *c* A high fiber diet produces a soft stool which is less mechanically irritating on passage past the hemorrhoidal tissue. A low-fiber diet predisposes the patient to constipation, which should be avoided.

38. *a* Asthma is an obstructive airway disease that is reversible with bronchodilating drugs. A common misconception is that asthma is a disease of childhood. Asthma is a chronic disease which is most commonly seen in childhood and adolescence, with a long period of remission and recurrence of symptoms in the 4th decade.

39. *d* Actinic keratoses are "pre-malignant" lesions typically found in sun-exposed areas of the skin. They may be black, brown, tan, or yellow. Approximately 20% of actinic keratoses, also called senile keratoses, develop into squamous cell carcinoma. Although the lesions rarely metastasize, removal is recommended for prophylaxis. Malignant melanoma is the 3rd most common type of skin cancer. It originates from a pigmented mole (nevus), may be flat or somewhat raised, has irregular borders and variegated color, and is highly metastatic. Seborrheic keratoses are chronic benign lesions that are raised, oily but flaky, waxy, wart-like, and erythematous, without association with sun exposure.

40. *b* Ham, cheese, and milk are high in sodium content, contributing to fluid retention and edema. Ham is also high in protein, which a cirrhotic liver cannot effectively metabolize. Commercially canned foods are high in sodium content, therefore, fresh vegetables and fruits are preferred.

41. *c* The dose of colchicine for treatment of an acute gout attack is 1 to 2 tabs (strength 0.5 to 0.6 per tab) to start, and then 1 tab every hour until pain is relieved, GI side effects appear, or the 8 mg/day maximum is reached.

42. *b* Local heat compresses provide comfort and facilitate healing by increasing perfusion to the area. Incision and drainage (I&D) of the furuncle will facilitate eradication of the infectious microorganism and speed healing. Recurring infection may be an indicator of impaired immunity or diabetes mellitus. Good skin hygiene is necessary, but prophylactic antibiotics are not indicated because of the potential for microbial resistance.

43. *c* Patients in chronic liver failure may be expected to have nausea due to gastrointestinal vascular congestion, shortness of breath due to ascites, and fatigue due to anemia of chronic disease. Although shortness of breath may be expected, many other serious conditions can cause shortness of breath and these must be investigated provided it is consistent with the patient's advance directives.

44. *b* Iron deficiency anemia is a microcytic and hypochromic anemia. Folic acid deficiency is a macrocytic normochromic anemia. Pernicious (vitamin B-12 deficiency) anemia is a macrocytic, megaloblastic, and normochromic anemia. The anemia of chronic disease is normocytic and normochromic.

45. *c* Abdominal bloating is not a clinical finding associated with pyloric stenosis. Left-to-right peristaltic waves may be visible on examination of the abdomen during and following feedings.

46. *d* Facial flushing, diplopia, pupillary dilation, polyuria, abdominal pain, and irregular pulse are signs and symptoms of hyperglycemia.

47. *c* Erythema and edema, but absence of vesicles, characterizes a 1st degree burn. A 2nd degree burn involves the dermis and epidermis, with edema and vesicles. Dry, waxy, leathery skin is characteristic of a 3rd degree burn. A 4th degree burn involves muscle and bone. Some organizations have discontinued use of the terms 1st, 2nd, 3rd, 4th degree burns.

48. *a* Elevation of the lower extremities, support stockings, and cool or cold environmental temperature further decrease arterial perfusion in patients with arterial insufficiency. Support stockings and frequent elevation of the lower extremities are indicated for venous insufficiency. Walking to the point of pain (claudication pain), resting until the pain subsides, and then resuming the walk facilitates arterial perfusion and enhances overall cardiovascular fitness.

49. *d* The anemia associated with folic acid deficiency is macrocytic (MCV > 100 fl) and normochromic.

50. *b* Intussusception and volvulus are surgical emergencies. Delayed release of the invaginated or "telescoped" bowel (intussusception), or delayed release of the twisted bowel (volvulus), may result in tissue death, gangrene, perforation, peritonitis, and/or sepsis, and fatality.

51. *c* Lab values diagnostic for iron deficiency anemia include increased TIBC, MCV < 80 fl, decreased MCHC, and Hgb < 14.0 g/dL in males and < 12.0 g/dL in females.

52. *c* Folic acid replacement therapy is usually 2 to 4 mg per day, but may be increased to 5 to 10 mg per day in the presence of chronic infection or alcohol use. Folic acid deficiency during pregnancy is associated with a high rate of neural tube defects. Supplemental folic acid during pregnancy should be 1 mg per day in the absence of folic acid deficiency anemia.

53. *a* Prescriptive authority varies from state to state. At this time, all 50 states have some form of prescriptive authority. Some are more restrictive than others. Some states allow prescription of controlled substances, others do not.

54. *d* Delirium is reversible, but dementia is not. The most common form of dementia is Alzheimer's disease.

55. *c* Diabetes mellitus is not a contraindication to breastfeeding for either the mother or the infant. More frequent monitoring of blood sugars will allow the patient to make medication adjustments as needed. Insulin does not pass into breast milk and so this may be the most appropriate management of the breastfeeding diabetic patient. Oral antidiabetic agents should be evaluated individually with consideration given to discontinuing the drug(s) and initiating insulin, or continuing the drug(s) with careful monitoring of the infant. Most oral sulfonylureas are excreted in breast milk.

56. *c* Research has demonstrated that insulin is absorbed most rapidly and consistently when injected in the subcutaneous tissue of the abdomen (with the exception of the area in a 1 inch radius around the umbilicus).

57. *a* Managed care systems are intended to integrate delivery of health care with financing of health care. This is typically done through a series of contracts with health care providers, diagnostic groups, and other support services.

58. *d* Propanolol is a beta-blocking agent. It has indications for management of hypertension, tachyarrhythmias, and essential tremor. It has a secondary effect of migraine prophylaxis. Other drugs associated with migraine prophylaxis are the calcium channel blockers, lithium, and amitriptyline.

59. *b* The patient with impaired parathyroid function is at risk for hypocalcemia. Hypocalcemia is characterized by increase in neuromuscular excitability. Clinical findings include: confusion, circumoral paresthesia, paresthesia of the fingers and toes, carpopedal spasms (muscle spasms in the hands and feet), positive Chvostek's sign (tapping on the facial nerve elicits twitching of the nose or lip), and positive Trousseau's sign (occlusion of the arterial blood flow to the arm for 5 minutes elicits contraction of the hand and fingers).

60. *b* Glucocorticosteroids promote protein catabolism. HRT and weight-bearing exercise, such as walking, are protective. An ADA weight loss diet is well-balanced in all of the essential nutrients. A postmenopausal female should include calcium supplementation of 1200 to 1500 mg per day. Calcium channel blockers have no effect on osteoporosis.

61. *a* Providing smaller, more frequent feedings, thickening the formula with rice cereal, frequent burping during feedings, and positioning the infant at 30 to 45 degrees reduces the risk of GER by decreasing gastric content volume and pressure on the lower esophageal sphincter (LES).

62. *b* The urine collection container should be kept immersed in a pan or bowl of ice with the lid securely closed during the collection period.

63. *d* As children grow, the lumen of the eustachian tube widens and becomes more diagonal, thus facilitating drainage and impeding movement of microorganisms into the middle ear.

64. *b* It may be difficult to differentiate testicular torsion from epididymitis on clinical examination alone. Doppler ultrasound is useful to detect disruption in arterial flow that occurs with testicular torsion.

65. *a* Pernicious anemia is a macrocytic (MCV > 100 fl), megaloblastic, and normochromic anemia, due to insufficient gastric mucosal secretion of intrinsic factor and resulting deficiency of vitamin B-12 absorption. Schilling test reveals renal excretion of radiolabeled B-12 reduced to less than 5% in patients with pernicious anemia. Characteristic clinical presentation includes a smooth, beefy red tongue, distal extremity paresthesias, unstable gait, and difficulty with fine motor finger movement. The rate is especially high among the elderly. Treatment with intramuscular vitamin B-12 injections is lifelong.

66. *a* Glucocorticosteroids, while effective mediators of the inflammation, are well known to cause demineralization of bone and decreased bone density. Steroids should be avoided or reserved only for short term use in osteopenic or osteoporotic patients. Bone density is not affected by DMARDS, NDAIDs, or COX-2 inhibitors.

67. *b* Testicular examination by a professional provider, and patient education regarding monthly testicular self-examination (TSE) to screen for testicular cancer, should be included in every annual physical examination. The highest incidence of testicular cancer is in men 20 through 35 years-of-age. Cryptorchidism places patients at significantly increased risk of testicular cancer.

68. *b* In contrast to Medicare, Medicaid services are state specific. Each state receives federal dollars to be used to take care of a group of individuals identified by each state. The individuals tend to be low income with no other payment source for medical expenses.

69. *c* Although all of the characteristics are associated with risk for cervical cancer, the highest incidence is among women of African-American descent and women in the lower socioeconomic group.

70. *d* Grave's disease is characterized by symptoms of sympathetic nervous system hyperstimulation (tachycardia, tremors, heat intolerance, weight loss), due to an excess of circulating thyroid hormone. Although not a common problem in the U.S., hypothyroidism may be caused by iodine deficiency. Hashimoto's disease, the most common cause of hypothyroidism, is also referred to as autoimmune thyroiditis.

71. *b* The most frequently occurring chronic conditions among the elderly are: arthritis (48%), hypertension (36%), heart disease (32%), hearing deficits (32%), cataracts (17%), and diabetes mellitus (11%).

72. *a* The most prevalent cause of action occurs in choice *a*. APRNs must refer patients in a timely manner when they see that their expertise will be exceeded—Lane v. Otis (1982), Azzolino v. Dingfelder (1994).

73. *b* Weeping ulcerations with irregular borders (particularly near the lateral malleolus) and edema are associated with venous insufficiency. Reduced cellular supply of oxygen and nutrients caused by chronically insufficient arterial perfusion is evidenced by loss of lean muscle mass and adipose tissue, thin dry skin, decreased or absent hair growth, and dry "punched out" ulcers (primarily over the PIP and DIP joints and medial malleolus).

74. *d* Senile keratoses, senile lentigines, cherry angiomas, senile purpura, and xerosis are normal benign skin variants associated with the aging process and require no pharmacotherapeutic treatment. Senile keratoses, also called seborrheic keratoses, are dark wart-like lesions. Senile lentigines ("liver spots") are flat brown macules. Cherry angiomas are small, round, red spots and senile purpura are purple patchy areas. Xerosis is dry, rough, scaly, pruritic skin commonly found on the anterior lower legs (the shins). Dermatophytosis refers to a tinea (fungal), infection of the skin, scalp, and/or nails which causes (depending on the site) pruritus, inflammation, hair loss, thickened discoloration of the nails, and requires treatment with an antifungal agent.

75. *a* Hypothyroidism is associated with an enlarged tongue (macroglossia). Cracked corners of the mouth (cheilosis) is common in the elderly, particularly when the patient is without teeth or dentures. The treatment is application of a topical lubricant at regular intervals. Insufficient production of intrinsic factor by the gastric mucosa decreases vitamin B-12 absorption, causing pernicious anemia. This anemia commonly presents with a very sore, smooth, beefy-red tongue.

76. *c* Kinesthesia (position change), stereognosis (identification of an object by touch), and graphesthesia (identification of a number drawn on the palm) are clinical tests of sensory neurological function. The Romberg test assesses cerebellar function. The patient is asked to stand with his eyes closed and feet together. He is assessed for his ability to not sway or fall.

77. *c* This is the classic clinical presentation of seborrheic dermatitis. Psoriasis, an autoimmune dermatological disorder, presents with thick, silvery plaques with erythematous bases, located primarily over the elbows, forearms, and knees. Tinea corporis presents with pruritic, annular lesions with central clearing, located on the face, trunk, arms, or legs. *Herpes zoster* (shingles), caused by the herpes II virus, presents as extremely painful vesicular lesions along one or more ipsilateral dermatomes.

78. *b* Bite wounds should be irrigated with 100 to 200 ml high-pressure jet fluid (usually sterile normal saline) per linear inch of wound to debride and reduce bacterial inoculation. A povidone-iodine/normal saline mixture is virucidal and is indicated when there is risk of rabies, hepatitis, or HIV transmission. Bite wounds which should not be sutured primarily include deep puncture wounds, lacerations less than 1.5 cm in length, wounds treated > 24 hours post-bite, wounds to the hand (especially those with joint involvement), extensive crush injuries, and injuries requiring extensive debridement. Primary closure is best delayed for 3 to 4 days or omitted altogether. An oral antibiotic should be considered for this patient.

79. *c* Presence of an S4 heart sound and lateral displacement of the PMI is associated with a diagnosis of hypertension. Displacement of the PMI reflects enlargement of the left ventricle secondary to hypertension.

80. *c* AV nicking is specifically seen in chronic, moderate hypertension. Microaneurysms are almost always associated with diabetes. Cotton wool spots are associated with any condition which damages the retinal microvasculature like diabetic hypertension. Dot and blot hemorrhages are most commonly seen in diabetes but may be seen in hypertension.

81. *a* This is the classic clinical presentation of basal cell carcinoma. Basal cell carcinoma is the most common skin cancer and is most often located on the nose, eyelid, cheek, neck, back, or back of the hands. It is slow growing and rarely associated with metastasis. The 2nd most common skin cancer, squamous cell carcinoma, is reddened, scaly, and wart-like with a depressed border, and is often found on sun-exposed areas of the skin such as the neck, ears, arms, and hands. It is slow growing and may potentially metastasize. The common nevus (mole) is a deposit of melanin, may be flat or raised, has a regular border, and may be located anywhere on the body (although it is not usually found on the palms of the hands or soles of the feet).

82. *d* Patients who take oral hypoglycemic agents should be switched to parenteral insulin and patients who take warfarin (Coumadin®) should be switched to parenteral heparin during pregnancy. Ibuprofen is not recommended during pregnancy and is category D in the third trimester. Fluoroquinolones (may interfere with development of articular cartilage) and tetracyclines (may be incorporated into developing teeth and bones) are contraindicated during pregnancy. Safer alternatives include penicillins and cephalosporins.

83. *d* The clinical presentation of this patient is typical of mononucleosis. Lymphadenopathy, splenomegaly, pharyngeal petechiae, and leukocytosis are common additional findings. Urinalysis, serum amylase, and LFTs would not yield information regarding the diagnosis. The confirmatory tests are throat culture and the heterophil antibody test.

84. *d* Pallor and cyanosis are typical of chronic bronchitis (type B COPD, the "blue bloater"). Emphysema (type A COPD, the "pink puffer") is not associated with pallor or cyanosis. Increased AP diameter produces a "barrel chest." The normal chest is elliptical whereas the barrel chest is round. The muscles of the thorax appear thin and wasted while the accessory muscles of respiration are hypertrophied. Breath sounds are diminished and cough is weak and ineffective.

85. *b* This clinical presentation is classic subluxation of the radial head ("nursemaid's elbow"). The injury is caused by sudden and sharp, or prolonged, forceful extension of the elbow, such as with forceful removal of clothing over the head, dangling while suspended by the hands, or sudden grabbing and jerking the child by the hand. The dislocation may be reduced clinically with immediate relief of pain and return of full range of motion.

86. *c* Beta-blockers, along with calcium channel blockers and most recently, ACE inhibitors are known to produce endothelial stabilizations and serve as excellent migraine prophylactic agents. Other prophylactic agents are amitriptyline, lithium, and SSRIs.

87. *c* When impetigo lesions are few and minor, a topical antibiotic (e.g., mupirocin) is sufficient. Multiple lesions, particularly when they are confluent, usually require an oral antibiotic as well. Keeping the lesions covered reduces further trauma from scratching and reduces transmission of this highly communicable disease.

88. *a* Tall stature, long thin arms with extended arm span, joint laxiety and hyperextensibility, bluish sclera, long and thin fingers (arachnodactyly), and excavatum/carinatum pectus deformity are presenting Marfan's syndrome features. Associated cardiovascular abnormalities include aortic and mitral valve regurgitation, aortic root dilation and aortic dissection, and hypertension. Marfan's syndrome is associated exclusively with male gender.

89. *c* Home health agencies cannot discriminate against Medicare beneficiaries who are economically less desirable because they are deemed heavy users of services. Termination of medically necessary home health services because the client is a heavy user, without affording the client reasonable notice, constitutes "dumping" and abandonment. The Rehabilitation Act of 1973 provides handicapped persons with the right to sue if they are denied benefits, are excluded from participation, or are otherwise subjected to discrimination by any program that receives federal government monies.

90. *c* Kyphosis (convex curvature of the thoracic spine) is a common finding in adolescence and is most often due to poor posture (functional kyphosis). Structural kyphosis may occur in isolation or may be associated with scoliosis (kyphoscoliosis). Lumbar spinal curvature may also be associated with scoliosis (lordoscoliosis). When all 3 structural deformities occur together, the condition is termed kypholordoscoliosis.

91. *b* Injection with PPD results in a delayed hypersensitivity reaction in patients who have been previously exposed to TB. In the absence of the reaction, immunocompromised states must be suspected. These include specific diseases such as HIV, use of steroids, and poor nutritional states such as occurs in anorexia nervosa.

92. *c* Macular degeneration is characterized by loss of central vision with preservation of peripheral vision. It is not a normal consequence of diabetes although other macular problems like microaneurysms and hard exudates may be present on the macula of diabetic patients.

93. *b* The temporomandibular joint (TMJ) is located just anterior to the tragus of the ear.

94. *a* Because of the abrupt onset and acuity, this condition may be attributed to retinal detachment or a hypercoagulation disorder resulting in microemboli. Immediate referral to an ophthalmologist is warranted with dilated retinal exam and fluorescein angiography as soon as possible. Detachment of the retina may be a painless, spontaneous, occurrence, and may be due to underlying diabetes mellitus.

95. *d* Presbycusis is gradual and progressive sensorineural hearing loss. Impaired ability to hear high-pitched sounds occurs initially and then lower pitched hearing is affected. Prevalence increases with advancing age and is more common in men than women. Speech discrimination is problematic, especially with the clutter of background noise.

96. *d* Tinnitus may be audible to both the patient and the examiner when the source is a vascular bruit. Tinnitus caused by excess aspirin, furosemide, or intravenous lidocaine, is a sign of drug ototoxicity and is usually reversible by stopping the drug.

97. *a* Infants must be placed in a rear facing infant car seat in the backseat until they reach 20 lbs. The safest place is the center of the backseat. Infants and young children should never be left unattended in a motor vehicle.

98. *a* A minor may not legally receive an immunization without consent of a parent or guardian unless the minor is emancipated. Consent is considered informed when the patient's mental age is at least 7 years. Consent is invalid when the patient has received a consciousness-altering drug such as a narcotic analgesic. Written consent is always preferred, although verbal consent (e.g., via telephone) may be given with 2 witnesses.

99. *d* HPV is a viral infection which produces warts on the genital area. They are generally benign. However, certain types have oncogenic potential. They are types 16, 18, 31, and 33. It may be transmitted sexually or through fomites.

100. *a* Thyrotoxicosis is characterized by positive chronotropic myocardial activity (tachycardia) caused by excessive SNS activity. Digitalis and beta-blockers are negative chronotropes (slow heart rate). Hypervolemia and hypertension are primary causes of excessive afterload and left ventricular failure (LVF), but not of diminished cardiac output.

101. *c* In order to assess the infant's development at this time, it is important to know gestational age at birth. A PKU test should have been done in the hospital and a follow up within 1 week. The umbilical cord stump usually falls off several days after birth.

102. *a* A breastfeeding infant often exhibits hyperbilirubinemia after the 3rd day of life. It is thought to be due to an enzyme found in breast milk that causes increased absorption of unconjugated bilirubin from the intestine. Pathological causes of hyperbilirubinemia should be ruled out, but the infant should continue to breastfeed until then.

103. *d* An audible clicking during breastfeeding probably indicates that the nipple is improperly positioned in the infant's mouth. The mother should break the suction with her finger and push the nipple and areola farther into the infant's mouth. Audible swallowing during breastfeeding is normal.

104. *c* This patient's glucose record indicates consistent morning hypoglycemia. This indicates he is probably receiving too much NPH insulin in the evening for his daytime caloric intake. The evening NPH insulin dose should be decreased by 2 units and blood sugars re-evaluated in about a week.

105. *d* Right heart failure exacerbation manifests clinically with jugular vein distension (JVD) when the patient's head and trunk are raised approximately 45% from supine. Arteriosclerosis causes decreased elasticity of the arteries and arterioles. Aortic regurgitation presents clinically with visible carotid artery pulsations and auscultated aortic murmur. Pulmonary hypertension does not manifest with either carotid or jugular vessel clinical findings.

106. *b* Cranial nerves III, IV, and VI are responsible for control of eye movement. CN II is the optic nerve and is responsible for vision. CN VII, the facial nerve, is implicated in Bell's palsy.

107. *a* The ELISA may be negative in the first 6 to 12 weeks postexposure. This patient's exposure occurred several months ago. The Western blot is a confirmatory test and should only be performed after a positive blood or saliva test. Generally, informed consent should be obtained prior to testing.

108. *b* This patient takes theophylline, a drug which is metabolized by the cytochrome P450 system. Clarithromycin is also metabolized by the CYP450 system. The addition of a second drug which competes with theophylline in the CYP450 system slows metabolism of theophylline causing the serum level to rise. Therefore, theophylline level should be monitored closely and/or the dosage reduced to avoid the risk of theophylline toxicity.

109. *b* Between 18 and 32 weeks, there is good correlation between fundal height and gestational age of the fetus. The expected heights are:
    10-12 weeks: fundus slightly above the symphysis pubis
    16 weeks: fundus midway between the symphysis pubis and umbilicus
    20-22 weeks: fundus at the level of the umbilicus
    28 weeks: fundus 3 fingerbreadths above the umbilicus
    36 weeks: fundus just below the xiphoid process

110. *c* Dieting is contraindicated in all trimesters. An average increase of 300 calories per day is recommended. Sexual intercourse generally causes no harm to the mother or the fetus unless there is preterm labor or threatening abortion. Aerobic exercise such as jogging is not contraindicated if the mother is accustomed to it. Beginning vigorous aerobic activity is not recommended.

111. *c* A pruritic lesion with silvery scales on an erythematous base is the classic description of psoriasis, a chronic skin disorder characterized by rapid proliferation of epidermal cells. The treatment of choice for psoriasis is topical steroids during periods of exacerbation and daily emollients to keep the skin well hydrated.

112. *d* Satellite lesions are a common finding in infants with a candidal diaper rash. They resemble pustules. They are not associated with psoriasis. When psoriatic lesions are gently scraped, tiny droplets of blood appear (positive Auspitz sign).

113. *c* The HMG CoA-reductase inhibitors, frequently called the "statins," lower LDL cholesterol, raise HDL cholesterol, and decrease overall cholesterol synthesis. Rhabdomyolysis is characterized by marked elevation of serum CPK, myoglobinuria, myalgias, muscle tenderness, weakness, and malaise with fever. A patient taking a "statin" who reports any of these complaints must be evaluated for rhabdomyolysis.

114. *d* A newborn should double his birth weight by 6 months-of -age and triple his birth weight by 12 months-of-age. Some infants will commonly triple their birth weight at an earlier age if the birth weight was 6 pounds or less.

115. *a* Thiazide diuretics given in higher doses are associated with mildly elevated serum lipids and glucose. In lower doses, these elevations are less likely.

116. *b* Atenolol is a beta-blocker. It should be avoided in patients with asthma or other bronchospastic conditions. These patients often require beta stimulation, not beta blockade. Although atenolol is a beta 1-selective agent, at higher doses beta 2 receptors (bronchial and vascular) are blocked. Beta-blockers, specifically atenolol, are beneficial post-myocardial infarction because they have demonstrated reduction in morbidity and mortality.

117. *c* Children with a total cholesterol greater than 170 mg/dL are known to be at increased risk for coronary artery disease (CAD). Total daily dietary intake of fat should be < 30% of total daily caloric intake for children and adults with < 7% from saturated fat. Reduction of daily dietary fat intake is not recommended for children under 2 years-of-age.

118. *b* Aortic stenosis (AS) is a systolic ejection murmur frequently auscultated in the elderly. The murmur of AS often radiates to the clavicles and neck and is often associated with a systolic thrill. The murmur of pulmonic stenosis is quieter and does not radiate. The murmur associated with mitral valve insufficiency radiates toward the left axilla. A hypertrophic obstructive cardiomyopathy murmur usually does not radiate to the neck but does increase in intensity with standing or the Valsalva maneuver.

119. *a* Visual acuity is screened by using the Snellen eye chart. Vision, which is 20/20, is considered normal. "Legally blind" is defined as 20/200 vision in the better eye with corrective lenses. A person with 20/40 vision has better vision than a person with 20/60 or 20/80 vision.

120. *a* The condition described is a noncommunicating hydrocele. This occurs in about 1% of adult males and may be associated with infection, neoplasm, or trauma. The scrotum should transilluminate if fluid is present. A solid mass will not transilluminate. The fluid may be monitored or surgically drained.

121. *c* Lymph node size is important. Nodes > 1 cm are significant and should be assessed carefully. Nodes > 5 cm are almost always neoplastic. Node tenderness usually suggests inflammation. Cancerous nodes frequently are larger, nontender, and stone-like in consistency. Shotty nodes are pea-sized, nontender, mobile, discrete and reflect pre-existent infection.

122. *c* Since this patient has a history of glaucoma, it is reasonable to assume he uses daily ophthalmic drops to maintain normal eye pressure. The most commonly prescribed drug for this purpose is an ophthalmic beta-blocker. Propanolol is a beta-blocker. If prescribed together, these 2 drugs can have an additive effect and may cause severe hypotension and/or bradycardia. If the patient is using an ophthalmic beta-blocker, it may be wise to avoid prescribing an oral beta-blocker.

123. *c* The red reflex represents light that is reflected from the retina. Absence of a red reflex can be indicative of several serious ophthalmic conditions. Three of the most noted are cataracts, detached retina, and retinoblastoma. Retinoblastoma is a rare retinal tumor with a strong family history component. Leukokoria, a white reflex, is often a clinical clue. The infant should be referred to an ophthalmologist immediately. A red reflex is present in a patient with iritis.

124. *d* This is most likely a benign normal variant especially common in infants of African-American, Native-American, southern European, and Asian descent. The bluish-black macule (termed Mongolian spot), resembles a bruise, is typically between 2 and 8 cm, presents over the sacrum or buttocks at birth, and usually disappears during early childhood.

125. *b* Crying without tearing is an indication of dehydration. Herpangina is characterized by multiple, painful, tiny ulcerations in the mouth. Dehydration is an important complication to teach caregivers about. This child will require rehydration with IV fluids to prevent further deterioration of his condition.

126. *c* Females in the peri-menopausal period have decreased vaginal lubrication, which results in itching, discharge, bleeding, and increased risk of urethritis. Vasomotor instability ("hot flashes" and "hot flushes") is the most common symptom during this period. Other symptoms include nervousness, palpitations, depression, and headache.

127. *b* Hematuria is very likely. Presence of nitrites in the urine may indicate a urinary tract infection. The PSA (prostate specific antigen) is expected to be elevated greater than 10.0 ng/ml. PSA 4.0 to 10.0 ng/ml is typically associated with BPH or prostatitis. Generally, the palpated prostate is nontender when a malignancy is present. If the patient complains of pain with digital rectal exam (DRE), the examiner should consider an infectious etiology as well.

128. *b* Amoxicillin is a good choice of antibiotic for this child. The most likely etiologic agent is *Streptococcus pneumonia* and amoxicillin provides the necessary coverage. Unless there is worsening of symptoms or presence of discharge from the external canal, fever and pain relief may not occur for another 24 to 48 hours. Once antibiotic therapy is started, generally 48 to 72 hours is needed to assess antibiotic failure.

129. *b* This is a description of arcus senilis, commonly associated with the aging process. It should be considered a possible indicator of atherosclerotic disease when it presents in individuals younger than 40 years-of-age. There is no epidemiological data to support an association with atherosclerotic disease after 40 years-of-age.

130. *a* According to Erikson, the developmental stage of young adulthood is "intimacy vs. isolation." The tasks of this stage are to select a life partner, choose an occupation or career, establish independence from parents, establish a social network, and establish intimate relationships. A young adult who does not achieve these tasks often becomes self-focused and excessively concerned with his own needs.

131. *b* If the patient has received protection from the immunization, he will produce positive hepatitis B surface antibody and will have a negative hepatitis core antibody. Generally, measuring a surface antibody is sufficient to determine immunity.

132. *d* Risk factors for osteopenia and osteoporosis include Caucasian race, hyperthyroidism or hyperparathyroidism, Cushing's disease, glucocorticosteroids and anticonvulsant medications, estrogen deficiency, hyperphosphatemia (such as occurs with renal disease), and inadequate intake of calcium and/or vitamin D. Estrogen replacement at menopause is osteoprotective.

133. *d* Perineal pain is a common symptom of acute bacterial prostatitis that differentiates it from urinary tract infection. Epididymitis doesn't produce dysuria and urgency.

134. *d* A varicocele is a collection of abnormally dilated veins in the scrotum and is not associated with a mass. It can produce a feeling of heaviness in the scrotum and increases in size with standing or with Valsalva maneuver. The patient's complaint most closely describes an inguinal hernia, but the other diagnoses must be excluded.

135. *b* On rare occasions, a child will experience a vasovagal episode related to fear during immunizations or other frightening situations. This should not dissuade the parents from future immunizations. If this had been an allergic reaction, it would not have occurred so quickly and would not have resolved without intervention.

136. *b* Bell's palsy is paresis or paralysis of cranial nerve VII. Complete resolution of a patient's symptoms may take weeks, months, or may never completely resolve. Though some improvement is expected a few days after steroids are initiated, it is not unusual for the patient to be unable to close his eye. The nurse practitioner should order an ophthalmic lubricant until the patient is able to completely close the eye.

137. *b* These characteristics of physical development correspond to particular Tanner stages. Pubic hair in a reverse triangular shape is Tanner stage 5. Development of breast buds describes Tanner stage 2. Onset of menses is not associated with any particular Tanner stage but does not precede the development of breast buds. The secondary mound appears in Tanner stage 4.

138. *b* Many systemic diseases such as diabetes, hypo and hyperthyroidism, and Cushing's syndrome can cause erectile dysfunction (ED, impotence). Many medications can cause ED, particularly the antihypertensives (e.g., Vasotec®) and the antidepressants (e.g., Paxil®). Other factors which may cause ED include smoking, drug abuse, alcohol use, hypertension, and peripheral vascular disease (PVD).

139. *d* This patient's laboratory results demonstrate primary hypothyroidism. Patients with hypothyroidism may exhibit lethargy, weight gain, intolerance to cold, constipation, menstrual irregularities, coarse, dry skin, and hair loss from scalp and body. In extreme cases, bradycardia, hypotension, and coma can result.

140. *c* If 2 consecutive tablets are missed, take 2 as soon as remembered and 2 the next day. If 3 are missed, the risk of pregnancy is greatly increased and an additional form of contraception should be used for the remainder of the pill pack if pregnancy is not desired.

141. *b* The patient's complaints are related to estrogen excess. A contraceptive pill containing less estrogen could be prescribed. Other symptoms related to estrogen excess include bloating, cervical mucorrhea, hypertension, migraine headache, and edema.

142. *c* A patient with moderate persistent asthma has symptoms daily. He is best managed with a daily inhaled corticosteroid and short- or long-acting bronchodilator. An oral leukotriene blocker may also be added to this regimen, but would be ineffective in completely eradicating the patient's daily symptoms.

143. *c* Peak flow is measured in liters per minute and is based on the patient's personal best or a peak expiratory flow table. The values in the table are calculated according to the patient's height in inches.

144. *c* This patient has genital herpes. During pregnancy, she should be treated with an oral antiviral agent such as acyclovir. Even with treatment of an initial episode, symptoms may persist for 14 to 21 days. Subsequent outbreaks are usually 7 to 10 days when treated. Cesarean section is indicated if genital herpetic lesions are present during labor.

145. *b* About half of patients with renal artery stenosis have an audible bruit. Renal artery bruits have a high sensitivity for renal artery stenosis, but poor specificity. Bruits may be auscultated in patients who are hypertensive without evidence of renal artery disease.

146. *c* Malnutrition in the elderly is not an uncommon problem. Many elders who live alone, who live on fixed incomes, who are depressed, or who have a medical disease or disability may eat only 1 or 2 main meals a day. Loss of appetite, lethargy, fatigue, and weight loss may be signs of disease process or depression. However, it cannot be assumed that the patient is malnourished. Elevated serum BUN and RBC count typically reflect inadequate hydration. The earliest and, therefore, most sensitive indicator of general nutritional deficiency (malnutrition or starvation) is decreased serum pre-albumin. Normal serum albumin is 3.5 g/dL and a decreased level reflects malnutrition that may have been present for some time.

147. *b* A breast lesion associated with neoplasm is typically a single ipsilateral mass that is firm, nontender, fixed or immobile (attached to adjacent tissue), with an irregular contour. One common benign breast condition is fibrocystic breast disease. Breast tissue feels "rope-like" and is more or less tender depending on the phase of the ovulatory cycle and exposure to "triggers" (such as caffeine and chocolate). This condition presents bilaterally. Breast cyst, another type of benign breast condition, typically has well-defined edges, is movable, and feels "fluid filled." Evaluation of a breast cyst includes fine needle aspiration.

148. *b* Hepatic enzymes are released in response to hepatic injury. Alcohol ingestion depresses synthesis of alanine aminotransferase (ALT) more than aspartate aminotransferase (AST). Therefore, in acute hepatic injury due to alcohol ingestion, AST is greater than ALT (AST:ALT ratio > 2.0). Acute hepatitis secondary to drug ingestion or a viral agent can cause significant injury to the liver and thus release hepatic enzymes, but generally the AST:ALT ratio is 1.0 or less.

149. *a* Choices *b*, *c*, and *d* are associated with systemic inflammatory changes as evidenced by elevated body temperature and changes in laboratory values. Typical changes in labs include: increased erythrocyte sedimentation rate (ESR), elevated hepatic enzymes (AST and ALT), presence of rheumatoid factor (RF), and/or presence of antinuclear antibodies (ANA). Osteoarthritis does not have inflammation as a clinical or subclinical feature.

150. *d* Dizziness is associated with a sensation of body movement when there is no actual body movement occurring (i.e., the person is spinning and the room is not). Vertigo is the sensation that the person is still and the room is spinning. There is no associated muscle weakness or visual disturbance with either of these conditions. The most common causes are related to drug ingestion, hypotension, inner or middle ear pathology, and positional vertigo. Dizziness is an adverse reaction associated with certain antibiotics (e.g., gentamicin and streptomycin) and high-dose salicylates. Vertigo is associated with certain inner ear pathology such as labyrinthitis and Meniere's disease. Meclizine is a long-acting antihistamine which is used to treat acute and chronic vertigo.

Practice Exam IV

_____ 1. After hearing the news that she is pregnant, an overweight patient remarks, "I'm not in good enough shape to have a baby. How can I get in shape?" The nurse practitioner would appropriately advise her to:

  a. join an aerobic exercise class.
  b. begin walking about 3 times per week with a family member or friend.
  c. take yoga or tai chi lessons for mental and physical relaxation.
  d. avoid physical exertion, as adequate rest is more important.

_____ 2. Expected spirometry readings when the patient has chronic bronchitis include all of the following _except_:

  a. increased residual volume (RV).
  b. decreased vital capacity (VC).
  c. decreased forced expiratory volume (FEV-1).
  d. decreased total lung capacity (TLC).

_____ 3. A 2-year-old child is brought to the clinic by his adoptive mother. She reports that he has frequent crying spells, "as if he is hurting real bad" and refuses to be held during these periods. She was told the child's biological mother may have the sickle cell trait and she wonders if the child has inherited the disease. The nurse practitioner would respond appropriately by saying:

  a. "I will order the Sickledex to screen for sickle cell anemia."
  b. "He is probably just testing you. Hold him anyway to show him he is loved."
  c. "I will order a test called hemoglobin electrophoresis, because you are probably right."
  d. "Just ignore him and the behavior should eventually stop."

_____ 4. A 30-year-old patient walks into the family practice clinic requesting treatment for a puncture wound received while swimming in a river. He is offered a Td vaccination. This is an example of:

  a. tertiary prevention.
  b. early case finding.
  c. primary prevention.
  d. secondary prevention.

_____ 5. A 36-year-old female presents to the clinic requesting oral contraceptive pills. She reports a sedentary lifestyle, a smoking history of 30-pack years and currently smoking 1 PPD, and daily medication for type 2 diabetes mellitus. Her body mass index is 35. Oral contraceptives are an absolute contraindication for this patient because she:

    a. is obese.
    b. has type 2 diabetes mellitus.
    c. is a smoker.
    d. leads a sedentary lifestyle.

_____ 6. A patient states "I just found out my old boyfriend died of AIDS." She is worried that she has contracted the illness and wants to be tested. The nurse practitioner correctly offers this patient the:

    a. ELISA as the initial screening test.
    b. ELISA as the confirmatory test.
    c. Western blot as the initial screening test.
    d. Western blot as the confirmatory test.

_____ 7. A first time mother asks the nurse practitioner when she should start feeding her baby cereal. The nurse practitioner replies:

    a. not before 4 to 6 months-of-age.
    b. at 2 months-of-age if the baby is taking 20 ounces of milk per 24-hour day.
    c. when the baby does not sleep through the night.
    d. as soon as the baby begins teething.

_____ 8. A mother brings her 14-year-old daughter to the clinic for a sports physical. They both have questions about puberty and the first gynecological visit. The adolescent reports that she has not yet started her menstrual periods. She denies ever having sexual intercourse. Physical examination reveals normal sexual development at Tanner stage 4. The nurse practitioner would be correct to tell the mother and daughter all of the following *except*:

    a. she should plan to have her first Pap smear when she is 21 years-of-age or when she becomes sexually active.
    b. she needs a consultation with an endocrinologist as her menstrual periods should have started by now.
    c. sexual intercourse utilizing barrier contraception is essential even now as protection from pregnancy and sexually transmitted diseases.
    d. the onset of menses will probably occur very soon.

____ 9. A 44-year-old patient complains of stiffness and soreness in his hands, hips, and knees. There is noticeable PIP and DIP joint enlargement in his hands. The nurse practitioner suspects arthritis. All of the following questions are helpful in the differentiation between rheumatoid arthritis (RA) and osteoarthritis (OA) *except*:

    a. "Do the joints of your fingers ever feel particularly warm or hot?"
    b. "Tell me about your usual energy level."
    c. "Does the soreness and stiffness get better or worse as the day progresses?"
    d. "Have you noticed decreased joint movement or flexibility?"

____ 10. A 19-year-old female is diagnosed with secondary amenorrhea. Findings in her history which may account for the cessation of menses include all of the following *except* she:

    a. has undiagnosed anorexia nervosa.
    b. leads a 1½-hour aerobic dance class 10 times each week.
    c. frequently uses the designer drug ecstasy or smokes marijuana on the weekend with friends.
    d. receives a Depo Provera® injection every 3 months at the family planning clinic.

____ 11. A 48-year-old female presents to the clinic with chest pain. She is examined by the nurse practitioner and is thought to have acute cholecystitis. Of the following choices, what is the *least* likely differential diagnosis?

    a. Gastroesophageal reflux disease (GERD)
    b. Angina secondary to ischemic heart disease
    c. Peptic ulcer disease (PUD)
    d. Chest wall syndrome

____ 12. Physical examination of the patient presenting with acute cholecystitis will be positive for:

    a. Murphy's sign.
    b. rebound tenderness at McBurney's point.
    c. pain localized to the left upper quadrant of the abdomen.
    d. pain radiating to the right shoulder area.

_____ 13. Which of the following may predispose the insulin dependent patient to hypoglycemia?

    a. Nonselective beta-adrenergic blockers
    b. Thiazide diuretics
    c. phenytoin
    d. Glucocorticosteroids

_____ 14. It is clear that in Alzheimer's disease, environmental factors as well as genetic factors exert considerable influence. One potentially treatable risk factor currently receiving much attention is:

    a. testosterone deficiency.
    b. estrogen deficiency.
    c. history of hypertension.
    d. sedentary lifestyle.

_____ 15. Which of the following is *not* associated with type 2 diabetes mellitus?

    a. Gestational diabetes, delivery of a macrosomic infant
    b. Hispanic, African-American, or Native-American descent
    c. Alcohol or other drug abuse
    d. Obesity, hypertension, hypertriglyceridemia

_____ 16. Which of the following is a *false* statement regarding battered women?

    a. Battered women are safer when they are pregnant.
    b. Battering often occurs for the first time during pregnancy.
    c. Many family members believe the battered woman is the cause of the abuse.
    d. Battering is more common in families with more than 3 children.

_____ 17. A patient is being started on treatment for iron deficiency anemia with a daily ferrous sulfate supplement. Which of the following indicates a need for further patient teaching?

    a. "My body absorbs the iron pill better when I take it with my orange juice at breakfast or with my vitamin C pill in the evening."
    b. "When I come back to the clinic in a month, the hemoglobin finger stick test will show if my anemia is getting better."
    c. "I take my iron pill with a glass of milk so it won't upset my stomach."
    d. "I take my iron pill in the morning and my milk of magnesia laxative at night."

_____ 18. A young female reports onset of right flank pain 2 days ago that is now severe. Last night she discovered a "burning rash" in the same area. The nurse practitioner identifies papular fluid filled lesions that are confluent and follow a linear distribution along the T-8 dermatome. The nurse practitioner would appropriately order:

   a. an oral antibiotic.
   b. a topical antifungal.
   c. an oral antiviral.
   d. a topical steroid cream.

_____ 19. A 23-year-old female presents with scaly hypopigmented macular lesions on her trunk, shoulders, and upper arms. The lesions fluoresce under Wood's lamp. Which of the following is an appropriate treatment for this condition?

   a. Apply selenium sulfide lotion 2 to 3 times per week and rinse off about 15 minutes later.
   b. Apply lindane from the chin to the tops of the feet and rinse off 8 hours later.
   c. Apply mupirocin (Bactroban®) to the affected areas 3 to 4 times per day.
   d. Take oral acyclovir 5 times per day for 5 days.

_____ 20. Which of the following is *not* a risk factor for transient ischemic attack (TIA)?

   a. Age
   b. Hypertension
   c. Common migraine headache
   d. Smoking

_____ 21. The nurse practitioner is providing follow up care for a 12 month old who had a febrile seizure 3 days ago. There has been no additional seizure activity and the febrile illness has resolved. The child's parents want more information about the seizure. The nurse practitioner replies:

   a. "Your child should be placed on anti-seizure medication to prevent a future recurrence of seizures."
   b. "Febrile seizures may cause developmental delays and behavioral abnormalities."
   c. "Seizures are usually caused by sudden, high fever and central nervous system irritability."
   d. "The recurrence risk of another febrile seizure is 90% within the first year after this seizure."

_____ 22. Which of the following patients is at *lowest* risk for secondary hypertension?

    a. A 38-year-old with untreated Graves' disease
    b. An 18-year-old with a cocaine addiction
    c. A 62-year-old with untreated depression
    d. A 29-year-old with untreated Cushing's disease

_____ 23. The nurse practitioner palpates an enlarged right epitrochlear lymph node. The next action is to assess the:

    a. throat, face, and right ear.
    b. right neck and supraclavicular region.
    c. right axilla and breast.
    d. right forearm and hand.

_____ 24. Which of the following is *not* a characteristic of the S3 heart sound?

    a. The sound is high-pitched and occurs just prior to the S1 heart sound.
    b. It is best auscultated in the mitral area at the 4th or 5th left ICS, MCL.
    c. It is produced by vibration during rapid ventricular filling pressure and is associated with right-sided heart failure.
    d. An S3 is fairly common in children, young adults, and females in the third trimester of pregnancy.

_____ 25. A 26-year-old female is informed that her pregnancy test is positive and that her due date is in approximately 8 months. The nurse practitioner is very concerned about the patient's half a pack per day cigarette smoking habit and correctly tells the patient that approximately half of the babies born to women who smoke:

    a. have pulmonary complications in the neonatal period.
    b. are born prematurely.
    c. are macrosomic.
    d. are small for gestational age.

_____ 26. A patient reports development of a painful "red eye" 2 days ago. Now both eyes are painful and red. On awakening this morning, her eyelids were crusted and stuck together. On examination, the nurse practitioner finds bilateral swelling and inflammation of the lids and conjunctiva. The ophthalmic treatment of choice for this condition is:

    a. a mast cell stabilizer.
    b. as antibiotic/steroid combination.
    c. a steroid.
    d. an antiviral.

____ 27. A 28-year-old female presents with a palpable breast mass in the upper outer quadrant which is semi-firm, nontender, and firmly attached to the adjacent skin. What is the most likely diagnosis?

    a. Adenocarcinoma
    b. Paget's disease
    c. Fibroadenoma
    d. Intraductal papilloma

____ 28. A 73-year-old patient has hypertension, CHF, and atrial fibrillation. The patient's adult daughter phones the nurse practitioner to report that her mother has been nauseated for several days and has vomited for the past 18 hours. She is confused but has no other neurological deficits. The nurse practitioner should:

    a. order oral rehydration fluids, such as Pedialyte®, and an antiemetic suppository.
    b. arrange for immediate transfer to the emergency department.
    c. arrange for admission to the hospital and order a CT scan of the head.
    d. have the patient come in to the clinic for further assessment.

____ 29. Breast cancer:

    a. is the most common cancer in females.
    b. is lobular more often than intraductal.
    c. develops in 1 out of every 50 women.
    d. is a fast growing cancer.

____ 30. A 22-year-old, healthy, college student is 62 inches tall and weighs 110 lbs. To maintain this weight, the patient with average activity should consume:

    a. about 1200 calories per day.
    b. about 1500 calories per day.
    c. 30 kcal/kg/day.
    d. 40 kcal/kg/day.

____ 31. The nurse practitioner receives a call from a 23-year-old patient who is 10 weeks pregnant. She reports that a few days after spending the day baby-sitting a friend's toddler, the toddler developed a "rash". The nurse practitioner would be *least* concerned if the patient was exposed to:

    a. meningitis.
    b. scarlet fever (scarlatina).
    c. poison ivy.
    d. varicella.

_____ 32. Which of the following patients is *least* likely to develop osteoporosis secondary to a comorbid condition?

a. A 45-year-old male with chronic renal failure
b. A 28-year-old female with type 2 diabetes mellitus
c. A 31-year-old female with rheumatoid arthritis taking a daily oral corticosteroid
d. A 44-year-old male with a seizure disorder taking an anticonvulsant medication since 8 years-of-age

_____ 33. A 22-year-old patient reports a 5 to 6 year history of stuffy nose with clear rhinorrhea, sneezing, and itchy watery eyes. The problem gets better in the wintertime and worse in the summer, "but never really goes away." Based on this information, the most appropriate treatments are:

a. an oral antihistamine and/or nasal mast cell stabilizer.
b. an oral steroid and/or ophthalmic steroid.
c. an oral antihistamine and nasal decongestant.
d. an oral steroid and nasal antihistamine.

_____ 34. A mother has been breastfeeding her infant since giving birth 6 weeks ago. Her right breast is engorged, erythematous, hot to touch, and very painful. She says the problem began 48 hours earlier. She has been feeding exclusively with the left breast. The nurse practitioner diagnoses acute mastitis and recommends all of the following *except*:

a. taking ibuprofen and applying moist heat compresses.
b. completely emptying the affected breast at least every 4 hours by breastfeeding or using a breast pump.
c. taking cephalexin TID for 7-10 days.
d. discontinuing breastfeeding from the affected breast and wearing a bra until the pain and engorgement have resolved.

_____ 35. The early stage of chronic renal failure is characterized by:

a. nausea, vomiting, oliguria.
b. weight gain, hypertension, and anuria.
c. proteinuria and hematuria.
d. thirst, polyuria, and low urine specific gravity.

_____ 36. Which of the following patients would appropriately be diagnosed with isolated systolic hypertension (ISH)?

a. A 69-year-old female with BP 160/65
b. A 43-year-old male with BP 188/108
c. A 39-year-old female with BP 148/92
d. An 78-year-old male with BP 204/112

_____ 37. A 21-year-old patient presents with abdominal guarding, rigid abdominal musculature, rebound tenderness at McBurney's point, and leukocytosis. What is the most likely diagnosis?

    a. Ulcerative colitis
    b. Cholecystitis
    c. Appendicitis
    d. Pancreatitis

_____ 38. A 57-year-old patient presents for an annual physical exam. He reports having 3 attacks of acute gout during the past year. He does not take any medication except NSAIDs during the attacks which help "a little bit." The nurse practitioner would appropriately recommend:

    a. daily colchicine for prophylaxis.
    b. Allopurinol® prn acute attack.
    c. a low purine diet and avoidance of alcohol.
    d. avoidance of NSAIDs.

_____ 39. A 45-year-old obese premenopausal female complains of indigestion, flatulence, and RUQ and epigastric "crampy pain" that radiates to the right scapula. Symptoms are exacerbated by a high fat meal. What is the most likely diagnosis?

    a. Hepatitis
    b. Chronic cholecystitis
    c. Acute pancreatitis
    d. Myocarditis

_____ 40. A characteristic of elders which affects the pharmacokinetics of drug therapy in that population is their relative increased:

    a. total body water.
    b. lean muscle mass.
    c. hepatic blood flow.
    d. percent of body fat.

_____ 41. Following the finding of prostate gland abnormalities on DRE, the nurse practitioner orders appropriate labs. When preparing to review lab reports with the patient, the nurse practitioner knows all of the following are true *except*:

    a. normal PSA is 10 ng/ml or less.
    b. PSA is elevated in the presence of malignant prostate epithelium.
    c. PSA is elevated in the presence of benign prostatic hyperplasia.
    d. positive serum acid phosphatase reflects malignancy of the prostate gland with bone metastasis.

_____ 42. A 75-year-old female complains that she awakens 3 to 4 times each night sensing bladder fullness, but is unable to "hold it" until she can get seated on the bathroom toilet. This type of urinary incontinence is termed:

a. overflow incontinence.
b. stress incontinence.
c. functional incontinence.
d. urge incontinence.

_____ 43. An 83-year-old man has a resting hand tremor. What disease process is this type of tremor most commonly associated with?

a. Multiple sclerosis (MS)
b. Parkinson's disease
c. Diabetic neuropathy
d. Huntington's chorea

_____ 44. A 43-year-old male has chronic gout. He has come to the clinic for the 3rd time in as many months for treatment of an acute exacerbation. Dietary counseling should include avoidance of all of the following *except*:

a. alcoholic beverages.
b. sardines, anchovies, and shellfish.
c. green leafy vegetables.
d. organ meats.

_____ 45. Swan neck and boutonniere deformities are typical clinical findings in the later presentation of:

a. gout.
b. rheumatoid arthritis (RA).
c. osteoporosis.
d. osteoarthritis (OA).

_____ 46. The nurse practitioner suspects that a 9-year-old child in her practice has attention deficit hyperactivity disorder (ADHD). After discussing the child's behavior with the parents, the nurse practitioner should:

a. start treatment with methylphenidate (Ritalin®).
b. arrange for a psychoeducational evaluation.
c. educate the child and parents about dietary restrictions.
d. talk to the child's siblings.

_____ 47. The nurse practitioner is performing a routine assessment of a 47-year-old female who wants to lose weight. She has truncal obesity with relatively slender forearms and lower legs. Her BMI is 38. Upon review of her history, physical examination, and laboratory reports, the nurse practitioner diagnoses "syndrome X." This diagnosis is based on the previous findings plus all of the following *except*:

    a. HDL < 35 mg/dL and triglyceride > 250 mg/dL.
    b. hyperinsulinemia.
    c. hypertension.
    d. atrial fibrillation.

_____ 48. Oral and parenteral contraceptive methods:

    a. stimulate secretion of LH.
    b. inhibit secretion of estrogen and progesterone.
    c. inhibit secretion of FSH.
    d. inhibit hCG.

_____ 49. Psychogenic cough:

    a. most commonly presents after the sixth decade of life.
    b. is a diagnosis solely of exclusion, made only after all other potential causes have been ruled out.
    c. is commonly associated with social anxiety disorder in young adults in their twenties or thirties.
    d. is commonly associated with a clinical diagnosis of generalized anxiety disorder and panic attack.

_____ 50. A 7-year-old child has acute otitis media and acute bacterial sinusitis. The treatment which is *least* likely to contribute to resolution is an:

    a. oral antihistamine.
    b. oral mucolytic.
    c. oral decongestant.
    d. anti-inflammatory agent.

_____ 51. A 51-year-old postmenopausal female, requests guidance regarding osteoporosis risk. The nurse practitioner would be correct to recommend all of the following *except*:

    a. moderate weight-bearing exercise 3 times per week.
    b. 1200 to 1500 mg calcium daily.
    c. avoidance of alcoholic beverages.
    d. weight loss.

_____52. A 57-year-old patient with known diverticulosis presents with sudden onset fever, leukocytosis, and bright red rectal bleeding. The patient is diagnosed with acute diverticulitis. All of the following are appropriate interventions at this time *except*:

    a. initiate antibiotic therapy.
    b. change the patient's diet to clear liquid during the acute phase.
    c. monitor the patient for hemostasis and anemia.
    d. reinforce the importance of a low fiber diet for management of the chronic condition.

_____53. Which of the following conditions requires partner treatment?

    a. Trichomoniasis
    b. Leiomyoma
    c. Bacterial vaginosis
    d. Candida vaginitis

_____54. The nurse practitioner correctly diagnoses iron deficiency anemia in a female patient whose lab report reveals:

    a. an increased reticulocyte count.
    b. a mean corpuscular volume (MCV) > 100 fl.
    c. hemoglobin (Hgb) 12.0 g/dL.
    d. an increased total iron binding capacity (TIBC).

_____55. A call is received from a nursing home reporting that an 86-year-old resident has become weak, dizzy, and short of breath over the past several hours. The patient has tachycardia, tachypnea, crackles, a "wet" cough, generalized pallor, and circumoral cyanosis. The most likely diagnosis is:

    a. congestive heart failure (CHF).
    b. pneumonia.
    c. foreign body aspiration.
    d. stroke.

_____ 56. A 49-year-old male presents for a pre-employment physical examination. He is a 60-pack year smoker with chronic emphysema. Findings would most likely reveal which of the following descriptions of the thorax and lungs?

    a. AP chest diameter equal to transverse chest diameter, decreased tactile fremitus, decreased diaphragmatic excursion, hyper-resonance to percussion, wheezes

    b. AP chest diameter less than transverse chest diameter, increased tactile fremitus, decreased diaphragmatic excursion, hypo-resonance to percussion, rhonchi

    c. AP chest diameter equal to transverse chest diameter, increased tactile fremitus, increased diaphragmatic excursion, hyper-resonance to percussion, wheezes and rhonchi

    d. AP chest diameter less than transverse chest diameter, decreased tactile fremitus, increased diaphragmatic excursion, hypo-resonance to percussion, productive cough

_____ 57. A 31-year-old female is informed that her pregnancy test is positive and that she is about 6 weeks pregnant. The nurse practitioner is very concerned about the patient's reported history of alcohol use. She correctly tells the patient that babies born to women who drink alcohol during pregnancy are at risk for all of the following *except*:

    a. having cognitive impairment.

    b. post-maturity delivery.

    c. small for gestational age (SGA).

    d. having characteristic facies.

_____ 58. Signs and symptoms of anemia, regardless of the specific cause or type, include all of the following *except*:

    a. weakness, dizziness, fatigue.

    b. headache and impaired concentration.

    c. dyspnea on exertion.

    d. shakiness or jitteriness.

_____ 59. A patient with uncontrolled primary hypertension presents with a complaint of frequent headaches. Headaches which may be attributed to blood pressure elevation are typically described as:

    a frontal, occurring during waking hours.

    b. temporal, presenting in the late afternoon or evening.

    c. occipital, presenting on awakening in the morning.

    d. facial, exacerbated by recumbent position.

_____ 60. What is a Tzanck test used to diagnose?

    a. Mastoiditis
    b. Trichomoniasis
    c. Hyphema
    d. Herpes virus

_____ 61. Which of the following patients is most likely to have a diagnosis of type 2 diabetes mellitus?

    a. An underweight 9-year-old with frequent staphylococcal infections, glucosuria, and ketonuria.
    b. A 49-year-old male with impotence and HbA_{1C} 10%.
    c. A 35-year-old obese female with frequent vaginal yeast infections and 110 mg/dL fasting serum glucose.
    d. A 55-year-old female with hypertension, hyperlipidemia, and 130 mg/dL (2 hour/75 g) glucose tolerance test.

_____ 62. A patient with a history of alcohol abuse presents with acute nausea, vomiting, and severe retrosternal pain which radiates to the back. Based on the most probable diagnosis, the nurse practitioner would appropriately order a CBC, chemistry profile, and:

    a. serum amylase and lipase, and liver function studies.
    b. serum BUN and creatinine, and 24 hour urine for creatinine clearance.
    c. serum bilirubin and liver function studies.
    d. flat plate of the abdomen followed by gastric endoscopic examination.

_____ 63. A middle-aged female complains of insomnia, night sweats, feeling intensely hot, emotional lability, extreme nervousness, and impatience. It would be *least* likely that her signs and symptoms are due to:

    a. thyrotoxicosis.
    b. menopausal vasomotor instability.
    c. alcohol or other drug withdrawal.
    d. new onset type 2 diabetes mellitus.

_____ 64. Which of the following drugs may potentiate hyperkalemia in a patient taking a potassium sparing diuretic?

    a. A thiazide diuretic
    b. An angiotensin converting enzyme inhibitor
    c. A beta-adrenergic blocker
    d. A calcium channel blocker

____ 65. The components of the Denver II Developmental Screening Test (DDST-R) are:

    a. personal/social, fine motor, gross motor, language.
    b. intelligence, motor performance, language development.
    c. vocabulary, clarity of speech, abstract thinking.
    d. problem solving, speech, gross motor, fine motor.

____ 66. Which of the following most accurately characterizes illness care among U.S. citizens age 65 years and older?

    a. The largest area of expenditure is nursing home care.
    b. Approximately 50% of all health care expenses are covered by health insurance plans.
    c. Elders account for approximately 10% of all acute care hospital admissions.
    d. Approximately 1/3 of total health care expenditures are accounted for by persons 65 years-of-age and older.

____ 67. A 53-year-old postmenopausal female, with a BMI of 38 and gastric esophageal reflux disease, takes a daily calcium supplement for protection against osteoporosis. All of the following are appropriate teaching points for this patient *except*:

    a. take the calcium supplement with milk to facilitate absorption.
    b. the addition of HRT may further decrease osteoporosis risk.
    c. take an OTC calcium-containing antacid to increase calcium intake.
    d. avoid caffeine-containing beverages.

____ 68. The nurse practitioner would be correct to tell a 27-year-old newly diagnosed hypertensive patient that:

    a. "isolated systolic hypertension is typical of young adults who are drug abusers."
    b. "the older you are, the more difficult it is to control blood pressure with medication."
    c. "lifestyle modifications such as losing excess weight, exercising, limiting salt and alcohol intake, and reducing stress will help to maintain a normal blood pressure."
    d. "for about 10 to 20 percent of people with primary hypertension, the cause is unknown."

_____ 69. Infants born to women who smoke are at risk for:

    a. premature delivery.
    b. congenital anomalies.
    c. low birth weight.
    d. nicotine withdrawal symptoms.

_____ 70. The differential diagnoses for transient episodes of dizziness would appropriately include all of the following *except*:

    a. hypoglycemia.
    b. transient ischemic attacks (TIAs).
    c. allergic rhinitis.
    d. serous otitis media.

_____ 71. A debilitated 77-year-old has had vomiting and diarrhea for 24 hours. The patient is at risk for consequences of hyponatremia which include all of the following *except*:

    a. seizures.
    b. hypertension.
    c. loss of consciousness.
    d. disorientation.

_____ 72. A mother presents with a 3-year-old who has croup. The plan for home care would appropriately include:

    a. a warm mist vaporizer.
    b. a cool mist vaporizer.
    c. breathing hot steam in an enclosed bathroom.
    d. cool, non-humidified air.

_____ 73. Appropriate meal planning for the patient with diabetes mellitus includes:

    a. total daily intake of 30% fat.
    b. total daily intake of 50% carbohydrate.
    c. 3 well-balanced meals and no snacks.
    d. total daily intake of 20% protein.

_____ 74. Appropriate nutritional guidance for the pregnant patient is:

    a. maintain usual caloric intake and add a daily multivitamin.
    b. increase caloric intake by 300 cal/day and add iron and folic acid supplementation.
    c. increase daily calories by 500 cal/day and add a daily multivitamin.
    d. if the daily diet is nutritious and well-balanced, vitamin supplementation is not necessary.

_____ 75. A 59-year-old male complains of decreased range of joint motion "everywhere," that gets better after the first two hours in the morning. Spinal x-rays reveal joint space narrowing. What is the most likely diagnosis?

    a. Osteoarthritis (OA)
    b. Rheumatoid arthritis (RA)
    c. Polymyalgia rheumatica
    d. Gout

_____ 76. Serology testing for syphilis is planned for pregnant patients because:

    a. syphilis during pregnancy predisposes the fetus to spontaneously abort or the newborn to have congenital syphilis.
    b. hormonal changes associated with pregnancy may trigger activation of latent syphilis.
    c. syphilis may be passed to the fetus beginning in the 3rd trimester.
    d. syphilis may be transmitted to the infant at the time of delivery.

_____ 77. A patient presents with sudden onset of "crushing chest pressure," diaphoresis, pallor, and extreme weakness. Electrocardiogram and serum enzyme changes support a diagnosis of acute myocardial infarction (AMI). The nurse practitioner would expect:

    a. widened QRS intervals, AV dissociation, elevated CPK-MB and LDH, and negative cardiac troponin I.
    b. ST changes, prominent Q waves, elevated CPK-MB and LDH, and elevated cardiac troponin I.
    c. prolonged PR interval, bradycardia, and increased CPK-MB and LDH.
    d. peaked T waves, tachycardia, elevated CPK-MB and LDH, and elevated cardiac troponin I.

_____ 78. A 48-year-old female complains of pain and stiffness in her right hip and knee that is mild on awakening in the morning, gets worse at the end of the day, and is relieved with hot baths and ibuprofen. Crepitus is palpable on range of motion of the knee. Signs of inflammation are notably absent. What is the most likely diagnosis?

    a. Rheumatoid arthritis (RA)
    b. Gout
    c. Osteoarthritis (OA)
    d. Osteoporosis

_____ 79. Which of the following is the current recommendation for cholesterol screening in children?

    a. All children should be screened annually after 5 years-of-age.
    b. All children should be screened every 5 years after 2 years-of-age.
    c. Children with a family history of hypercholesterolemia or premature cardiovascular disease should be screened.
    d. There is no current recommendation for cholesterol screening in children.

_____ 80. What is the marker for asthma in the WBC differentiatial?

    a. Elevated neutrophils
    b. Decreased basophils
    c. Elevated eosinophils
    d. Decreased monocytes

_____ 81. Which of the following statements most accurately characterizes elders in the United States?

    a. Most reside in nursing homes.
    b. The primary source of financial support is retirement pensions and life savings.
    c. Most are widowed females.
    d. This age group represents 5% of the total U.S. population.

_____ 82. The anemia associated with chronic disease is:

    a. normocytic and normochromic.
    b. macrocytic and hyperchromic.
    c. microcytic and hypochromic.
    d. macrocytic and normochromic.

_____ 83. Which of the following patients is at *lowest* risk for osteoporosis?

    a. A 56-year-old male with a 35-year history of smoking and alcohol abuse
    b. A 57-year-old menopausal female with a BMI of 18
    c. A 28-year-old female with a 10-year history of anorexia nervosa
    d. An obese 40-year-old female who walks 2 miles every day

_____ 84. Stress incontinence:

    a. is associated with the normal aging process.
    b. may be caused by anticholinergic or antidepressant medication.
    c. is due to detrusor muscle instability.
    d. may be aggravated by caffeine or alcohol.

_____ 85. The result of the Weber tuning fork test is lateralization of sound to the right ear. This finding indicates a:

    a. conduction problem in the left ear.
    b. conduction problem in the right ear.
    c. sensorineural problem in the right ear.
    d. sensorineural problem in the left ear.

_____ 86. Yesterday, a patient got sand in his eye during a volleyball game at the beach. Today, he presents with an exquisitely painful left eye, photophobia, and constant tearing. The nurse practitioner removes a tiny speck of sand from under the lid and notes vertical corneal abrasions. The treatment of choice is:

    a. patching the injured eye only; no medication is needed.
    b. an ophthalmic steroid to reduce swelling, inflammation, and pain.
    c. an ophthalmic antibiotic ointment, eye patch, and pain medication.
    d. normal saline drops only; eye patching is not necessary.

_____ 87. A 13-year-old patient complains that he fell while running during football practice. Now his knee hurts and sometimes "locks." The nurse practitioner performs McMurray's test. Which of the following is true about this test?

    a. An audible or palpable "click" is positive for a torn meniscus.
    b. A varus stress is applied to the flexed knee.
    c. The straight leg is internally rotated with the patient supine and flat.
    d. The knee is grasped with the examiner's fingers placed laterally.

_____ 88. A 26-year-old female presents with vaginal itching and a malodorous vaginal discharge. Wet prep is positive for budding hyphae and flagellated protozoa and negative for WBCs and clue cells. KOH is positive. Based on these lab and microscopy findings, the most likely diagnoses are:

    a. gonorrhea and genital herpes.
    b. trichomoniasis and vaginal candidiasis.
    c. genital herpes and trichomoniasis.
    d. vaginal candidiasis and bacterial vaginosis.

_____ 89. A 57-year-old postmenopausal female presents with a complaint of vaginal burning, pruritus, and painful intercourse. On examination, the nurse practitioner would be most concerned about finding:

    a. a thin, pale, dry vaginal mucosa.
    b. absence of rugae.
    c. a friable cervix with petechiae.
    d. raised yellowish cervical lesions.

_____ 90. A patient with diabetes mellitus calls the clinic reporting signs and symptoms of viral syndrome. She asks, "should I skip my diabetes medicine until I get my appetite back?" The nurse practitioner reviews the sick day guidelines, which include all of the following *except*:

    a. monitor fingerstick glucose checks more often.
    b. take all diabetes medications as prescribed.
    c. maintain adequate fluid hydration.
    d. hold all diabetes medications until eating habits have returned to normal.

_____ 91. What is the most common causative pathogen found in cystitis, pyelonephritis, and prostatitis?

    a. *Escherichia coli*
    b. *Proteus mirabilis*
    c. *Enterobacter*
    d. *Klebsiella*

_____ 92. A palpable thyroid nodule is benign. How does it feel on palpation?

    a. Smooth
    b. Hard
    c. Nontender
    d. Fixed

_____ 93. The nurse practitioner is initiating NPH insulin therapy in a 40-year-old patient with diabetes. Fasting glucose ranges from 225 to 300 mg/dL. Which of the following is the most appropriate initial dosing regimen?

    a. 10 units in the morning and 10 units in the evening.
    b. 1 u/kg/day divided into 2 doses with 2/3 in the morning and 1/3 in the evening.
    c. 1.25 to 1.5 u/kg/day divided into 2 doses with 2/3 in the morning and 1/3 in the evening.
    d. 20 units in the morning and 10 units in the evening.

_____ 94. The reason beta-adrenergic blockers should be avoided in patients with asthma is that they may:

    a. interfere with the action of oral and inhaled beta-agonists.
    b. potentiate pulmonary inflammation.
    c. increase the tenacity of pulmonary secretions.
    d. inhibit the cough reflex.

_____ 95. Which of the following is appropriate to include in a breast cancer awareness seminar for women?

    a. All women should have an initial mammogram by 40 years-of-age and annually beginning at 50 years-of-age.
    b. A palpable breast lump that is suspicious for breast cancer is usually round, soft, and tender or painful when palpated.
    c. Menopause at a later age decreases the risk of breast cancer.
    d. Breast examination performed annually by a professional health care provider is an adequate substitute for monthly self breast examination.

_____ 96. Electrocardiogram markers of hypokalemia include all of the following *except*:

    a. tachyarrhythmias.
    b. ST segment depression.
    c. peaked T waves.
    d. premature ventricular contractions.

_____ 97. The nurse practitioner knows that the frail elderly are at high risk for malnutrition. Indicators of malnutrition in this population include all of the following *except*:

    a. hunger and increased appetite.
    b. glossitis.
    c. delayed wound healing.
    d. cachexia.

_____ 98. Which of the following may predispose the patient to hyperkalemia?

    a. insulin
    b. ramipril
    c. hydrochlorothiazide
    d. furosemide

_____ 99. What advice should be given to the parents of an infant at risk for SIDS?

    a. "Position the baby prone for sleeping."
    b. "Place the baby in supine or side-lying position for sleeping."
    c. "Monthly physical exams will pick up new risk factors."
    d. "An apnea monitor will prevent SIDS from occurring."

_____ 100. A mother presents with her 12-year-old son who has chills, fever, headache, malaise, and myalgias. On examination, the nurse practitioner finds an erythematous lesion, 7.5 cm in diameter, with annular edges and central clearing. The boy first noticed the lesion when he was preparing to go back home from a 2 week summer camp in the mountains. Of the following, which is the most likely diagnosis?

    a. Pityriasis rosea
    b. Impetigo
    c. Lyme disease
    d. Tinea corporis

_____ 101. Which patient is at *highest* risk for sudden infant death syndrome (SIDS)?

    a. A 14-month-old infant with sleep apnea.
    b. A well-developed 2-month-old infant.
    c. A 12-month-old infant with asthma.
    d. A 7-month-old infant who sleeps in the supine position.

_____ 102. A 48-year-old female presents with a chief complaint of insomnia. On further investigation, she reports fatigue, nervousness and agitation during the daytime, and feeling hot most of the time. Which of the following would *not* be included in the differential diagnoses?

    a. Menopause
    b. Hyperthyroidism
    c. Anxiety disorder
    d. Parkinson's disease

_____ 103. A widowed 85-year-old was recently moved from her home of 65 years to a bedroom in her daughter's home. According to reports by family members, she is now "cantankerous," gets "mixed up" easily, and cries for no apparent reason. Factors in the patient history that are consistent with delirium may include all of the following *except*:

    a. insidious onset and chronic progressive course.
    b. a new anticholinergic medication.
    c. dehydration and/or malnutrition.
    d. recent changes in surroundings and routines.

_____104. Frequent throat clearing with or without cough is *least* likely explained by:

a. foreign body in the ear.
b. vasomotor rhinitis.
c. allergic rhinitis.
d. acute sinusitis.

_____105. Which of the following may worsen symptoms of urgency in a patient with benign prostatic hyperplasia (BPH)?

a. Beta-blockers
b. Alpha-adrenergic blockers
c. Alcohol and caffeine
d. Anticholinergic medications

_____106. On clinical assessment of a 1-month-old infant, the nurse practitioner suspects congenital hip dislocation. All of the following are associated with this diagnosis *except*:

a. asymmetry of the gluteal folds and skin creases of the legs.
b. negative Ortolani's and Barlow's signs.
c. limb length discrepancy.
d. limited abduction of the thigh with the hip flexed.

_____107. A 44-year-old male reports gradual hearing loss over the past 3 months. Results of the Rinne tuning fork test are: AC > BC in both ears. This indicates:

a. bilateral sensorineural hearing loss.
b. sensorineural hearing loss in the left ear.
c. bilateral conductive hearing loss.
d. conductive hearing loss in the left ear.

_____108. A patient complains of "very puffy feet" since shortly after beginning a new medication 3 months ago. There is no underlying physiological cause for this condition. Which medication is most likely causing the problem?

a. nifedipine (Procardia®)
b. hydrochlorothiazide (HCTZ)
c. enalapril (Vasotec®)
d. metoprolol (Toprol®)

_____109. Microscopic examination of expressed prostatic secretions (EPS) and post-prostate massage urine is positive for WBCs > 10 to 20/HPF and negative for bacteria. The most likely diagnosis is:

    a. chronic nonbacterial prostatitis.
    b. benign prostatic hyperplasia (BPH).
    c. acute bacterial prostatitis.
    d. carcinoma of the prostate gland.

_____110. The most appropriate medications for elderly patients:

    a. are highly protein-bound.
    b. may be dosed once daily.
    c. have a narrow therapeutic index.
    d. have anticholinergic effects.

_____111. Which of the following statements about atopic dermatitis is *false*?

    a. It is frequently associated with allergic conjunctivitis, allergic rhinitis, and asthma.
    b. It presents in genetically predisposed individuals.
    c. Symmetrical lichenification is typically on the flexor surfaces and xerosis is generalized.
    d. It is a disease of adulthood.

_____112. To reduce skin cancer risk associated with ultraviolet light and ionizing radiation, sun exposure should be avoided between the hours of:

    a. 10 am and 12 noon.
    b. 12 noon and 2 pm.
    c. 10 am and 3 pm.
    d. 12 noon and 3 pm.

_____113. A patient complains of chronic rhinorrhea, nasal stuffiness and throat clearing, and cough. This constellation of symptoms is most *likely* explained by:

    a. acute sinusitis.
    b. allergic rhinitis.
    c. allergic conjunctivitis.
    d. asthma.

_____114. Herniated nucleus pulposus typically presents clinically by all of the following *except*:

    a.   numbness and paresthesia along the distribution of the involved dermatome.
    b.   listing away from the unaffected side toward the affected side.
    c.   decreased mobility and motor function.
    d.   local tenderness to palpation.

_____115. All of the following interventions with pediatric patients are appropriate *except*:

    a.   allowing a parent-figure to remain with the patient during unpleasant or painful procedures.
    b.   preparing the patient before treatments and procedures with explanations, demonstrations, or forms of play to reduce stress and fear.
    c.   consoling the patient following unpleasant or painful interventions.
    d.   premedicating the patient prior to all painful interventions.

_____116. A male patient schedules a wellness visit on his 50th birthday. The nurse practitioner appropriately recommends all of the following *except*:

    a.   stool for occult blood.
    b.   digital rectal examination (DRE) and prostate specific antigen (PSA).
    c.   annual lipid profile.
    d.   annual ECG and chest x-ray.

_____117. Therapeutic international normalized ratio (INR) for a patient taking warfarin (Coumadin®) for chronic atrial fibrillation is expected to be:

    a.   increased.
    b.   decreased.
    c.   the same as the PTT.
    d.   3 times the expected PT.

_____118. Approximately 70% of the organisms found in canine oral and nasal fluids, and consequently in fresh dog bite wounds, are:

    a.   *Staphylococcus* and *Pasteurella multocida.*
    b.   *Klebsiella* and *Moraxella sp.*
    c.   *Escherichia coli* and *Proteus mirabilis.*
    d.   *Beta streptococci* and *Brucella canis.*

_____119. A patient recovering from a recent stroke is starting warfarin therapy. The nurse practitioner should teach the patient to avoid all of the following *except*:

    a. broccoli and cauliflower.
    b. milk and milk products.
    c. mustard greens and collard greens.
    d. alcohol and licorice.

_____120. All of the following affect the action of warfarin (Coumadin®) *except*:

    a. oral antibacterials.
    b. alcohol.
    c. NSAIDs.
    d. sulfonylureas.

_____121. The reason beta-adrenergic blockers should be avoided in patients with diabetes is because they may:

    a. potentiate hyperglycemia.
    b. interfere with the action of insulin and oral hypoglycemics.
    c. mask symptoms of hypoglycemia.
    d. stimulate hepatic glucose secretion.

_____122. A female patient asks "How do I calculate my ideal body weight?" The nurse practitioner appropriately answers:

    a. "Start with 100 pounds, and add 5 pounds for every inch in height over five feet."
    b. "Add 6 pounds for every inch over 5 feet, then add 100 pounds."
    c. "Start with 100 pounds, and add 10 pounds for every inch in height over five feet."
    d. "Multiply your height in inches times 2."

_____123. Salicylates and other NSAID agents have all of the following actions *except*:

    a. anti-inflammatory effects via inhibition of prostaglandin synthesis.
    b. antiemetic effects via suppression of gastric acid secretion.
    c. antipyretic effects via inhibition of heat production by the hypothalamus.
    d. analgesia via inhibition of prostaglandin synthesis.

____124. Patients should be encouraged to purchase brand name only for each of the following drugs *except*:

a. lanoxin.
b. phenytoin.
c. hydrochlorothiazide.
d. levothyroxine.

____125. Tricyclic antidepressants should be avoided in elderly patients because they have potentially disabling side effects. Which of the following is *least* likely to be an adverse side effect of TCAs?

a. Nausea and urinary retention
b. Confusion, sedation, and memory impairment
c. Unsteady gait and orthostatic hypotension
d. Potentiation of seizures

____126. Characteristics of prescription and OTC drug use in the elder population include all of the following *except*:

a. a high incidence of drug reactions.
b. multiple prescribers and polypharmacy.
c. increased tolerance to drug effects.
d. decreased rate of metabolism and excretion.

____127. All of the following principles apply to drug therapy for elders *except*:

a. start with a low dose and increase as needed as slowly as possible to achieve the desired results.
b. encourage the elderly to continue self-medication administration to facilitate independence and self-sufficiency.
c. recommend medication dispensers organized by day and time.
d. review all medications at least twice a year and every time the drug regimen is changed.

____128. A pre-adolescent male expresses concern about his physical growth and development as compared to girls his age. The nurse practitioner correctly tells him that the pubertal growth spurt occurs about:

a. 1 year earlier in boys.
b. the same time for boys and girls.
c. 2 years earlier in girls.
d. 2 years earlier in boys.

_____129. Which of the following statements concerning informed consent is *false*?

    a. The risks, benefits, and alternatives must be explained in words the patient understands.
    b. It ensures the patient's right to choose or refuse an intervention.
    c. It is not legally binding if the patient cannot write his or her name.
    d. It may be signed by a surrogate decision-maker who has power of attorney for medical decisions.

_____130. Patients with renal calculi should be taught that the best prevention is:

    a. to maintain adequate hydration.
    b. restriction of dietary protein.
    c. restriction of dietary purine.
    d. to alkalinize the urine.

_____131. A patient with polycythemia secondary to COPD would be expected to have:

    a. a fluid volume deficit.
    b. dyspnea and activity intolerance.
    c. immune suppression.
    d. anemia.

_____132. Which immunization(s) is(are) contraindicated for patients who are allergic to eggs?

    a. Hepatitis B and varicella
    b. Poliomyelitis (IPV) and diphtheria/tetanus (Td)
    c. Influenza
    d. Pneumococcal

_____133. Which of the following drug classes poses the *lowest* fall risk for elderly patients?

    a. Antipsychotics
    b. Antihypertensives
    c. Antidepressants
    d. Antibiotics

_____134. Which of the following interventions does *not* contribute to the resolution, or shorten the course, of atopic dermatitis lesions?

    a. Tacrolimus ointment (Protopic®)
    b. Topical corticosteroid cream
    c. Antihistamines
    d. Avoidance of trigger factors

_____135. Changes in pulmonary air flow associated with asthma exacerbations and remissions is best assessed by monitoring:

    a. sputum characteristics.
    b. the number of different types of medications required for control.
    c. peak expiratory flow rate (PEFR) as measured by a peak flowmeter.
    d. frequency of rescue inhaler use.

_____136. Moderate weight loss, particularly of visceral adipose tissue, in patients with type 2 diabetes mellitus may have all of the following beneficial effects *except*:

    a. improved insulin sensitivity.
    b. increased glucose uptake and utilization by the cells.
    c. increased lean muscle mass.
    d. improved lipid profile.

_____137. Which of the following is *not* true about carpal tunnel syndrome?

    a. Symptoms present in the first 3½ fingers of the affected hand.
    b. Symptoms are absent in the 5th finger.
    c. Median nerve compression can result in decreased strength and impaired fine motor coordination.
    d. Phalen's and Tinel's tests are negative.

_____138. All of the following are associated with erectile dysfunction (ED) *except*:

    a. beta-adrenergic blockers, alpha-adrenergic blockers, and calcium channel blockers.
    b. NSAIDs and oral hypoglycemic agents.
    c. alcohol, marijuana, and opiates.
    d. diabetes mellitus and peripheral vascular disease.

_____139. "Pre-diabetes" is:

    a. early insulin resistance and hyperinsulinemia.
    b. complete pancreatic beta cell failure.
    c. diagnosed by fasting glucose greater than 126 mg/dL.
    d. caused by a sedentary lifestyle.

_____140. The obesity associated with type 2 diabetes mellitus is:

    a. a lower body (gynecoid) distribution.
    b. defined as BMI 30 or greater.
    c. defined as waist-to-hip ratio 0.5 or less.
    d. a truncal (android) distribution.

_____141. The first line treatment for allergic rhinitis is:

    a. an oral decongestant.
    b. an oral 1st generation antihistamine and an intranasal decongestant.
    c. a leukotriene blocker and/or nasal cromolyn.
    d. an oral 2nd generation antihistamine or intranasal antihistamine.

_____142. Which of the following is the *least* likely differential diagnosis for viral upper respiratory infection?

    a. Vasomotor rhinitis
    b. Seasonal allergic rhinitis
    c. Rhinitis medicamentosa
    d. Acute bacterial sinusitis

_____143. Which of the following statements about asthma is true?

    a. A negative methacholine challenge test has a positive predictive value of 100%.
    b. Patients with classic asthma typically demonstrate reversible airflow obstruction on spirometry in response to inhalation of a short-acting beta-agonist.
    c. Cough variant asthma (cough is the only symptom) accounts for about 10% of all asthma diagnoses.
    d. Asthma is a disease of childhood characterized by irreversible hyporesponsive airflow obstruction.

_____144. Chronic bacterial prostatitis (CBP) may be due to any of the following *except*:

    a. *Proteus mirabilis.*
    b. *Streptococcus pyogenes.*
    c. *Enterococcus faecalis.*
    d. *Escherichia coli.*

_____145. The leading cause of death from injury in childhood is:

    a. drowning.
    b. motor vehicle accident (MVA).
    c. cancer.
    d. poisoning.

_____146. At what age does chest circumference typically equal head circumference?

    a. 6 months
    b. 1 to 2 years
    c. 2½ years
    d. 3 years

_____147. A 3-year-old has enlarged, tender, cervical lymph nodes indicating:

    a. infection proximal to the nodes.
    b. a possible cancer diagnosis.
    c. shotty nodes, a common normal variant in children.
    d. an infectious process distal to the nodes.

_____148. On assessment, the nurse practitioner expects the infant to focus both eyes simultaneously, and track an object, by what age?

    a. 6 weeks
    b. 3 to 4 months
    c. 6 to 9 months
    d. 12 months

_____149. A 42-year-old male executive is diagnosed with depression. He is otherwise healthy. An appropriate initial treatment choice is a:

    a. monoamine oxidase inhibitor (MAOI).
    b. selective serotonin reuptake inhibitor (SSRI).
    c. benzodiazepine.
    d. non-tricyclic second generation antidepressant.

_____ 150. A 7-year-old female patient presents with injuries that are inconsistent with the explanation given for them. The nurse practitioner questions the mother about abuse. She admits that her husband, the child's father, beat the child. How should the nurse practitioner proceed?

    a. Inform the mother that the abuse must be reported to child protection services.
    b. Counsel the mother that if it happens again it will be reported to child protection services.
    c. Ask the child what she did to cause the punishment.
    d. Refer the family to the National Domestic Violence Hotline.

Practice Exam IV
Answers and Rationales

1. *b*   Walking is an excellent exercise to begin during pregnancy. Generally, pregnancy is not a good time to begin new aerobic exercise because pregnant women are more likely to have sprains and other ligament injuries. However, experienced exercisers may continue their usual aerobic activities. As a rule of thumb, activities which keep heart rates below 140 bpm are usually considered acceptable in pregnant patients.

2. *d*   RV is increased, VC is decreased, FEV-1 is decreased, and TLC remains normal or may be only slightly increased with chronic bronchitis. RV, VC, and FEV-1 spirometry readings are the same whether the COPD is due to chronic bronchitis or chronic emphysema, however, TLC is normal or only slightly increased with chronic bronchitis. Significant obstruction is present when FEV-1 is less than 70% of FVC (forced vital capacity).

3. *a*   The Sickledex® is a screening tool for sickle cell anemia. If the Sickledex® is positive, a hemoglobin electrophoresis is ordered for confirmation of sickle cell anemia or another anemia. The patient's behavior probably has nothing to do with sickle cell anemia.

4. *c*   Primary prevention consists of activities that decrease the probability of occurrence of specific illness. A tetanus (Td) vaccination decreases the probability that tetanus will develop after an injury.

5. *b*   In July 2000, the American College of Obstetricians and Gynecologists reported that age > 35 years and diabetes or hypertension were considered absolute contraindications to oral contraceptive use. Relative contraindications are heavy smokers > 35 years.

6. *a.*   The initial test to offer this patient is the ELISA, which is a screening test for infection with HIV. The Western blot, a confirmatory test for HIV infection, is only indicated when the ELISA is positive.

7. *a*   The introduction of solid food to a baby is not recommended before the baby is 4 to 6 months-of-age. Cereals are introduced first and fruits second.

8. *b*   This patient's stage of sexual development is appropriate for age. By 16 years-of-age, with or without development of secondary sexual characteristics, she should have begun menses. At that time, she should be referred if the first menstrual period has not started.

9. *d* Limited range of joint motion is characteristic of both types of arthritis. The soreness and stiffness associated with OA improves as the day progresses and joint range of motion improves with the performance of daily activities. Joint pain and stiffness associated with RA worsens with use. Loss of energy, malaise, and easy fatigability are constitutional symptoms associated with RA. RA is an inflammatory disease of the joints and flare-ups are characterized by very warm and erythematous joints relieved by anti-inflammatory medications such as NSAIDs, DMARDS, and glucocorticosteroids.

10. *c* Alcohol or illicit drug use is not associated with amenorrhea. Females with anorexia nervosa are often amenorrheic, but there is no association between amenorrhea and bulimia nervosa. Amenorrhea is a common finding in female athletes due to the high frequency and extremes of exercise. The most common cause of secondary amenorrhea is pregnancy.

11. *d* Angina and peptic ulcer disease may have similar clinical presentations, including nausea and intermittent "burning" retrosternal chest pain. The pain of PUD is relieved by ingesting an antacid. Stable angina is exacerbated by activity and relieved by rest. GERD is associated with ingestion of food. The pain of chest wall syndrome is reproduced with firm palpation of the intercostal spaces anywhere from the sternal margin to the mid-axillary line and is relieved with anti-inflammatory agents.

12. *a* McBurney's point is the anatomical landmark in the RLQ of the abdomen for locating the vermiform appendix. Pain associated with pancreatitis and duodenal ulcer commonly radiates to the anterior aspect of the RUQ and pain associated with cholecystitis commonly radiates to both the anterior and posterior aspects of the RUQ. Pain radiating to the right shoulder is typically caused by inflammatory liver disease. While the examiner presses over the gallbladder at the upper rib margin of the RUQ, the patient is asked to inhale fully. When the gallbladder is inflamed, as with acute cholecystitis, the patient suddenly ceases the inhalation as the gallbladder is pressed against the examiner's fingers (hence, "Murphy's sign").

13. *a* Glucocorticosteroids, thiazide diuretics, and phenytoin may predispose the patient to hyperglycemia. Nonselective beta-blockers may potentiate insulin-induced hypoglycemia as well as mask the signs and symptoms of hypoglycemia.

14. *b* Because women live longer than men, more women develop Alzheimer's disease. Some experts believe, however, that women have a higher risk of Alzheimer's disease independent of their average life span. This may be related to the fact that women stop producing estrogen, while men continue to produce testosterone.

15. *c* Development of type 2 diabetes mellitus is not associated with past or present history of alcohol or other drug use. All of the other patient characteristics are associated with insulin resistance, glucose intolerance, and type 2 diabetes mellitus. Another risk factor is positive family history of type 2 diabetes mellitus, particularly in a first degree relative (parent or sibling).

16. *a* Battering frequently occurs for the first time during pregnancy or worsens during pregnancy.

17. *c* Aluminum and magnesium preparations, such as antacids and milk of magnesia, bind with iron thereby decreasing absorption. Iron also binds with calcium (milk, milk products, calcium supplements) and should not be taken concurrently. Vitamin C facilitates absorption of iron.

18. *c* The lesions described are *herpes zoster* (shingles), a viral infection of the spinal nerve root. It is treated with an oral antiviral medication, such as acyclovir, within 4 days of the onset of symptoms. Beyond this period of time, there is little or no benefit to the patient. An antibiotic would be indicated only in the presence of a secondary bacterial infection.

19. *a* The condition described is tinea versicolor, a fungal dermatitis. The lesions will have a golden fluorescence under Wood's lamp. KOH will be positive for hyphae and spores. Distribution of the lesions is primarily on the chest, back, and shoulders and less commonly the groin, thigh, and genitalia. The condition typically presents in young adults and tends to be recurrent because the causative agent, *Malassezia furfur*, is a normal skin inhabitant.

20. *c* Other risk factors for transient ischemic attack (TIA) are cardiac disease, diabetes, family history of TIA, hypercoagulation state, and recent chiropractic manipulation.

21. *c* The most common cause of seizures in young children, ages 6 months to 5 years, is fever. They generally occur within the first 24 hours of the onset of the febrile illness and do not necessarily occur when the temperature is at its highest point. Febrile seizures are usually brief and are not a cause of developmental delay or behavioral abnormalities. The risk of recurrence is about 30% in a future febrile illness.

22. *c* Diseases and conditions which may cause hypertension include Graves' disease (hyperthyroidism), Cushing's disease, pheochromocytoma, coarctation of the aorta, and diseases of the renal parenchyma and renal artery. Hypertension may be a consequence of sympathetic nervous system stimulation (anxiety, panic). Drug-related causes of hypertension include cocaine use and withdrawal, alcohol withdrawal, opioid withdrawal, pseudoephedrine contained in OTC preparations, and steroids.

23. *d* Lymph drainage from the hand and forearm flows proximally through the epitrochlear lymph nodes. Inflammation, swelling, tenderness, or nodularity of epitrochlear lymph nodes may indicate a problem in the epitrochlear region or "upstream" in the forearm or hand.

24. *a* The S3 heart sound is low-pitched and occurs just after the S2 heart sound. It is produced by rapid ventricular filling and is best auscultated in the mitral area. It is a common finding with right-sided heart failure, rapid growth, and the third trimester of pregnancy.

25. *d* Women who smoke during pregnancy are at risk for delivering an infant who is small for gestational age. SGA is defined as less than 2500 grams. Babies who are macrosomic at birth are typically born to women who have diabetes. Alcohol consumption during pregnancy places the infant at risk for fetal alcohol syndrome (FAS), a syndrome of cognitive deficits and characteristic facies.

26. *b* The clinical condition described is bacterial conjunctivitis which is easily transmitted from one eye to the other. The morning crusting is dried purulent exudate. Ophthalmic steroids alone are contraindicated in bacterial conjunctivitis as they reduce ophthalmic resistance to the infective organism. An antibacterial/steroid combination reduces inflammation and edema while supplying the needed antibacterial agent. Ophthalmic antivirals are used for treatment of conditions such as ophthalmic *herpes zoster*, iritis, and uveitis.

27. *a* The most common breast carcinoma is adenocarcinoma and the most common site is the upper outer quadrant (tail of Spence) of the breast. Paget's disease, accounting for only 1% of all breast cancers, is a dermatitis or eczema-like skin presentation caused by skin invasion of a mammary duct carcinoma. Intraductal papilloma is usually a benign lesion which may develop into intraductal carcinoma and often presents with a sanguinous nipple discharge. Fibroadenoma is a benign disease of the breast which is usually painless and accompanied by a mobile mass.

28. *b* Digoxin is a drug commonly used in the treatment regimen for congestive heart failure. Anorexia, nausea, and vomiting are signs and symptoms of digitalis toxicity. Atrial fibrillation predisposes this patient to embolism and stroke is a possibility. The nausea, vomiting, and confusion may be an indication of increasing intracranial pressure or stroke. If she is taking warfarin (Coumadin®), her INR should be checked.

29. *a* One out of 8 women will develop breast cancer, the most common type of cancer in females. 80 to 85% of breast cancer is intraductal, 10 to 12% is lobular, and 1% is Paget's disease. Breast cancer is slow growing. Early diagnosis and treatment significantly increase breast cancer survival, making monthly self breast examination education and age appropriate screening mammography essential components of routine well woman care.

30. *d* To maintain the same weight in this patient, approximately 2000 calories, or 40 kcal/kg/day, is needed. If her physical activities increase, a concomitant increase of 10 kcal/kg/day are needed. For an inactive patient, a decrease of 10 kcal/kg/day would be needed to maintain weight.

31. *c* Meningitis, varicella, and scarlet fever are infectious diseases associated with fetal teratogenicity. Poison ivy is a relatively benign, self-limiting, dermatitis. A patient is not able to transmit poison ivy to another person by direct contact. Contact with oil from the plant is the mechanism of transmission.

32. *b* Osteoporosis is not associated with type 2 diabetes mellitus but is commonly associated with chronic renal failure and long term anticonvulsant or steroid use.

33. *a* The most likely diagnosis is perennial allergies, specifically allergic rhinitis. Second generation oral antihistamines, intranasal mast cell stabilizers, and intranasal antihistamines are the best choices for control of histamine reactions to allergens in the nasal passages. Topical nasal steroids are considered the gold standard.

34. *d* Application of moist heat provides comfort, increases blood flow to the breast, and facilitates the "let down" reflex. Ibuprofen is an appropriate anti-inflammatory analgesic. Cephalexin is safe during breastfeeding. The breast should be emptied on a regular schedule to alleviate engorgement and to continue breast milk production. A bra should be worn for support. Breastfeeding is not contraindicated with mastitis.

35. *d* Polyuria, low specific gravity, and thirst in the early stage of chronic renal failure is due to inability of the renal tubules to adequately concentrate urine.

36. *a* Isolated systolic hypertension (ISH) is defined as systolic blood pressure 140 mmHg or greater and concomitant diastolic BP less than 90 mmHg. This is a common cause of hypertension in the elderly. By about the 6th decade, diastolic pressure tends to remain static or decline while the systolic BP continues to rise.

37. *c* McBurney's point is the RLQ abdominal landmark for the appendix. Rigid abdominal musculature, rebound tenderness, and positive psoas sign (inflamed psoas muscle) indicates inflammation of the peritoneum. Cholecystitis presents with RUQ pain and positive Murphy's sign. Ulcerative colitis presents with LLQ pain. Pain associated with pancreatitis is typically in the epigastric region.

38. *c* Allopurinol® 100 mg qd to qid daily is the treatment of choice for chronic gout prophylaxis. Colchicine and NSAIDs are treatments of choice for acute attacks. Alcohol and purine-containing foods (organ meats, preserved seafood, shellfish) trigger attacks because they block uric acid secretion by the renal tubules which result in underexcretion.

39. *b* The "typical" patient with chronic cholecystitis is "female, fat, fertile, and (over) 40" years-of-age. Myocarditis produces retrosternal pain that is not related to diet. The pain of pancreatitis radiates to the back. The pain of hepatitis is nonspecific upper quadrant pain.

40. *d* As patients age, the percent of body fat typically increases compared to lean muscle mass and total body water. Because of this, pharmacokinetics and the pharmacodynamics of drugs are changed. This results in less efficient metabolism, another reason elders are more likely to experience adverse drug effects.

41. *a* Normal PSA is 4 ng/ml or less. PSA levels greater than 4 ng/ml and less than 10 ng/ml are associated with BPH. A PSA level greater than 10 ng/ml suggests prostate cancer. Positive serum acid phosphatase is associated with malignancy of the prostate gland with bone metastasis.

42. *d* The sensation of bladder fullness and urgency are characteristic of urge incontinence. Stress incontinence is characterized by incontinent periods after coughing, laughing, or sneezing. Overflow incontinence is seen in diabetic or paraplegic patients who are unable to sense a full bladder.

43. *b* A tremor with the limb relaxed or at rest is most commonly observed in Parkinson's disease. Intention tremor is typical of multiple sclerosis. Diabetic neuropathy does not typically produce tremor. Huntington's chorea produces irregular, jerking movements.

44. *c* Choices *a*, *b*, and *d* are high in purine content and should be avoided by patients with gout.

45. *b* Swan neck and boutonniere deformities of the joints of the hands are associated with later stages of rheumatoid arthritis.

46. *b* Before beginning treatment with medications, the child should have a psychoeducational evaluation for attention deficit hyperactivity disorder (ADHD). Dietary restrictions have not been shown to be effective for most children with ADHD.

47. *d* Common features of syndrome X include truncal obesity, HDL equal to or less than 35 mg/dL, triglyceride equal to or greater than 250 mg/dL, hyperinsulinemia, insulin resistance, and hypertension. Cardiac pathology is not part of the clinical presentation of syndrome X.

48. *c* The estrogen and progesterone in OCPs, and parenteral progesterone, inhibit pituitary production of follicle stimulating hormone (FSH).

49. *b* A diagnosis of psychogenic cough should only be made after other potential explanations, such as asthma, postnasal drip syndrome, foreign body aspiration, have been ruled out. This somatic cough disorder, with psychogenic origins, most commonly presents in patients younger than 18 years-of-age, and is often associated with anxieties and fears related to school attendance and other social stressors.

50. *a* A decongestant and anti-inflammatory agent will shrink the mucous membranes and a mucolytic will thin the secretions to facilitate evacuation of the sinus cavities and eustachian tubes. Antihistamines should be avoided in acute sinusitis and acute otitis media because they cause the secretions to become thicker and more tenacious, and often "trap" the microorganism.

51. *d* Estrogen deficiency, consumption of alcohol, smoking, and inadequate weight-bearing activity contribute to osteoporosis risk. For overweight women (BMI > 28), weight loss contributes to reduction in osteoporosis risk. Recommended calcium supplementation is 500 mg per day for premenopausal women without evidence of osteopenia and osteoporosis and 1200 to 1500 mg per day for menopausal women.

52. *d* Appropriate treatment for chronic diverticulosis includes a diet high in fiber. A daily supplement of bran or a psyllium hydrophilic mucilloid (Metamucil®) is strongly recommended.

53. *a* Gonorrhea, chlamydia, and trichomoniasis, are sexually transmitted diseases requiring partner treatment. Bacterial vaginosis and candida vaginitis are not sexually transmitted. Leiomyoma is an estrogen dependent benign tumor of the uterus which is an uncommon finding in the postmenopausal female unless she is receiving HRT.

54. *d* Normal hemoglobin is 12.0 g/dL for females and 14.0 g/dL for males. Iron deficiency anemia is characterized by an MCV < 80 fl, increased TIBC, decreased serum iron and ferritin. MCV > 100 fl is indicative of a macrocytic anemia.

55. *a* This is a clinical description of left-sided heart failure. The decreased level of consciousness, dizziness, and fatigue are caused by decreased oxygenation secondary to pulmonary congestion. Left ventricular failure causes a reduction in ejection fraction which allows fluid accumulation in the lungs. Pneumonia must always be considered in the elderly patient with cough and shortness of breath. Often there is absence of fever which makes the diagnosis more difficult. Signs of foreign body obstruction include acute onset of respiratory distress, stridor, a "croupy" sound on inspiration and/or expiration, or absence of breath sounds in one lung or a lobe of one lung.

56. *a* The two types of COPD are chronic emphysema and chronic bronchitis. Both are associated with a history of smoking. Typical physical examination findings for the patient with chronic emphysema include AP chest diameter equal to transverse chest diameter ("barrel chest"), decreased tactile fremitus, decreased diaphragmatic excursion, hyper-resonance to percussion, and wheezes. AP chest diameter equal to transverse chest diameter, increased tactile fremitus, decreased diaphragmatic excursion, hypo-resonance to percussion, wheezes, rhonchi, and productive cough are typical examination findings associated with chronic bronchitis.

57. *b* Women who drink alcohol during pregnancy are at risk for delivering an infant with fetal alcohol syndrome (FAS). FAS is a syndrome which includes size small for gestational age (SGA), permanent cognitive deficits and characteristic facies. The amount or frequency of alcohol consumption that is considered "safe" is unknown. Total avoidance is recommended.

58. *d* Regardless of the cause or type, anemia may often be mistaken for depression. All of the patient's mental functions may be delayed or impaired. Common signs and symptoms include generalized malaise, sluggishness, forgetfulness, lethargy, syncope, pallor, and problems associated with decreased tissue oxygenation. Central nervous system function is not increased. There is no associated nervousness or anxiety.

59. *c* Uncontrolled primary hypertension is usually asymptomatic. However, the headache associated with elevated blood pressure is typically occipital and presents on awakening in the morning. Other symptoms which may be associated with uncontrolled primary hypertension include tachycardia, palpitations, tinnitus, and fatigue. If target organ damage has occurred, signs and symptoms may present that can be attributed to target organ pathology.

60. *d* Herpetic lesions (*herpes simplex* or *varicella zoster*) are typically vesicular. To prepare a Tzanck prep, the vesicle is unroofed using a scalpel and then the base of the vesicle is scraped. The scrapings are fixed to a microscope slide using 95% alcohol and an appropriate stain. When positive, numerous multi-nucleated giant cells are visible.

61. *b* According to the American Diabetes Association's diagnostic criteria, the diagnosis of type 2 diabetes mellitus may be made when: (a) the result of a 2-hour glucose tolerance test (GTT), with 75 g of glucose, is equal to or greater than 200 mg/dL or (b) fasting glucose is 126 mg/dL or greater on 2 separate occasions. Target HbA_{1C} for diabetics is $\leq$ 6.5 %. Although glycosylated hemoglobin is not used for diagnosis, 10% represents consistently elevated glucose levels > 200 mg/dL. Ketonuria is associated with beta cell failure, as with uncontrolled type 1 diabetes mellitus or late stage type 2 diabetes mellitus.

62. *a* The patient's acute clinical complaints reflect probable pancreatitis which could be confirmed by elevated serum amylase, lipase, and liver function studies. Serum bilirubin would be ordered to rule out cholecystitis. Elevated serum BUN could reflect dehydration secondary to vomiting. Serum creatinine and 24 hour urine creatinine clearance reflect renal function. A flat plate of the abdomen and gastric endoscopy would be appropriate to investigate probable perforated peptic ulcer or duodenal ulcer, intussusception, volvulus, or other acute abdominal disorders.

63. *d* New onset diabetes produces elevated serum glucose levels less than 200 mg/dL and usually no clinical signs or symptoms. At higher levels, the patient may report lethargy, fatigue, weakness, weight loss, and polydipsia, polyuria, and/or polyphagia. Complaints of insomnia, night sweats, feeling intensely hot, emotional lability, and extreme nervousness may be caused by thyroxine excess, menopausal vasomotor instability, or withdrawal from alcohol or other drugs of addiction.

64. *b* Hyperkalemia has been associated with the use of all ACE inhibitors. Patients at greatest risk of hyperkalemia are those with CHF, renal insufficiency, and those taking potassium-sparing diuretics.

65. *a* The Denver II Developmental Screening Test revised (DDST-R, Denver II) is a screening tool used to assess the areas of personal/social, fine motor, gross motor, and language development from infancy through 5½ years-of-age. Interpretation of performance in each area is categorized "normal," "suspect," or untestable." It is not a measure of intelligence. Language development is the single best measure of cognitive development in early childhood.

66. *d* Approximately 35% of all health care expenditures are for persons in the 65 years and older age group, with the largest area of expenditure being hospitalization in acute care facilities. Approximately 25% of all health care expenses are not covered by insurance plans and must be borne by the individual.

67. *a* Calcium binds with milk and other dairy products, thereby decreasing absorption of supplemental calcium in the gastrointestinal tract. A high intake of caffeine containing beverages is associated with osteoporosis. Research has demonstrated that supplemental HRT decreases the risk of osteoporosis. Some OTC antacids contain calcium, providing both calcium supplementation and stomach acid neutralization.

68. *c* Primary (essential) hypertension, for which the cause is unknown, accounts for approximately 80 to 90 % of all hypertension. Isolated systolic hypertension (ISH) is associated with advancing age beginning in the 6th decade. The ease or difficulty of controlling blood pressure is dependent upon a variety of factors, but age is not necessarily one of them.

69. *c* For women who smoke during pregnancy, the risk of delivering an infant who is small for gestational age (SGA, < 2500 g) is approximately twice that of women who do not smoke during pregnancy. Smoking cessation should be strongly encouraged at the time of preconceptual counseling and smoking during pregnancy should be strongly discouraged.

70. *c* Hypoglycemia, TIA, Meniere's disease, migraine headache, and otitis media may present with dizziness and disturbances in balance and equilibrium. Allergic rhinitis, with characteristic enlarged, pale, boggy turbinates and clear rhinorrhea, is not associated with any of these symptoms.

71. *b* Neurological consequences of hyponatremia due to dehydration and volume depletion include confusion, disorientation, lethargy, coma, and seizures. Volume depletion causes hypotension. The treatment is IV fluid therapy with a hypertonic saline solution.

72. *b* Cool mist helps reduce inflammation and swelling as well as loosen secretions. Warm mist and hot steam aggravate pulmonary inflammation and swelling.

73. *b* Dietary food plans for diabetics should consist mainly of carbohydrates (50%) and limited amounts of protein (30%) and fats (20%). High fiber foods are important to a diabetic patient's diet because they slow absorption of carbohydrates and help prevent rapid rises in postprandial blood sugars.

74. *b* Recommendations during pregnancy include well-balanced and nutritious meals and snacks, an additional 300 calories per day, and supplemental folic acid, iron, and calcium.

75. *b* Almost 85% of adults over 50 years-of-age have some degree of osteoarthritis and 2 to 3% will have rheumatoid arthritis of several years duration. RA is an inflammatory disease affecting multiple joints bilaterally and producing a syndrome of constitutional symptoms. Joint pain and stiffness are worse on awakening in the morning and improvement is noticed after about 2 hours of activity. Treatment includes DMARDs, steroids, and NSAIDs.

76. *a* Syphilis is passed to the fetus in utero at any time beginning with the 2nd trimester (4th month of gestation) and carries the risk of spontaneous abortion or congenital syphilis.

77. *b* CPK begins to rise at 4 to 6 hours, peaks in 16 to 30 hours, and returns to normal in 3 to 4 days. CPK-MB is specific to myocardial tissue damage. LDH begins to rise within 24 to 48 hours, peaks in 3 to 6 days, and returns to normal in 7 to 10 days. ST segment depression indicates myocardial ischemia (early MI) and ST segment elevation indicates myocardial tissue death (AMI). Prominent Q waves reflect myocardial tissue damage (AMI). Cardiac troponin I elevates early and higher levels correlate with poorer outcomes.

78. *c* Osteoarthritis is characterized by morning stiffness lasting less than 1 hour, absence of constitutional symptoms, and negative laboratory inflammatory markers. It is seen more often in weightbearing joints such as the knee or hip and is often accompanied by crepitus.

79. *c* All children who have a parental history of hypercholesterolemia should be screened with a nonfasting cholesterol. Children with a value > 200 mg/dL should be screened with a fasting lipid profile. These are the recommendations by the National Cholesterol Education Program Expert Panel on Blood Cholesterol Levels in Children and Adolescents, the American Academy of Pediatrics, the Bright Futures guidelines, the AMA Guidelines for Adolescent and Preventive Services, and the American Academy of Family Physicians.

80. *c* An elevated eosinophil count reflects exposure and inflammatory reaction to an allergen trigger. It is commonly elevated during an acute asthma exacerbation, allergy exacerbation, or with parasitic infections.

81. *c* One out of every 8 Americans is 65 years-of-age or older, representing approximately 13% of the U.S. population. These statistics are increasing due to ever increasing longevity. The majority of elders are female, widowed, and reside with family members. Social security is the primary source of income (40%). The median annual income is approximately $15,000 for males and $9,000 for females.

82. *a* Anemia of chronic disease is normocytic and normochromic. Iron deficiency anemia is microcytic and hypochromic. Folic acid deficiency anemia and pernicious (vitamin B-12 deficiency) anemia are macrocytic and normochromic anemias.

83. *d* Smoking, alcohol abuse, anorexia nervosa, and low BMI are risk factors for osteoporosis.

84. *d* Stress urinary incontinence is not expected as a result of the normal aging process. The primary problem is sphincter incompetence. The ingestion of caffeine or alcohol decreases sphincter control. Anticholinergic and antidepressant medications are causative factors related to overflow incontinence. Detrusor muscle instability is the primary underlying problem causing urge incontinence.

85. *b* The Weber tuning fork test is a screening test of bone conduction of sound. In the presence of obstruction, such as cerumen impaction, otitis media, severe otitis externa, or presence of a foreign body, sound lateralizes to (is heard better in) the affected hear. The increased density of the obstruction facilitates conduction of sound, so the patient reports hearing sound "better" in the affected ear.

86. *c* Corneal abrasion is an extremely painful eye injury that is described as "aching" and "stabbing." Vertical abrasions indicate presence of a foreign body under the lid. An ophthalmic steroid alone is contraindicated with corneal abrasion as ophthalmic resistance to invasion by microorganisms would be decreased. An ophthalmic antibiotic ointment and eye patching will provide protection from secondary infection, relieve the photophobia, and protect the cornea from further irritation caused by blinking.

87. *a* Following trauma to the knee, when a patient complains of local pain with either locking or giving way, McMurray's test is indicated to rule out a torn meniscus. With the patient positioned supine and flat, and the examiner standing on the affected side, the affected leg is flexed approximately 90 degrees at the hip, knee, and ankle and the examiner grasps the knee with fingers on the medial side. Rotating the leg inward and outward relaxes and loosens the affected joint. Then the leg is rotated externally and the knee is slowly extended while a valgus (inward) stress is applied to the knee. An audible or palpable "click" is positive for a torn meniscus.

88. *b* On wet prep microscopic exam, the diagnosis of vaginal candidiasis is made on finding budding hyphae and the diagnosis of trichomoniasis is made on finding motile flagellated protozoa (trichomonads). A positive KOH whiff test and the presence of clue cells confirm a diagnosis of bacterial vaginosis. Genital herpes presents with painful vesicular lesions that may be closed (early lesions) or open and draining (more mature lesions). Opening and culturing lesions provides a laboratory confirmatory diagnosis. Diagnosis of gonorrhea requires culture.

89. *c* The normal postmenopausal vagina has a thin, dry vaginal mucosa associated with atrophy of the epithelium and an absence of rugae. This condition may be treated with intravaginal applications of estrogen cream. Raised yellowish lesions on the cervix are common benign lesions known as nabothian cysts. A cervix that is friable (bleeds easily when touched), with petechial hemorrhages (termed "strawberry cervix,") is usually observed with infection from *T. vaginalis*.

90. *d* When sick, patients who use insulin and/or oral diabetes medication should drink plenty of fluids to maintain adequate hydration, take their diabetes medication as usual, and monitor fingerstick glucose levels more closely, making adjustments only as needed.

91. *a* *E. coli* is the most common causative organism in upper and lower urinary tract infections and infection of the prostate gland.

92. *a*   A benign thyroid nodule is typically smooth, soft, easily mobile, and tender to palpation. A thyroid nodule that is suspicious for cancer is typically hard, nontender, and fixed with an irregular shape. Fine needle aspiration biopsy is the diagnostic test of choice.

93. *b*   The standard formula for calculating beginning NPH insulin therapy for a patient is 1 u/kg/day divided into 2 doses with 2/3 administered in the morning and 1/3 administered in the evening. Adolescents begin with 1.25 to 1.5 u/kg/day due to the accelerated metabolism and growth velocity characteristic of this age group.

94. *a*   Beta-blockers may interfere with the action of beta-agonist drugs (such as albuterol or salmeterol) but more importantly, they block beta-receptor sites in patients who need beta stimulation to avoid bronchoconstriction. Theoretically, selective beta-blockers in low doses are the safest beta-blockers to use in patients with bronchospastic disease like asthma.

95. *a*   A palpable breast lump that is irregularly shaped, firm or hard, nontender, and/or attached to adjacent tissue, is suspicious for breast cancer. Earlier onset of menses and later onset of menopause are risk factors for breast cancer. Both monthly self-examination and annual clinical examination by a professional health care provider are recommended for all women. Initial screening mammography is recommended for all women by 40 years-of-age.

96. *c*   ECG markers of hypokalemia (serum potassium < 3.5 mEq/L) include flattened T waves, depression of the ST segment, presence of "u" waves, tachyarrhythmias, and ventricular ectopic beats. Peaked T waves indicate hyperkalemia. Other markers of hyperkalemia (serum potassium > 5.0 mEq/L) include widened QRS complexes, prolonged P-R intervals, and ventricular ectopic beats.

97. *a*   The malnourished elder may be cachectic or obese. Vitamin B-12 deficiency (pernicious anemia) is a cause of glossitis. Hunger and appetite are absent, further compounding the problem since poor appetite is also common in the well-nourished elderly. Inadequate delivery of essential nutrients to the tissues increases the risk of tissue breakdown (pressure ulcers) and impairs tissue healing. Malnutrition may be misdiagnosed as depression in the elderly. Low serum albumin is a late indicator of malnutrition in the elderly.

98. *b*   ACE inhibitors are potassium-sparing. Ramipril is an ACE inhibitor. Drugs which end in "il" are often ACE inhibitors.

99. *b*   Infants should be placed in the supine or side-lying position for sleep. There are no physical clues evident on physical exam to identify a SIDS-prone infant. Apnea alarms are recommended for high risk infants but they must be used each time the infant sleeps, not just at nighttime.

100. *c* The 7.5 cm lesion described is typical of Lyme disease caused by *Borrelia burgdorferi,* transmitted by an infected deer tick. The lesion erythema migrans, appears within 1 month after infection (stage 1) along with this patient's other complaints of headache, malaise, myalgias, and arthralgias. If untreated, this will progress to stage 2 or 3 when treatment and eradication of symptoms is more difficult.

101. *b* SIDS is the unexpected death of an infant less than 1 year-of-age for which there is no explanation even after a thorough investigation and autopsy. Approximately 90% of SIDS deaths occur before 6 months-of-age and peak at 2 months-of-age. Having a sibling with SIDS greatly increases an infant's risk for SIDS.

102. *d* The patient's complaints are characteristic of menopause, hyperthyroidism, and anxiety disorder. Appropriate work-up would include CBC, serum FSH, serum TSH and fasting glucose. Parkinson's disease presents insidiously with social isolation, apathy, passivity, confusion, and blunted or flat affect which may be misdiagnosed as depression.

103. *a* Delirium has a rapid onset and limited course, and is reversible by correcting the underlying problem(s). Factors commonly associated with delirium include medication intoxication, fluid and electrolyte derangements (especially hyponatremia, hypoglycemia, hypokalemia), anticholinergics, benzodiazepines, cimetidine, CHF, uremia, and removal from familiar surroundings.

104. *d* Foreign body in contact with the tympanic membrane, such as a hair clipping or hair growing in the canal wall, can stimulate the sensation of matter in the throat and reflexive cough. Vasomotor rhinitis, a non-allergic form of rhinitis, and allergic rhinitis are common causes of cough. Acute sinusitis is most often characterized by tenacious bacteria-laden mucus that resists draining without a decongestant mucolytic medication.

105. *c* Alpha-adrenergic blockers are one of the nonsurgical treatments of choice for BPH. Anticholinergics are contraindicated because they cause urinary retention. Diuretics, alcohol, and caffeine can worsen symptoms of urgency and frequency.

106. *b* Congenital dislocation of the hip in infants is suspected when there is asymmetry of the gluteal folds and skin creases of the legs, limb length discrepancy, limited abduction of the thigh with the hip in flexion, and positive Ortolani's and Barlow's signs. Subluxation of the femoral head may occur as a consequence of ligament laxity. In ambulatory children, the presenting indication may be a positive Trendelenburg sign. Acetabular dysplasia may be a consequence if this condition is untreated.

107. *a* The Rinne tuning fork test is a screening test for sensorineural hearing impairment. A normal finding is AC > BC (air conduction greater than bone conduction) with the usual ratio 2:1 (air conduction 2 times longer than bone conduction). Results of the Rinne test for this patient reveal bilateral sensorineural hearing impairment. Conductive hearing loss is BC > AC.

108. *a* Mild to moderate peripheral edema is associated with arteriolar vasodilation and not necessarily due to left ventricular dysfunction. It is most commonly seen in patients taking felodipine and nifedipine.

109. *a* The signs and symptoms of chronic nonbacterial prostatitis and chronic bacterial prostatitis are nearly identical. However, with nonbacterial prostatitis there are no bacteria in the specimen, but inflammatory cells (oval fat bodies) can be found. There is no known cause.

110. *b* Once daily dosing improves compliance and in the elderly, may be safer. Highly protein-bound drugs as well as those with narrow therapeutic indices can become toxic in the elderly who have diminishing hepatic and renal function. Drugs with anticholinergic effects can produce incontinence and urinary retention.

111. *d* The majority of atopic dermatitis presents in the first year of life. It is a genetically transmitted alteration in immune function. Comorbid conditions include asthma, allergic rhinitis, and allergic conjunctivitis.

112. *c* The risk of skin cancer associated with ultraviolet light and ionizing radiation is greatest between the hours of 10 am and 3 pm. Patients who are unable to avoid sun exposure during this period should be encouraged to wear protective clothing (hat, long sleeves) and/or apply a sun block.

113. *b* Although nasal symptoms may aggravate and exacerbate asthma, the singular diagnosis of asthma is not associated with nasal symptoms. Allergic rhinitis commonly causes the symptoms described.

114. *b* When the nucleus pulposus (located in the center of the intervertebral disc) ruptures and herniates into the spinal canal, it causes pressure on the spinal root, with consequent numbness and paresthesia along the distribution of the involved dermatome. Mobility and motor function may be impaired. There is usually local tenderness to palpation. This injury occurs most often in men between the ages of 20 and 45 and most frequently due to lifting and/or twisting. Lumbar herniation most often affect the L4-L5 and L5-S1 intervertebral spaces and causes sciatic pain producible with straight leg raising (LaSegue's test). On standing, the patient typically lists away from the affected side toward the unaffected side.

115. *d* Premedication is not warranted prior to all painful interventions. For example, premedication is not warranted prior to routine immunizations but certainly is appropriate prior to suturing. Pain management should be an integral part of total patient care.

116. *d* Responses *a, b,* and *c* are currently recommended by most learned authorities and specialty organizations. Annual lipid profile may be appropriate for some patients, but there are no recommendations for annual ECG and chest X-ray outside the presence of specific disease states or risk factors.

117. *a* Warfarin (Coumadin®) therapy increases INR. Therapeutic levels vary according to the reason anticoagulation is needed. A patient with chronic atrial fibrillation requires a therapeutic INR of 2.0 to 3.0 whereas therapeutic INR for a patient with a mechanical heart valve is 3.5 to 4.5.

118. *a* All of these organisms are found in canine oral and nasal fluids, and cultured from fresh dog bite wounds, but the most common (70%) are *Staphylococcus* and *Pasteurella multocida*.

119. *b* Patients taking warfarin (Coumadin®) should avoid foods that are high in vitamin K. Warfarin interferes with hepatic synthesis of vitamin K-dependent clotting factors, thus delaying clot formation. Foods which are high in vitamin K are those listed as well as egg yolks, "cold water" fish (high in omega-3 fatty acids), and vegetables oils.

120. *a* Warfarin (Coumadin®) is 99% protein-bound and readily distributed to all the tissues. It has a narrow therapeutic index and is affected by a number of drugs and foods. Warfarin relies on multiple cytochrome systems in the liver for metabolism. Because of this, significant interactions occur with choices *b, c,* and *d.*

121. *c* Beta-blockers may potentiate insulin-induced hypoglycemia so they should be used cautiously in diabetic patients. Additionally beta-blockers may mask the signs and symptoms of hypoglycemia, another reason to use them cautiously in diabetic patients.

122. *a* The gross calculation of ideal body weight (IBW) begins with 100 lbs for the first 5 feet in height. Then, females add 5 lbs for every inch over 5 feet and males add 6 lbs for every inch over 5 feet.

123. *b* There are no antiemetic effects caused by salicylates or NSAIDs. In fact, they often produce GI upset related to inhibition of prostaglandin synthesis. Prostaglandins exert a GI protective effect.

124. *c* Lanoxin, phenytoin, and levothyroxine each have a narrow therapeutic index and side effects may potentially be toxic. Further, generic pharmaceutical lots vary in potency. Therefore, the patient should be advised to select brand names or to consistently purchase the generic manufactured by the same company.

125. *d* Seizures are a very infrequent and rare adverse effect of tricyclic antidepressants. The other noted side effects are common.

126. *c* With advancing age, patients become more sensitive to the effects of most drugs. Additionally, as drugs are added to a patient's regimen, the potential for drug interactions and slowed metabolism are increased. The rule of thumb when introducing a new drug to an elder patient's medication regimen is to "start low and go slow."

127. *b* With increasing impairment of functioning in activities of daily living related to vision, hearing, memory, and motor function, elders may need the assistance of family and/or caretakers to manage medication and other therapeutic regimens.

128. *c* Puberty is the time of onset of sexual maturation in both genders. Females typically experience onset of puberty prior to males of the same age. Manifestations of pubertal development are due to secondary sex hormones produced by the ovaries, testes, and pituitary gland.

129. *c* The ability or inability to write one's own name has nothing to do with informed consent. Informed consent is a legal requirement to insure that patients are fully advised of the purpose, nature, benefits, risks and possible adverse outcome of a procedure or treatment. Regardless of the nature of the treatment or procedure, lack of informed consent constitutes a violation of the patient's rights.

130. *a* Vigorous fluid therapy around the clock is beneficial for all forms of renal calculi. Fluid intake should be sufficient to assure urinary output of 2 to 3 liters per day. Milk and milk products should be limited with calcium stones. Alkalinization of the urine is beneficial with uric acid stones.

131. *b* Chronic hypoxia associated with COPD stimulates excess production of RBCs. The increase in blood viscosity increases patient risk for venous thrombosis. Fluid volume, immunity, and hemoglobin are not affected.

132. *c* According to the CDC, anaphylactic reaction to eggs is a contraindication for receiving the influenza immunization only. The other immunizations listed are safe for egg allergic patients.

133. *d* Antipsychotics, anxiolytics, antidepressants, and antihypertensives may potentially cause dizziness or orthostatic hypotension and, thus, may carry a fall risk for elderly patients. Antibiotics do not increase risk for falls.

134. *c* The underlying immune response of atopic dermatitis suggests cell-mediated immunity (production of IgE). Signs and symptoms are mediated by lymphocyte secretions, not histamine. Antihistamines provide sedation which may enhance rest. Tacrolimus (Protopic®) is an immune modulator produced by *Streptomyces tsukubaensis* that inhibits interleukin-2 (IL-2). The mode of action is the same as for cyclosporine.

135. *c* Patients with asthma should know their "personal best" during periods of asthma remission for comparison with periods of exacerbation (to assess seriousness of the exacerbation).

136. *c* Lean muscle mass may only be increased by exercise.

137. *d* Phalen's and Tinel's signs are positive and diagnostic of carpal tunnel syndrome. Another hallmark feature is nighttime awakening with symptoms. Symptoms follow the distribution of the median nerve which innervates the first 3 fingers and the thumb-side half of the 4th finger. There is no involvement of the 5th finger.

138. *b* Neither NSAIDs nor hypoglycemic agents are associated with erectile dysfunction (ED). Male diabetic patients frequently have ED. However, it is due to the disease, not the medications used to treat diabetes. Erectile dysfunction may also be caused by diuretics, spironolactone, antidepressants, peripheral neuropathy, and spinal injury at S2 to S4 or higher.

139. *a* "Pre-diabetes" is the new terminology used by the American Diabetes Association to describe a population of patients who are not diabetic but who are expected to be diagnosed with diabetes within 10 years.

140. *d* Excessive adipose tissue that accumulates in a truncal distribution is associated with more serious health risk than gynoid distribution. Truncal obesity is associated with diabetes, hypertension, and hyperlipidemia. BMI (body mass index) is used to diagnose obesity.

141. *d* According to the Joint Task Force on Practice Parameters in Allergy, Asthma, and Immunology, the first-line treatment for allergic rhinitis is either an oral 2nd generation antihistamine or intranasal antihistamine. The oral second generation antihistamines, which are fexofenadine (Allegra®), cetirizine (Zyrtec®), loratadine (Claritin®) and desloratadine (Clarinex®), are usually non-sedating. The intranasal antihistamine, also non-sedating, is azelastine (Astelin®). The 1st generation antihistamines have sedation as a major side effect. Oral decongestants do not provide relief from the histamine reaction.

142. *d* Vasomotor rhinitis, seasonal allergic rhinitis, and rhinitis medicamentosa are typically associated with nasal congestion, pale and boggy turbinates, and clear rhinorrhea. Acute bacterial sinusitis, a bacterial infection of the sinus cavities, presents with facial pain, a purulent nasal discharge, and halitosis.

143. *b* Asthma is a reversible, hyperresponsive, airflow obstruction disease which typically presents in childhood and may reappear in adulthood. A methacholine challenge test for asthma has a positive predictive value of 100% when the test is positive. About 50% to 60% of all asthma diagnoses are cough variant (cough is the only symptom).

144. *b* Causative microorganisms associated with chronic bacterial prostatitis (CBP) include *Proteus mirabilis*, *Klebsiella pneumoniae*, *Escherichia coli*, and *Enterococcus faecalis*. *Streptococcus pyrogenes* is associated with upper respiratory infection.

145. *b* The leading cause of death in childhood is due to accidents, motor vehicles in particular. Children should always use seatbelts when in a moving vehicle. Children should not ride in the front seat because of risk of injury or death from air bags.

146. *b* Other notable aspects of the physical exam are weight and height. The infant should have tripled his weight by 12 months-of-age. During the 12 to 24 month period, a child should gain 4 to 6 pounds and 3 to 5 inches in height.

147. *a* Size of lymph nodes is important. Nodes > 1 cm are significant and should be assessed carefully. Nodes > 5 cm are almost always neoplastic. Tenderness of a node usually suggests inflammation. Cancerous nodes frequently are larger, nontender, and stone like in consistency. Shotty nodes are pea sized, nontender, mobile, discrete and reflect pre-existent infection.

148. *b* Other expected milestones by 4 months: babbles, coos, smiles, rolls from prone to supine, reaches for objects and controls head well. The infant may be able to track an object 45 to 90° by 1 month-of-age.

149. *b* Selective serotonin reuptake inhibitors (SSRIs) or tricyclic antidepressants (TCAs) are the drugs of choice for initial treatment of depression. Benzodiazepines are used for the treatment of anxiety and can be used for short-term use in depression with an anxiety component if other drugs have failed. Non-tricyclic second generation antidepressants are not used for initial treatment due to their limited safety.

150. *a* Reporting abuse is mandated by law when the victim is a child or an elderly adult.

Bibliography

Albers, G., Alter, M., Caplan, L., & Silverstein, P. (1996). Recognize a TIA & help prevent a stroke. *Patient Care, 30*(11), 38-60.

ACIP. (1996). ACIP issues recommendations on the prevention of varicella. *American Family Physician, 54*(8), 2578-2581.

American Diabetes Association. (2002). Report of the expert committee on the diagnosis and classification of diabetes mellitus. *Diabetes Care*, 25: S5-S20.

American Nurses Association (1996). *Scope and standards of advanced practice registered nursing.* Kansas City, MO: American Nurses Association.

American Nurses Association. (1994). *ANA scope of practice of the primary health care Nurse Practitioner.* Washington, DC: American Nurses Publishing.

American Psychological Association. (1996). *American psychological association practice guidelines.* Washington, DC: American Psychological Association.

Andrews, B.C. (1995). *Office orthopedics for primary care: Diagnosis and treatment.* Philadelphia: Saunders.

Anderson, B.C. (1995). *Office orthopedics for primary care.* Philadelphia: Saunders.

Arnold, G.J., & Neiheisel, M. (1997). A comprehensive approach to evaluating nipple discharge. *The Nurse Practitioner, 22*(7), 96-111.

Barker, L.R., Burton, J.R., & Zieve, P.D. (1999). *Principles of ambulatory care* (5th ed.). Philadelphia: Lippincott Williams & Wilkins.

Benenson, A.S., & Chin, J. (1999). *Control of communicable diseases manual* (17th ed.). Washington, DC: American Public Health Association.

Beers, M.H. and Berkow, R. (2004). *The Merck manual of diagnosis and therapy* (17th ed.). Whitehorse Station, NJ: Merck.

Bigos, S., Bowyer, O., Braen, G., et al. (1994). *Acute low back problems in adults.* Clinical Practice Guideline, No. 14. (AHCPR Pub. No. 95-0643). Rockville, MD: U.S. Department of Health and Human Services, Public Health Service, Agency for Health Care Policy and Research.

Blackburn, W.D. (1999). *Approach to the patient with musculoskeletal disorder.* Birmingham: Professional Communications.

Botoman, V.A., Bonner, G.T., & Botoman, N.A. (1998). Management of inflammatory bowel disease. *American Family Physician, 57*(1), 57-68.

Branch, W.T. (2003). *Office practice of medicine.* Philadelphia, PA: Saunders.

Brandt, E., Hadley, S., & Holtz, H. (1996). Family violence: A covert health crisis. *Patient Care, 30*(14), 138-165.

Braunwald, W., Fauci, A.S., & Kasper, D.L., Hauser, S., Longo, D. & Jameson, J. (2001). *Harrison's principles of internal medicine* (15th ed.). Blacklick, OH: McGraw Hill.

Burke, M.M., & Laramie, J.A. (2000). *Primary care of the older adult: A multidisciplinary approach.* St. Louis: Mosby

Burns, C.E., Barber, N., Brady, M.A., & Dunn, A.M. (2000). *Pediatric primary care: A handbook for nurse practitioners* (2nd ed.). Philadelphia: Saunders.

Carson, S. (1997). Human papillomatous virus infection update: Impact on women's health. *The Nurse Practitioner, 22*(4), 24-37.

Centers for Disease Control and Prevention. (2001). Revised guidelines for HIV counseling, testing, and referral and revised recommendations for HIV screnning of pregnant women. *MMWR, 50*(RR-19).

Centers for Disease Control and Prevention. (2002). 2002 sexually transmitted diseases treatment guidelines. *MMWR, 51*(RR-6).

Centers for Disease Control and Prevention. (1997). USPHS/IDSA guidelines for the prevention of opportunistic infections in persons infected with human immunodeficiency virus. *MMWR, 46*(RR-12).

Clinical guidelines on the identification, evaluation and treatment of overweight and obesity in adults. (1998). Retrieved December 1, 2003 from http://nhlbi.nih.gov/guidelines/obesity/ob_gdlns.pdf.

Clough, J., & Miller D. (1996). The new thinking on osteoarthritis. *Patient Care, 30*(14), 110-137.

Crowther, C.L. (1999). *Primary orthopedic care.* St. Louis: Mosby.

Cunningham, F.G. (2001). *Williams' obstetrics* (21st ed.). Norwalk, CT: Appleton & Lange.

Dajani, A.S., Taubert, K.A., Wilson, W., Boler, A.F., et al. (1997). Prevention of bacterial endocarditis: Recommendation by the American Heart Association. *Journal of the American Medical Association, 277,* 1794-1801.

D'Alonzo, G.E., & Tolep, K.A. (1997). Salmeterol in the treatment of chronic asthma. *American Family Physician, 57*(2), 558-562.

Dambro, M.R. (2003). *Griffith's 5 minute clinical consult.* Baltimore: Williams & Wilkins.

Davis, T., Meldrum, H., Tippy, P., Weis, B., & Williams, A. (1996). How poor literacy leads to poor health care. *Patient Care, 30*(16), 94-127.

DeGowin, R.L., & Brown, D.D. (2000). *DeGowin's Diagnostic Examination* (7th ed.). New York: McGraw Hill.

Donovan, D.A., & Nicholas, P.K. (1997). Prostatitis: Diagnosis and treatment in primary care. *The Nurse Practitioner, 22*(4), 144-156.

Elliott, K.A. (1998). Managing patients with vulvovaginal candidiasis. *The Nurse Practitioner, 23*(3), 44-53.

El-Sadr, R., Oleske, J.M., Agins, B.D., et al. (1994). *Evaluation and management of early HIV infection.* Clinical Practice Guideline No. 7. (AHCPR Publications No. 94-0572). Rockville, MD: Agency for Health Care Policy and Research, Public Health Service, U.S. Department of Health and Human Services.

The Expert Committee on the Diagnosis and Classification of Diabetes (1997). Report of the expert committee on the diagnosis and classification of diabetes mellitus. *Diabetes Care, 20*(7), 1183-1197

Fiore, M.C., Bailey, W.C., Cohen, S.J., et al. (1996). *Smoking cessation.* Clinical Practice Guideline No. 18. (AHCPR Publication No. 96-0696). Rockville, MD: U.S. Department of Health and Human Services, Public Health Service, Agency for Health Care Policy and Research.

Fischbach, F. (2003). *A manual of laboratory and diagnostic tests* (7th ed.). Philadelphia: Lippincott.

Fonte, D.R. (1997). The basics of natural family planning. *Advance for Nurse Practitioners, 5*(3), 37-42.

Forster, J. (1996). Two ways to prevent neonatal group B strep. *Patient Care, 30*(12), 22-26.

Frederickson, H.L., & Wilkins-Haug, L. (1997). *OB/GYN secrets* (2nd ed.). Philadelphia: Hanley and Belfus.

Gates, S.J., & Mooar, P.A. (1995). *Musculoskeletal primary care.* Philadelphia: Lippincott Williams & Wilkins.

Goldman, L. & Ausiello, D. (Eds.). (2004). *Cecil's textbook of medicine* (22nd ed.). Philadelphia: Saunders.

Goolsby, M.J. (2002). *Nurse practitioner secrets.* Philadelphia: Hanley & Belfus.

Goolsby, M.J. (1998). Screening, diagnosing, and management of prostate cancer. *The Nurse Practitioner, 23*(3), 11-32.

Goroll, A.H., et al. (Eds.). (1999). *Primary care medicine: Office evaluation and management of the adult patient* (4th ed.). Philadelphia: Lippincott.

Graber, M.A., & Lanternier, M.L. (2001). *The family practice handbook* (4th ed.). St. Louis: Mosby.

Griffith, C.J. (1996). Evaluation and management of anemia. *Advance for Nurse Practitioners, 4*(5), 29-35.

Griffith, H.W. (2002). *Instructions for patients.* (7th ed.). Philadelphia: Saunders.

Guide to clinical preventive services Third edition: Periodic updates. AHRQ Publicaton No. 04-1P003, January 2004. Agency for Healthcare Research and Quality, Rockville, MD.

Guidelines for the diagnosis and management of asthma-update on selected topics 2002 (2002). Retrieved Jan. 8, 2004, from http://www.nhlbi.nih.gov/guidelines/asthma/ asthmafullrpt.pdf.

Guido, G.W. (2001). *Legal and ethical issues in nursing* (3rd ed.). Upper Saddle River, NJ: Prentice Hall.

Ham, R.J., & Sloan, P.D. (2001). Primary care geriatrics: A case-based approach (4th ed.). St. Louis: Mosby.

Hansen, M.F. (1996). Acute otitis media in children. *The Nurse Practitioner, 21*(5), 72-80.

Hara, J.H. (1996). The red eye: Diagnosis and treatment. *American Family Physician, 54*(8), 2423-2430.

Health Care Finance Administration. (1996). *Medicare issues.* Title XVIII Public Law, 89-97. Health Care Finance Administration Medicare Services.

Hektor-Dunphy, L.M. (1999). Management guidelines for adult nurse practitioners. Philadelphia: Davis.

Hueston, W.J., & Mainous, A.G. (1998). Acute bronchitis. *American Family Physician, 57*(6), 1270-1276.

Imke, S. (1998). Parkinson's disease: A medical management update. *Advance for Nurse Practitioners, 6*(1), 24-28.

Ivey, J.B. (1997). The adolescent with pelvic inflammatory disease: Assessment and management. *The Nurse Practitioner, 22*(2), 78-91.

Jacobs, D.S., Oxley, D.K., & DeMott, W. R. (2001). *Laboratory test handbook* (5th ed.). Hudson, Ohio: LexiComp Inc.

Junila, J., & Larsen, P. (1998). Testicular masses. *American Family Physician, 57*(4), 685-692.

Kass-Annese, B. (1999). *Management of the perimenopausal & menopausal woman: A total wellness program.* Philadelphia: Lippincott.

Kendig, S. (2002). Managing managed care. *Women's health care: A practical journal for nurse practitioners, 1*(1), 15-20.

Knox, G.W., & McPherson, A. (1997). Meniere's disease: Differential diagnosis and treatment. *American Family Physician, 55*(4), 1185-1190.

Konstam, M., Dracup, K. Baker, D., et al. (1994). *Heart failure: Evaluation and care of patients with left-ventricular systolic dysfunction.* Clinical Practice Guideline No. 11. (AHCPR Publication No. 94-0612). Rockville, MD: Agency for Health Care Policy and Research, Public Health Service, U.S. Department of Health and Human Services.

Lawrence, R.A. (1994). *Breastfeeding: A guide for medical professionals* (4th ed.). St. Louis: Mosby-Year Books.

Leccese, C. (1997). A promising horizon. *Advance for Nurse Practitioners, 5*(10), 60-62.

Leiner, S. (1997). Acute bronchitis in adults: Commonly diagnosed but poorly defined. *The Nurse Practitioner, 22*(1), 104-117.

McConnell, J.D., Barry, M.J., Bruskewitz, R.C., et al. (1994). *Benign prostatic hyperplasia: Diagnosis and treatment.* Clinical Practice Guideline, No. 8. (AHCPR Publication No. 94-0582). Rockville, MD: Agency for Health Care Policy and Research, Public Health Service, U.S. Department of Health and Human Services.

Majeronie, B.A. (1998). Bacterial vaginosis. *American Family Physician, 57*(6), 1285-1289.

Martini, F.H., & Timmons, M.J. (2000). *Human anatomy.* Upper Saddle River, NJ: Prentice Hall.

Mashburn, J., & Scharbo-DeHaan, M. (1997). A clinician's guide to pap smear interpretation. *The Nurse Practitioner, 22*(4), 115-143.

Mellion, M.B. (1999). *Sports medicine secret* (2nd ed.). Philadelphia: Hanley and Belfus.

Meredith, P.V., & Horan, N.M. (2000). *Adult primary care.* Philadelphia: Saunders.

Mezey, M., & McGivern, D. (1993). *Nurses, nurse practitioners.* New York: Springer.

Mladenovic, J. (Ed.). (1999). *Primary care secrets* (2nd ed.). Philadelphia: Hanley and Belfus.

Morrison, E. (1997). Controversies in women's health maintenance. *American Family Physician, 55*(4), 1283-1286.

Murray, R., & Zentner, J. (2001). *Nursing assessment and health promotion* (7th ed.). Norwalk, CT: Appleton & Lange.

Naegle, M.A., & D'Avanzo, C.E. (2001). *Addictions and substance abuse: Strategies for advanced practice nursing.* Upper Saddle River, NJ: Prentice Hall.

National Heart, Lung, and Blood Institute. (1997). *Guidelines for the diagnosis and management of asthma. National asthma education program expert panel report 2.* Public Health Services. Bethesda:MD: National Heart, Lung, and Blood Institute.

National Institutes of Health. (1997). *Screening for prostate cancer.* [On-line]. Available: www.nci.nih.gov.

Nelson, W. (2003). *Textbook of pediatrics.* (17th ed.). Philadelphia: Saunders.

Nemeroff, C.B., & Schatzberg, A.F. (1999*). Recognition and treatment of psychiatric disorders: A psychopharmacology handbook for primary care.* Washington, DC: American Psychiatric Press.

Olds, S.B., London, M.L., & Ladewig, P.W. (1996). *Maternal-infant nursing: A family-centered approach* (5th ed.). Menlo Park, CA: Addison-Wesley Nursing.

Onion, D.K. (1999). *The little black book of primary care: Pearls and references* (3rd ed.). Malden, MA: Blackwell Science.

Pagana, K.D., & Pagana, T.J. (2001). *Mosby's diagnostic and laboratory test reference* (5th ed.). St. Louis: Mosby.

Pasui, K., & McFarland, K.F. (1997). Management of diabetes in pregnancy. *American Family Physicians, 55*(8), 2731-2738.

Perna, W. (1996). Mastalgia: diagnosis and treatment. *Journal of the American Academy of Nurse Practitioners, 8*(12), 579-584.

Perry, L.E. (1996). Preconception care: A health promotion opportunity. *The Nurse Practitioner, 21*(11), 24-41.

Peter, G. (Ed.). (2003). *2003 red book: Report of the committee on infectious diseases* (26th ed.). Elk Grove, IL: American Academy of Pediatrics.

Peters, S. (1996). After baby: Choosing a contraceptive method. *Advance for Nurse Practitioners, 4*(9), 31-34.

Peters, S. (1997). For men only: an overview of three top health concerns. *Advance for Nurse Practitioners, 5*(4), 53-58.

Rakel, R.E. (1998). *Essentials of family practice* (2nd ed.). Philadelphia: Saunders.

Rakel, R. & Bope, E.T. (2004). *Conn's current therapy*. Philadelphia: Elsevier Science.

Ransom, S.B., & McNeeley, S.G. (1997). *Gynecology for the primary care provider*. Philadelphia: Saunders.

Rapid differential diagnosis (2002). Philadelphia: Lippincott Williams & Wilkins.

Recommended childhood and adolescent immunization schedule-United States, January-June 2004 (2004). Retrieved February 6, 2004 from http://cispimmunize.org/2004IZSchedule.pdf.

Richer, S. (1997). A practical guide for differentiating between iron deficiency anemia and anemia of chronic disease in children and adults. *The Nurse Practitioner, 22*(4), 82-98.

Rifat, S., & Micking, D. (1996). Practical methods of preventing ankle injury. *American Family Physician, 53*(8), 2491-2497.

Riley, K.E. (1997). Evaluation and management of primary nocturnal enuresis. *Journal of the American Academy of Nurse Practitioners, 9*(1), 33-39.

Ruppert, S. (1996). Differential diagnosis of common causes of pediatric pharyngitis. *The Nurse Practitioner, 21*(4), 38-48.

Schlenk, J. (1997). Advance directives: Role of nurse practitioners. *Journal of the American Academy of Nurse Practitioners, 9*(7), 317-321.

Schilling, J. (1997). Hyperthyroidism: Diagnosis and management of Graves' disease. *The Nurse Practitioner, 22*(6), 72-90.

Schwartz, M.W. (Ed.) (2004). *The 5 minute pediatric consult.* Baltimore: Williams & Wilkins.

Seidel, H.M., Ball, J.W., Dains, J.E., & Benedict, G.W. (1999). *Mosby's guide to physical examination* (4th *ed.).* St. Louis: Mosby-Year Books.

Seller, R.H. (1996). *Differential diagnosis of common complaints* (3rd ed.). Philadelphia: Saunders.

Seventh report of the joint national committee on prevention, detection, evaluation, and treatment of high blood pressure (JNC7) Express (2003). Retrieved August 13, 2003 from http://www.nhlbi.hib.gov/guidelines/hypertension/express.pdf.

Shine, J.W. (1997). Microcytic anemia. *American Family Physician, 55*(7), 2455-2462.

Sickle Cell Disease Guideline Panel. (1993). *Sickle cell disease: Screening, diagnosis, management, and counseling in newborns and infants.* Clinical Practice Guideline No. 6. (AHCPR Pub. No. 93-0562). Rockville, MD: Agency for Health Care Policy and Research, Public Health Services, U.S. Department of Health and Human Services.

Steinberg, G.G., Akins, C.M., & Baran, D.T. (1999). *Orthopedics in primary care* (3rd ed.). Philadelphia: Lippincott Williams & Wilkins.

Strickland, K., & Dempster, J.S. (1996). The primary care management of leiomyoma-induced abnormal uterine bleeding. *Journal of the American Academy of Nurse Practitioners, 8*(11), 541-545.

Third report of the expert panel on detection, evaluation, and treatment of high blood cholesterol in adults (Adult Treatment Panel III) (2002). Retrieved Feb 4, 2004 from http://nhlbi.hin.gov/guidelines/cholesterol/atp3full.pdf.

Uphold, C.R., & Graham, M.V. (2002). *Clinical guidelines in family practice* (4th ed.). Gainesville: Barmarrae Books.

U. S. Department of Health and Human Resources (1994). *Clinician's handbook of preventive services: Putting prevention into practice.* (1994). Washington, DC: U.S. Department of Health and Human Services, Public Health Service, Office of Disease Prevention and Health Promotion.

Vail, B., (1997). Management of chronic viral hepatitis. *American Family Physician, 55*(8), 2749-2752.

Wegener, S. (1996). *Clinical care in rheumatic disease.* Atlanta, GA: American College of Rheumatology.

Wexler, R.K. (1998). The injured ankle. *American Family Physician, 57*(3), 474-480.

White, J.E., Linhart, J., & Medley, L.E. (1996). Culture, diet, and the maternity patient: Issues for reflection and education. *Advance for Nurse Practitioners, 4*(9), 26-29.

Zalar, G.L., & Warmuth, I.P. (1996). Common cutaneous viral infections. *Hospital Medicine, 32*(11), 13-22.

Zollo, A.J. (Ed.). (2001). *Medical Secrets.* Philadelphia: Hanley and Belfus.

Audio Review Course
Available on Tapes and CDs
It's the next best thing to being there!

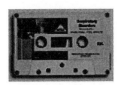 Cassettes
$179.95

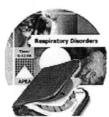 CD's
$219.95

Updated annually!

Produced from live review courses
Our audio cassettes and CD's provide you with a comprehensive review of the material covered. Over 15 hours of lecture on 12 audio tapes or 20 CD's. Comprehensive syllabus included.

Digital recording for the ultimate clarity
Our courses have been digitally recorded using state-of-the-art technology and are reproduced on quality audio cassette tapes and CD's. Our audio review course is the best on the market; one listen and you'll know what we're talking about!

Most thorough review available
Students who attend our live review course have a 98-99% passing rate on the AANP and ANCC exams. If you cannot attend an APEA review course in person, hearing the course on our audio casettes or CD's will be the next best thing to being there.

Question & Answer session included
Each section of our audio review course ends with a question and answer session that will help you retain what you have learned.

Dynamic speaker
Our review course is taught by Amelie Hollier, MSN, APRN, BC, a nationally certified family nurse practitioner and one of the most dynamic speakers in the healthcare industry. You will love her informative style, personable delivery, and accurate real-life anecdotes. She is joy to listen to!

Call us at 800-899-4502 or visit our website @ www.apea.com

Pediatric Antibiotic Dosage Cards

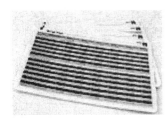

$6.00
(add $2 shipping)

Never calculate a dose again! You'll appreciate this amazing set of four pocket sized cards arranged by class: penicillins, cephalosporins, macrolides, et cetera -- they give the correct dose by weight and the concentration so you know exactly what to prescribe. Back side gives information about the antibiotics. *Indispensable!*

Advanced Practice Education Associates
103 Darwin Circle
Lafayette, LA 70508

Please send _____ Copy of _Pediatric Dosage Cards_ for $8.00.

Please send _____ Copy of _Audio Review Course_ on Tape for $233.95

Please send _____ Copy of _Audio Review Course_ on CDs for $184.95.

(Prices includes packaging).

Payment: ☐Check ☐VISA ☐MasterCard ☐American Express

Credit Card Number: _____

Name on card: _____ Exp. Date: _____/_____

Shipping Address:

Name_____

Address_____

City_____State _____Zip _____

Please allow 2 weeks for delivery. Prices and availability subject to change without notice.

Advanced Practice Education Associates
http://www.apea.com
1-800-899-4502

VISIT OUR ON-LINE TESTING CENTER
@ www.apea.com.

Test your readiness for the certification exam. Identify your strengths and weaknesses! Adult and Family NP options available!

APEA is today's premier automated NP testing solution. APEA's online testing is student oriented, easy to use, and presents users with a logical testing methodology robust enough to assist you with the complexity of preparing for the NP Certification Exam.

APEA offers two types of Online Prep Exams:

- **Interactive Practice Mode** (Family or Adult Options Available*)
- **Full Exam Mode** (Family or Adult Options Available*)

*The family option includes pediatric questions.

The sample questions presented are **randomly selected** from our database of thousands of prep exam questions. Using our system can help you to become familiar with the question types you will find on the Certification Exam.

Interactive Practice Mode consists of **60** questions. The Practice Mode questions are organized by content category and will provide you with immediate feedback on your answers. Our questions represent the types of questions included in the Certification Exam.

Full Exam Mode consists of **150** questions. It is designed to give users the experience of a complete practice certification exam. Upon completion of the exam, your percentage of correct answers will be calculated as well as your percentage within each category of the exam and will be displayed for your reference. Questions that are answered incorrectly will also be displayed at the end of the exam along with the rationale.

We look forward to helping you prepare for the Family or Adult Nurse Practitioner Certification Exams.

We look forward to helping you prepare for the Family or Adult Nurse Practitioner Certification Exam.

www.apea.com   800-899-4502

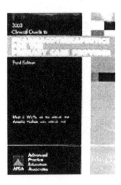

Clinical Guide to Pharmacotherapeutics for the Primary Care Provider

By

Mari J. Wirfs, MN, PhD, BC, FNP
Amelie Hollier, MSN, APRN, BC FNP

**Excellent pocket medication reference for the primary care provider.
Only prescribing reference arranged by diagnosis.**

Clinical Guide to Pharmacotherapeutics for the Primary Care Provider is a useful pocket-sized, clinical guide for physicians, nurse practitioners and other advanced practice RNs, physician assistants and other primary care providers. This clinical guide is arranged by diagnosis with each commonly prescribed medication listed and explained. The bulleted format allows for quick and easy access to current comprehensive information. The clinical guide is divided into two sections.

Section One:
· Generic/brand names for drug
· Drug categories and dosages
· Age and population dosing
   considerations
· Contraindications, dose timing
   regarding food, need for lab
   work, common adverse effects

Section Two:
· Generic/brand names
   cross-reference
· Pregnancy risk categories
· Potency categories for topical
   steroids
· Immunization schedules for
   children and adults

**Advanced Practice Education Associates
103 Darwin Circle
Lafayette, LA 70508**

Please send _____ Copy of *Clinical Guide to Pharmacotherapeutics for the Primary Care Provider* for $44.95 (includes packaging).

Payment: ☐Check   ☐VISA   ☐MasterCard   ☐American Express

Credit Card Number: _____

Name on card: _____ **Exp. Date:** _____/_____

Shipping Address:

Name _____

Address _____

City _____**State** _____**Zip** _____

Please allow 2 weeks for delivery. Prices and availability subject to change without notice.

Advanced Practice Education Associates
http://www.apea.com
1-800-899-4502

APEA

Advanced Practice Education Associates

Presents

Family Nurse Practitioner
Certification Review Book

By

Amelie Hollier, MSN, APRN, BC, FNP

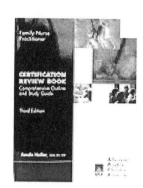

The *Family Nurse Practitioner Certification Review Book* is written for FNP students preparing for the AANP or ANCC certification exam. This study guide offers a comprehensive review of all common diseases arranged by body system, growth and development, and professional issues. Chapters are organized by subjects and diseases in an outline format to facilitate studying and reinforce learning of similar subject areas. Considerations for treating adult, pediatric, pregnant, and lactating patients are integrated throughout.

> *"An excellent study tool and resource for the FNP student!"*
> *"A great clinical guideline reference for the practicing NP!"*

• •

Advanced Practice Education Associates
103 Darwin Circle, Lafayette, LA 70508

Please send _____ *Family Nurse Practitioner Certification Review Book* for $54.95
Please send _____ **COMBO PACKAGE:**
    Family Nurse Practitioner Certification Review Book and *Family*
    Nurse Practitioner Certification Prep Exams for $97.90.
      Prices include packaging.

Payment: ☐Check   ☐VISA   ☐MasterCard   ☐American Express

Credit Card Number: _____ **Exp. Date:** _____ / _____

Shipping Address:

Name _____

Address _____

City _____ **State** _____ **Zip** _____

Please allow 2-3 weeks for delivery. Prices and availability subject to change without notice.

Advanced Practice Education Associates
http://www.apea.com
1-800-899-4502

APEA